ELEMENTARY PHARMACEUTICAL CALCULATIONS

ELEMENTARY PHARMACEUTICAL CALCULATIONS

D. K. Tripathi
M. Pharm, Ph.D
Professor and Principal
Rungta College of Pharmaceutical Sciences and Research,
Bhilai, Chhattisgarh.

Formerly Professor & Principal of Sri Jayadev College of Pharmaceutical Sciences, Bhubaneswar.
H. C. Garg Institute of Pharmacy and Technology
Kolkata, (Presently NSHM)
Bengal School of Technology
Chinsura, West Bengal.

PharmaMed Press
An imprint of Pharma Book Syndicate
A unit of BSP Books Pvt. Ltd.
4-4-309/316, Giriraj Lane,
Sultan Bazar, Hyderabad - 500 095.

Elementary Pharmaceutical Calculation ***by D. K. Tripathi***

Published by

PharmaMed Press

An imprint of Pharma Book Syndicate

A unit of BSP Books Pvt. Ltd.

4-4-309/316, Giriraj Lane, Sultan Bazar, Hyderabad - 500 095.

Phone: 040-23445600, 23445688; Fax: 91+40-23445611

E-mail: info@pharmamedpress.com

ISBN: 978-93-8681-991-8 (HB)

CONTENTS

Chapter 4

Density, Specific Gravity and Specific Volume

Chapter 5

Calculation Related to Capsule Filling, Suppository Molds, Dry Powders and Doses

Chapter 10

Radiopharmaceuticals

Chapter 11

Calculations Related to Plant Extracts and Drug Molecule

Chapter 12

Biostatistics

Chapter 13

Dissolution Tests

PREFACE

Calculation in pharmacy is wide and broad-based starting from dispensing to manufacturing, quality control, research and development in pharmaceutical industries. This is an important subject area for any student pursuing pharmacy course irrespective of level of the course. Thus, the students during their course of studies and pharmaceutical technologists during their work need to know calculations related to (1) Physical and chemical properties of active ingredients and excipients, (2) Rate of absorption, (3) Biological activity, and (4) Rate of degradation of the drug substances. There is need to have such book on pharmaceutical calculations that can fulfill the needs of Institutions as well as industries. The book, *Elementary Pharmaceutical Calculations* has been designed so that it can meet the needs of students. The content of the book has been divided into 13 chapters. Each chapter begins with introductory description of concept, relevant formulas with derivation and then examples to explain how the formula can be used to solve problems; finally at the end there are problems given to solve.

Although the metric system or SI units are in use, the FPS system is still being practiced in some cases or by some people. Hence, both the systems have been described and explained with the help of relevant examples.

It is expected that this book will be able to cater the needs of students and of those who are engaged in industries or in academic profession.

This is being the first edition of the book needs to be revised in accordance with the specific need or suggestion, if any. The author sincerely desires to have comments for further development of the book.

D. K. Tripathi

ACKNOWLEDGEMENT

At the beginning the author begs the blessing from his teachers who have taught and guided to walk on the right path. Hence, the author of this book honestly grateful to all the teachers.

The author is sincerely thankful to the Management of Santosh Rungta Group of Institutions, Bhilai for extending facility for preparation of the book. The author also thanks to his colleagues for their cooperation being extended especially to Dr. Amit Alexander and Sri Hemant Bandhasir. Finally the author is thankful the members of his family for their cooperation.

D. K. Tripathi

1

SYSTEMS OF UNITS

Foot-Pound-Second (FPS) System

Since long, the foot-pound-second (fps) system of units has been used to measure dimensions and quantities of material. The fundamental units are the foot for length, the pound for weight, and the second for time. The FPS system has two variants, known as the American version and the Imperial version. Now-a-days none of the systems is being used by scientists (after implementation of SI units). The International System of Units (SI) is preferred because it is simple and convenient. However, FPS units are still used to some extent by the general public, especially in the United States and in India also.

Units of Length

There are different units such as thou, inch, hand, foot, yard, rod, pace, mile, furlong, fathom, etc. used to measure length. However, the conversion factors are not simple.

Thou

One thousandth of an inch is called ***thou***. In the United States it is called **mil**. The plural of thou is thou' and of mil is 'mils'.

Inch

An inch was originally defined as the width of a man's thumb, but later on it was defined as *the length of three barleycorns placed end to end*. The word inch comes from the Latin word for one-twelfth (*uncia*). The Romans, when invaded in the year 43, brought the concept of the 12 inch-foot to England and since then it had been used. Earlier the inch was subdivided into halves, quarters, eighths, sixteenths, and other powers of two; and also into hundredths (as in the caliber of fire-arms) or thousandths (called thou in the UK and mils in the US). After introduction of SI system, one inch is defined as 0.0254 m (or 2.54 cm).

Hand

A hand is considered as *the width of a man's hand measured across the palm and including the thumb*. It was mostly used to measure the height of horses; not for other purposes. A standard hand is 4 inches.

Foot

A foot was defined as the length of a man‘s foot. *A standard foot is 12 inches*. Foot (ft) is the fundamental unit of length in FPS system. One foot (1 ft) represents a length of 12 inches. The inch was originally defined as the length of three typical barleycorns laid end-to-end. A foot was also approximately equal to three hand widths or 2/3rd of a cubit (the distance from an average person's elbow to the tips of the fingers). Nowadays, a foot is considered to be 0.3048 meter, where the meter is the fundamental unit of distances in the metric system and International System of Units (SI).

Cubit

The cubit is an ancient unit. *The distance between the elbow and the tip of the middle finger on a man's arm is called cubit.* The term was derived from the Latin word *cubitum* (elbow). It has been differently expressed at different places over different times. For example, the Roman cubit was 17.47 inches long, the Greek 18.20 inches, the Sumerian 20.42 inches, the Egyptian 20.6 to 20.8 inches and the English cubit is 18 inches.

Yard

Yard is an Old English word for staff, rod, or stick. *The length from the King's nose to his outstretched hand was considered as a yard.*

Afterwards, a stick measuring same length was marked and was considered as the standard stick of the kingdom. The word, yardstick was derived from this. *A standard yard is 3 feet long.*

Pace

The term, pace has originally arrived from Rome. The *passus* was measured *from the heel of one foot to the heel of the same foot when it next touched the ground* (one normal walking step). This is a convenient unit for measuring walking distances (again, for men with feet). A standard pace is 5 feet long.

Fathom

The word fathom has its roots in the Old English word used for embracing arms (*foeom*). It is also a unit used to measure the length, commonly used by the navigators. It refers to *the length between two arms of a man at extended position*. Usually it was used to measure the ropes used to determine the depth of navigable waters. *A standard fathom refers to a length of 6 feet.*

Rod

One rod measures the length of 16½ feet or 5½ yards. It is also called a pole or a perch.

Chain

Chains are commonly used by the surveyors for measuring distances. The English mathematician

Edmund Gunter developed the chain and is commonly called as Gunter's chain. The links of Gunter's chain are $7\frac{92}{100}$ inches long. One chain measures one hundred links that make a total length of 792 inches or 66 ft or 22 yards.

Furlong

The concept of a furrow (furlong) originally came from the trench made in the ground by a plow. *A*

Standard furrow is 220 yards long or 1/8 mile.

Mile

One mile referred to the distance of a thousand paces – in Latin, mille passus. A pace measures 5 feet; thus, one mile is roughly 5000 feet. Actually one mile was defined as 5280 feet (1760 yards) by the decree of the English parliament during the reign of Elizabeth I. Since this was a legal definition, it became known as the statute mile. Statute is a legal word for law.

But, the value of a mile varies from country to country and from time to time; for example, in Austria 1 mile is 8297 yards; *in England, India and in US, 1 mile is 1760 yards*; in Hungary 1 mile is 9139 yards; in Brunswick, 1 mile is 11816 yards; in Italy 1 mile is 2025 yards; in Netherlands 1 mile is 1094 yards In Norway 1 mile is 12182 yards; in Poland 1 mile is 8,100 yards, in Prussia 1 mile is 8238 yards, in

Spain 1 mile is 1552 yards, in Sweden 1 mile is11660 yards, and in Switzerland 1 mile is 8548 yards.

Nautical mile

Originally a nautical mile was defined as the distance of arc covered by one minute. It was measured on a meridian of the Earth; basically 1/60 of 1/360 of the Earth's circumference from one pole to another and back. Thus, the circumference of the Earth becomes 21600 nautical miles.

The Earth is slightly flattened sphere (an oblate spheroid). The distance around the equator is 0.2% longer than that around the poles. This difference seems to be small; but is important to ships, planes, and spacecrafts travelling long distances. A 0.2% error over the width of the Pacific Ocean is about 20 miles (20 statute miles). Hence, a nautical mile is defined as 1852 m exactly, which is equal to 6076.115 feet approximately.

Conversion of the length units of the English system is given below

Units	Equivalent unit	Units	Equivalent unit
1 thou	0.001 inch (in)	1 fathom	2 yd = 6 ft = 72 in
1 hand	4 in	1 rod	$5\frac{1}{2}$ yd = $16\frac{1}{2}$ ft = 198 in
1 foot (ft)	12 in	1 chain	4 rods = 22 yd = 66 ft
1 cubit	18 in	1 furlong	10 chain = 220 yd = 660 ft
1 yard (yd)	3 ft = 36 in	1 statute mile (mi)	8 furlongs = 1760 yd = 5280 ft
1 pace	5 ft = 60 in	1 nautical mile	1852 m (exactly) = 6076.12 ft (approx)
		1 league	3 miles = 5280 yd = 15840 ft

Units of Mass or Weight

In fact, the english unit for mass and unit for weight for same mass under a standard gravitation force (9.80665 m/sec^2) are same. This part of the English system may be called the French system; because many of the units have come to England from France. There are two sub-systems or paths – avoirdupois and troy or apothecaries.

Apothecaries system or Troy system	Avoirdupois system
Troy system was used for Troyes, France to deal in precious metals, gems, and medicines. This system came from Cairo during crusades and apothecaries system came from France. The name, apothecaries was derived from the French word – 'apotecaire' referred to shopkeeper dealing in medicines. One pound = 12 ounces.	The term Avoirdupois came from the French phrase –""*aveir de pois"* or "aver de peis" which means "goods of weight" or "goods (sold) by weight", not "goods sold by piece". Avoirdupois system is used as mass units for most commodities. One pound = 16 ounces.

Grain

A grain was said *equal to the mass of an average grain of wheat* taken from the middle of an ear. One avoirdupois pound is equal to 7000 grains and in troy one pound is equal to 5760 grains.

Scruple

This term is derived from the Latin word *scrupus*, a small rough pebble or a chip of stone basically, something small. *A scruple is* 20 *grains*.

Pennyweight

At some time in England, 1 English *penny was considered to be 24 grains*.

Dram

This word is derived from the Greek word, drachma. It is a fraction of an ounce, its maybe 1/8th or 1/16th depending on the system. One drachma weighed about one dram. Dram also refers to serving of whiskey.

Ounce

The word ounce referred to one twelfth. It has the meaning similar to inch, the old English word for one twelfth, uncial. One inch is $1/12^{th}$ of a foot and ounce is $1/12^{th}$ of a pound. However, sometimes one ounce may be $1/6^{th}$ of a pound.

Pound

The term pound came from the Latin word pondus' for weight and its abbreviation _lb' came from the Roman unit libra' which means $3/4^{th}$ of an English pound. The word _libra' again came from the Latin word, _libro' meaning to weigh. One pound (1 lb) is the force that produces an acceleration of 32.1740 feet per second square (32.1740 ft/sec^2) when applied against a known standard mass. The acceleration of 32.1740 ft/sec^2 is approximately the value of the earth's gravitational acceleration at 45 degrees north latitude.

Stone

This unit usually used for bulk agricultural commodities and officially 1 stone = 14 pounds. In practice, the value of a stone depends on the article weighed. For example, for glass one stone is equal to 5 lbs; for fish, meat, sugar, or spices one stone is equal to 8 lbs; for wax one stone is equal to 12 lbs; for cheese one stone is equal to 16 lbs. the word stone stands for both singular and plural; that is, 1 stone, 10 stone, etc.

Hundredweight

By name it should be a hundred of something; in fact, hundredweight was adopted for hundred pounds in England in long back. Since stone was considered as the basic unit and 1 stone = 14 pounds, nearest multiple of one hundredweight (100 pounds) is 112 pounds or 8 stone. As a result, 100 pound hundredweight is called short hundredweight and 112 pound hundredweight is called long hundred weight.

Ton

The word 'ton' came from the English word 'tunne' which means 'a big container'. The word was used to refer the capacity of a big container. Thereafter, it was considered as a unit of both weight and volume Use as volume-unit is restricted in railroad and shipping industries; but, as weight-unit it became popular and it was defined as the unit to represent 2000 pounds. Later on in England the value of one ton was changed from 2000 lbs to 2240 lbs; because 2240 lbs is a multiple of stone (160 stone); while 2000lbs is not a multiple of stone. However, American ton represents 2000 lbs. American ton (2000 lbs) is called short ton and English ton (2240 lbs) is called long ton.

Unit of Time (Second)

One second (1 s or 1 sec) is the time that elapses during 9.192631770×10^9 cycles of the radiation produced by the transition between two levels of Ce133 (Cesium). It is also $\frac{1}{86400}$ of a mean solar day. (60 seconds constitute a minute, 60 minutes constitute an hour, and 24 hours constitute a day; that is

$$1 \text{ day} = 60 \times 60 \times 24 = 86{,}400 \text{ sec})$$

International System of Units (SI)

As per the *United States Pharmacopeia or National Formulary,* the International System of Units (SI) is the official system for weights and measures. The International System of Units (SI) is the decimal system of weights and measure. It was internationally recognized and earlier known as the metric system. In late eighteenth century this system was developed in France and in 1988 it was implemented worldwide.

The base units of the SI are Meter – Kilogram - Second. Meter was originally defined as $\frac{1}{40000000}^{\text{th}}$ the Earth's polar circumference. Subsequently it has been redefined as the distance travelled by light in a vacuum in $\frac{1}{299792458}^{\text{th}}$ of a second. One meter is generally considered as 39.37 inches. The mass of a kilogram was originally defined as the mass of one liter of water. Later on the standard mass of platinum-iridium alloy representing one kilogram has been preserved in a vault in France. According to FPS system one kilogram is almost equal to 2.2 lbs. The relative value of the International System of Units (SI) and their prefixes are given below:

Relative values	Prefix	Unit
One quintillionth (10^{-18}) of meter, liter or	atto-	Attometer/Attoliter/Attogram
gram	femto-	Femtometer/Femtoliter/Femtogram
One quadrillionth (100^{-15}) of meter, liter	pico-	Picometer/Picoliter/Picogram
or gram	nano-	Nanometer/Nanoliter/Nanogram
One trillionth (10^{-12}) of the meter, liter or	micro-	Micrometer/Microliter/Microgram
gram	milli-	Millimeter/Milliliter/Milligram
One billionth (10^{-9}) of meter, liter or	centi-	Centimeter/Centiliter/Centigram
gram One millionth (10^{-6}) of meter, liter	deci-	Decimeter/Deciliter/Decigram
10 times of meter, liter or gram	deka-	Dekameter/Dekaliter/Dekagram
100 times (10^2) of meter, liter or gram	hecto-	Hectometer/Hectoliter/Hectogram
1000 times (10^3) of meter, liter or gram	kilo-	Kilometer/Kiloliter/Kilogram
10,000 times (10^4) of meter, liter or gram	myria-	Myriameter/Myrialiter/Myriagram
1 million times (10^6) of meter, liter or gram	mega-	Megameter/Megaliter/Megagr
1 billion times (10^9) of meter, liter or gram	giga-	Gigameter/Gigaliter/Gigagram
1 trillion times (10^{12}) of meter, liter or gram	tera-	Tetrameter/Teraliter/Teragram
1 quadrillion times (10^{15}) of meter, liter or gram	peta-	Petameter/Petaliter/Petagram
1 quintillion times (10^{18}) of meter, liter or gram	exa-	Exameter/Exaliter/Exagram

The base or primary SI unit for length is **meter**, for mass is **gram** and for time is **second**. However, historically and technically the base unit of mass is kilogram. The units for other quantities are derived. For example, volume is cubic length or mass by density. Its base unit is **liter**.

There is another system of SI units – centimeter-gram-second (CGS system).

The standard subdivisions and multiples of the base units are called **Denominations** and the number used in conjunction with a denomination is termed a **denominate number**.

There are certain rules or guidelines for correct use of SI units. In some cases, variation in writing is found. Hence, the guidelines for correct use of SI units are mentioned in a tabular form.

Correct use	Incorrect use	Remarks
5 *l*, 5L, 4g, 21 mm	4 G, 21 Mm	The symbol of liter may be L or l, the name of a unit should not be in capital form except at the beginning or heading of a sentence.
10.5 mL, 10.5 mL (U.S.)	10.5 mL (non-U.S.) or 10-5 mL	In USA the decimal point is placed on the line with the denomination and denomination number.
6 mL and 5 g	6 mL and 5 g.	Periods are not used following SI symbols except at the end of a sentence.
9 mL/h or 9 $mL.h^{-1}$	9 mL per hour	Compound unit indicated by solidus (/) or a negative exponent can only be used.
15 mg/mL	15 mg/milliliter	Symbols should not be combined with full terms.
1 mL or 1milliliters	1 mL	When full term is written plurals of unit name can be used.
mcg or μg	-	Both the symbols are valid.
cm^3,etc	cc	For cubic centimeter cc is not a valid SI symbol.
3.5 g	31/2 g	Decimal fractions are accepted, not common fractions.
0.75 g	0.75 g	Zero must be put before the decimal point, to avoid error.

It is most important to realize that a misplaced or misread decimal point can lead to an error in calculation. There are certain ways by which this can be eliminated or reduced greatly. The guidelines to be followed are mentioned below;

- After a whole number trailing zeros should *not* be put. For example, 25 mg, not 25.0 mg.

  Although in some cases to indicate exactness to a specific number of decimal places trailing zeros is often put. For example, 50.0 mg.

- While using symbols of unit dimensions the unit suitable for numeric value up to 1000 should be used. For example, write 750 g, not 0.75 kg; similarly write 500 mL, not 0.5 L.

Equivalence of units between SI (CGS) and other Systems of Measurement

As per the *United States Pharmacopeia National Formulary* the International System of Units (SI) is the official system for weights and measures.

The **Apothecaries' system of measurement** is the traditional system used in pharmacy. It has now become historic one, the components of this system are occasionally found even on prescriptions.

The **Avoirdupois system** is the common system of commerce, used in the United States along with the SI. Through this system, goods are purchased and sold in terms of ounce and pound. Thus, it is necessary to know the quantitative relationships among these systems and the means for inter system conversion. For example, conversion of temperature between the Fahrenheit and Celsius (or centigrade) scales, or conversion of concentration of alcohol from proof strength to %v/v. The FPS (foot-pound-second) system had been used in the US and in the British ruled countries till SI system came into effect.

Measurement of Volume

Over the definition of gallon the English and American units differed in 1824. According to the British Weights & Measure Act a gallon was defined as the volume of water that weighs 10 pounds; while the Americans accepted the old definition one gallon of water weighs 8 pounds. As a result, the English units for volume became 20% larger than the American units. The units set before 1824 are called English units and the units set after 1824 are called Imperial units. The English units that were continued in the United States are called US customary units.

Below in the table the units of the English and Imperial systems have been mentioned, not of the US customary system.

Unit & Abbreviation	English System	Unit & Abbreviation	Imperial System
1 cubic foot (cu ft)	1728 cubic inch (cu in)	1 dram (dr)	60 minim (min)
1 cubic yard (cu yd)	27 cu ft = 46656 cu in	1 teaspoon (tsp)	100 min
1 register ton	100 cu ft	1tablespoon (tbsp)	3 tsp = 300 min
1 cord	128 cu ft	1 ounce (oz)	$1\frac{3}{5}$ tbsp = $4\frac{4}{5}$ tsp = 8 dr = 480 min

Table *contd...*

Unit & Abbreviation	English System	Unit & Abbreviation	Imperial System
1 acre foot	$1613\frac{1}{3}$ cu yd = 43560 cu ft	1 gill (gi)	5 oz
1 cubic mile	5451776000 cu yd = 147197952000 cu ft	1 cup (c)	8 oz
		1 pint (pt)	$2\frac{1}{2}$ c = 20 oz
		1 quart (qt)	2 pt = 5 c = 40 oz
		1 gallon (gal)	4 qt = 8 pt = 20 c = 160 oz = 4.54609 liters
		1 peak (pk)	2 gal = 8 qt = 16 pt
		1 bushel (bu)	4 pk = 8 gal = 32 qt = 64 pt
		1 quarter (qr)	8 bu = 64 gal = 256 qt
		1 barrel (bbl)	$26\frac{1}{4}$ gal (wine) = 36 gal (beer)
		1 hogshead	$52\frac{1}{2}$ gal (wine) = 54 gal (beer)

Measurement of weight by the British Systems

Unit	Abbreviations Avoirdupois system ( ) Apothecaries' system [ ]	Avoirdupois system	Apothecaries'/Troy system
1 grain	(gr) [G]	1/7000 pound	1/5760 pound
1 scruple	[Ǝ]		20 grains
1 pennyweight	[dwt]		24 grains
1 dram	(dr) [ʒ]	1/256 pound	3 scruples = 60 grains
1 ounce	[℥]	16 drams = 437.5 grains	8 drams = 480 grains
1 pound	(lb, ℔, #) [lb, ℔, #]	16 ounces = 7000 grains	12 ounces = 5760 grains
1 stone	(st)	14 pounds	
1 short hundred weight	(cwt)	100 pounds	
1 long hundred weight	(cwt)	112 pounds	
1 short ton	(tn)	2000 pounds	
1 long ton	(tn)	2240 pounds	

Conversion between the Systems

Sometimes it is necessary to convert a weight or measurement from units of one system to another system. Conversion of denomination of one system to that of another needs a *conversion factor* or *conversion equivalent.* The practical and precise conversion equivalents for measurement of weight, length and volume are there. Some useful equivalents are given below.

Unit	Equivalent unit	Unit	Equivalent unit
1 inch (in)	2.54 cm	1 fluidounce (fl. oz.)	29.57 mL
1 meter (m)	39.37 in	1 pint (16 fl. oz.)	473 mL
1 pound (lb, Avoirdupois)	454 g	1 quart (32 fl. oz.)	946 mL
1 kilogram (kg)	2.2 lb	1 gallon, US (128 fl. oz.)	3785 mL
		1 gallon, UK	4545 mL

Example

Convert 65765 mcg to g

Solution

1000 mcg = 1 mg

1 mcg = 65765 mcg 1000 mcg = 65.765 mg

1000 mg = 1 g

1 mg = 65.765 mg1000 mg

Ans. 0.066965 gm

Example

Convert 57668 μl to liter.

Solution

1000 μl = 1 ml

57668 μl = 57668 μl×1 ml 1000 μl = 57.668 ml

1000 ml = 1L

1 ml = 57.668 ml1000 ml

Ans. 0.057668 L

Example

Add 5 kg 457 mg, 76 mg and 8.75 g. Express the total in kg-g-mg.

Solution

1 kg = 1000 g, 1 g = 1000 mg.

1 kg = 1000000 mg

5 kg 457 mg = 5000000 mg + 457 mg = 5000457 mg

+ 76 mg

+ 8.75 g = 8.75 × 1000 mg = 8750 mg

Total = 5009283 mg

= 5009283 mg ÷ 1000 = 5009283 g

= 5009.283g ÷1000 =

Ans. 5 kg 9 g 283 mg

Example

As per record 5 g 95 mg of Cyanocobalamine was issued from a stock of 7.475 g. Calculate the balance amount and express in terms of milligrams.

Solution

Stock of Cyanocobalamine = 7.475g = 7.475 × 1000 mg = 7475 mg

(-) Quantity issued = 5g 95 mg = 5×1000 mg + 95 mg = 5095mg

Balance amount of Cyanocobalamine

Ans. 2380 mg

Example

A mixture contains substances of different weights; 0.075 g, 20 mg, 0.0005 g, 4 mg, and 500 μg. What is the total weight (in mg) of the mixture?

Solution

0.075 g + 20 mg + 0.0005g + 4 mg + 500μg

= (0.075g × 1000) + 20 mg + (0.0005g×1000) + 4 mg + (500μg ÷ 1000)

= 75mg + 20mg + 0.5mg + 4mg + 0.5mg

= 100 mg

The total weight of mixture is

Ans. 100 mg

Example

During manufacturing of a formulation 103 kg of a drug was initially issued. Based on IPQC report another amount of 573 g 35 mg was issued. The stock of the drug after second issue was 74 kg 865 g 75 mg. Find out the opening stock.

Solution

Quantity issued initially = 103 kg = 103kg×1000 = 103000g × 1000 = 103000000 mg

(+) Quantity issued second time = 573 g 35 mg = 573g×1000+35mg = 573035 mg

Total quantity issued = 103573035 mg

Balance after issue = 74 kg 865 g 75 mg = (74×1000 + 865)g 75 mg = 74865g 75 mg

= (74865 ×1000) mg +75 mg = 74865075 mg

Opening stock = Quantity issued + Balance = 103573035 mg + 74865075 mg

= 178438110 mg

Ans. 178kg 438g 110mg

Example

A shopkeeper purchased 24 lbs (avoir.) of olive oil. Out of which he sold 3kg and 25 g. How much stock he should have?

Solution

Olive oil purchased = 24 lbs (avoir.) = 24×454 g = 10896 g

(-) Olive oil sold = 3 kg + 25 g = 3×1000g + 25 g = 3025 g

Balance of olive oil = 7871 g = 7871 ÷ 1000 kg

= 7.871 kg

Ans. 7 kg 871 g

Example

Three-fourth liter of a solution for intravenous infusion contains 2.5 g of drug. How many milliliters of the solution would contain 75 mg of drug?

Solution

1 liter (1000 ml) of solution contains 2.5 g

$3/4^{th}$ liter of the solution = $\frac{3 \times 1000}{4}$ ml = 750 ml

That is, 750 ml of the solution contains 2.5 g of drug

In other words, 2.5 g (2.5 g × 1000 = 2500 mg) of the drug is present in 750 ml.

$$75\text{mg of the drug is present in } \frac{750\text{ml} \times 75\text{mg}}{2500\text{mg}}$$

Ans. 22.5 ml

Example

A 60ml suspension of Ampicillin contains 250 mg/5 mL. Find out the volume of the suspension (milliliters) that contain 400 mg of Ampicillin.

Solution

The suspension contains 250mg of Ampicillin in 5 ml

That is, 1ml of suspension contains $\frac{250\text{mg}}{5}$ = 50 mg of Ampicillin

In other words, 50 mg of Ampicillin is present in 1 ml of suspension

So, 400 mg of Ampicillin is present in $\frac{400\text{mg}}{50\text{mg/ml}}$

Ans. 8 ml of suspension

Example

An injection contains 70 mg of drug in 2 mL. To administer 0.02 g of drug how many milliliters of the injection should be injected?

Solution

70 mg of drug is present in 2 ml of injection

1 mg of drug is present in $\frac{2ml \times 1mg}{70mg}$ = 0.0286 ml

0.02 g = 0.02 g × 1000 = 20 mg of drug should be present in 0.0286 ml × 20

Ans. 0.572 ml

Example

A patient is administered dose of 21mg of drug per day for 6 weeks, followed by 14 mg per day for 2 weeks, and then 7 mg per day for 2 more weeks. Calculate the total quantity, in grams, of the drug administered to the patient during this course of treatment.

Solution

1 week = 7 days

6 weeks = 6 × 7 days = 42 days

In one day 21 mg of the drug is administered

In 42 days, 21 mg × 42 = 882 mg of drug is administered during 6 weeks

2 weeks = 2 × 7 days = 14 days

In one day 14 mg of the drug is administered

In 14 days, 14 × 14mg = 196 mg of drug is administered during 2 weeks

In one day 7 mg of the drug is administered

In 14 days, 14 × 7mg = 98 mg of drug is administered during 2 weeks

Total drug administered = 882mg + 196mg + 98mg = 1176 mg

1176 mg = 1176mg ÷ 1000

Ans. 1.176g of drug is administered during 10 weeks

Example

A solution contains 250 mg of drug in each 25 mL. Express the concentration of solution in terms of μg of drug per μL.

Solution

1 mg = 1000 μg

250 mg = 250 × 1000 μg = 250000 μg

1 ml = 1000 μL

25 ml = 25 × 1000 μL = 25000 μL

So, 25000μL contain 250000μg of drug

Or, each μL contains $\frac{250000\mu g}{25000}$ = 10 μg/mL

The concentration of solution is

Ans. 10 μg/ μL

Example

If an inhaler contains 9 mg of salbutamol, how many inhalation doses can be delivered if each inhalation dose contains 90μg?

Solution

The dose of the drug = 90 μg

1 mg = 1000 μg

9 mg = 9000 μg

Number of doses present in 9 mg = 90 × 1000 = 9000 μg

Each dose contains 90μg

The number of doses in 9000 μg = $\frac{9000}{90}$

Ans. 100 doses

Equivalence between Different Systems

There are three systems of measurement:

- International System,
- Avoirdupois and
- Apothecaries 'systems.

The avoirdupois system had been widely used in the United States in measuring body weight and in selling goods (ounce or pound). However, the system is being replaced by the international system. Earlier, in pharmacy the apothecaries' system had been the predominant system to measure volume and weight. Now it has largely been replaced by the SI.

For the sake of knowledge one must know the relationship between the various systems of measurement.

Sometimes, the quantities in units of the Apothecaries' or of the Avoirdupois systems of measurement are to be converted to equivalent quantities in SI units and vice versa for the purpose of calculation. Some important and useful equivalents are given below ***Equivalents of Length*** 1 inch = 2.54 cm 1 meter (m) = 39.37 inch ***Equivalents of Weight*** 1 pound (lb, Avoirdupois) = 454 g 1 kilogram (kg) = 2.2 lb	***Equivalents of Volume*** 1 fluidounce (fl. oz.) = 29.57 mL 1 pint (16 fl. oz.) = 473 mL 1 quart (32 fl. oz.) = 946 mL 1 gallon, US (128 fl. oz.) = 3785 mL 1 gallon, UK = 4545 mL

Example

A container has the capacity to contain 58 gallons, US of water. Calculate the capacity of the container in terms of liters.

Solution

1 gallon, US = 3785 ml

58 gallons, US = 58 × 3785 ml

= 219530 ml

$$= \frac{219530\text{ml}}{1000}$$

Ans. 219.53 L

Example

The volume of a container is 25 gallons, UK. What would be the volume in liter?

Solution

1 gallon, UK = 4545 ml

25 gallon, UK = 25 × 4545 ml

= 113625 ml

Ans. 113.625 L

Example

In a warehouse there are many drums of light liquid paraffin under different systems of measurement. These are listed as 2 drums of 10 gallons, UK; 5 drums of 21 gallons, US; 4 drums of 100 L and a drum containing 4 quarts 1 pint of light liquid paraffin. Find out how many liters of light liquid paraffin are there?

Solution

2×10 gallons, UK = $2 \times 10 \times 4545$ ml = 90900 ml

5×21 gallons, US = $5 \times 21 \times 3785$ ml = 397425 ml

4×100 L = $4 \times 100 \times 1000$ ml = 400000 ml

4 quarts 1 pint = 4×946 ml + 473 ml = 4257 ml

Total = 892582 ml = 892582ml ÷ 1000

Ans. 892.582 L

Example

There was a stock of 15 kg glycerin. An order for 16 bottles of one pound each is to be supplied after repacking. Find out the balance quantity.

Solution

1 kg = 2.2 lb and 1 lb = 454 g

15 kg = 15×2.2 lb = 33 lb

To be supplied = 16 bottles of 1lb = 16 lbs

Balance stock = 33 lbs – 16 lbs = 17 lb

= 17 lbs × 454.5 = 7726.5 g

= 7718 ÷ 1000 = 7.718 kg; or

Ans. 7 kg 718 g

Example

The dimensions of a transdermal patch are 4.5 cm by 3.8cm. Express the dimensions in corresponding inches. [1 inch is equivalent to 2.54 cm]

Solution

2.54 cm = 1 inch

$$4.5 \text{ cm} = \frac{1 \times 4.5}{2.54} = 1.77 \text{ in}$$

$$3.8 \text{ cm} = \frac{1 \times 3.8}{2.54} = 1.50 \text{ in}$$

Area of the patch = 4.5 cm × 3.8 cm = 1.77 in × 1.50 in

Ans. 2.655 sq in

Example

The dose of a drug is 0.36 mg/kg/day. This is equivalent to which of the following?

(a) 360 cg/lb/day

(b) 360 mg/lb/day

(c) 163.6 mcg/lb/day

Solution

(a) 1 mg = 110 cg = 0.1 cg [1cg is = 1 centigram = 10 mg]

0.36 mg = 0.36 × 0.1cg = 0.036 cg

1kg = 2.2 lb

The daily dose 0.36 mg/kg = 0.0362.2 cg/lb = 0.163 cg/l

(b) The daily dose 0.36 mg1kg = $\frac{0.36 \text{ mg}}{2.2 \text{ lb}}$ = 0.163 mg/lb

(c) 1 mg = 1000 mcg

The daily dose 0.36 mg1kg = $\frac{0.36 \times 1000 \text{ mcg}}{2.2 \text{ lb}}$ = 163.63 mcg/lb

The equivalent dose of 0.36 mg/kg/day is

163.6 mcg/lb/day

Ans. that is (c)

Example

An average speed of air is 414 miles per hour. Which is the closest equivalent air speed?

(a) 6 mi/min

(b) 257 km/h

(c) 666 km/h

(d) 180 m/sec

Solution

1 mile = 1.6093 km

414 mile = 1.6093 × 414 km = 666.25 km

(a) The speed of air = 414 miles/hour = 414/60 mi/min = 6.9 mi/min

(b) The speed of air = 414 mi/h = 666.251 km/h = 666.25 km/h

(c) The speed of air = 414 mi/h = $\frac{666.25 \times 1000}{60 \times 60}$ = 185.07 m/sec

The nearest equivalent air speed is **666.25 km/h**

Ans. (c)

Conversion of Temperature

In 1709, Gabriel Fahrenheit, the German scientist marked the melting temperature of ice at 32° on a thermometer, and boiling temperature of water at 212°; the difference between the two temperatures was 180°.

In 1742, Anders Celsius, a Swedish astronomer, recommended a scale showing 0° for the freezing point of water and 100° for the boiling point of water, a difference of 100°.

As a result, the *Fahrenheit* (°F) and the *Celsius,* or *centigrade,* (°C) thermometers were established. Both types of thermometers measure the difference of temperature of same activities (boiling and freezing of water). Thus, 100°C is equivalent to 180°F; each degree centigrade is the equivalent of 1.8 or 9/5 degree Fahrenheit.

$$°F = \frac{9}{5}°C + 32 \text{ and } °C = \frac{5}{9} \times (°F - 32)$$

Example

Convert 60 °C to corresponding degrees Fahrenheit.

Solution

$°F = \frac{9}{5}(60\ °C) + 32 = 140$

Hence, 60 °C

Ans. 140°F

Example

Convert 128°F to corresponding degrees Centigrade.

Solution

$$°C = \frac{5}{9} \times (128\ °F - 32) = \frac{5}{9} \times 96 = 40\ °C$$

Hence, 128 °F

Ans. 40 °C

Example

The body temperature was recorded as 37 °C when a *Celsius* thermometer was used. If a Doctor's thermometer were used what would had been the temperature?

Solution

Doctor's thermometer reads the temperature in *Fahrenheit* scale.

Say, the equivalent temperature in *Fahrenheit* scale was x°F

$$\text{Then, } x = \frac{9}{5}(37°C) + 32 = (37 \times \frac{9}{5} + 32)°F$$

Ans. 98.6°F

Storage temperatures

In manufacturing, shipping, and storage of pharmaceutical products temperature plays an important role. At high temperature physicochemical instability of a therapeutic agent or its product may takes place. For better stability of drug products, the manufacturer needs to specify the appropriate storage temperature in the label of each pharmaceutical product, this includes temperature range under which the product should be stored. The *United States Pharmacopeia* provides the following definitions for the storage of pharmaceuticals.

Storage condition	Temperature
Freezer:	Between -25°C and -10°C (-13°F and 14°F)
Cold:	Within 8°C (46°F)
Refrigerator:	Between 2°C and 8°C (36°F and 46°F)
Cool:	Between 8°C and 15°C (46°F and 59°F)
Warm:	Between 30°C and 40°C (86°F and 104°F)
Excessive Heat:	Above 40°C (104°F)
Controlled Room Temperature:	Between 20°C and 25°C (68°F and 77°F)

Calculation Involving Units

Many of the pharmaceutical products are derived from biological sources. The potency of such product is based on *units of activity*. Specific biologic standards are used to determine the units of activity and the units of activity vary among the products.

The units of activity is determined and expressed in terms of a measurable quantity, such as units per milligram or units per milliliter. For example, as per the USP the sterile penicillin G sodium must contain not less than 1500 and not more than 1750 Penicillin G Units per milligram. The potency of the USP Reference Standard of the antibiotic is 1590 USP Units of penicillin G sodium per milligram. The potency of antibiotics may also be designated in terms of µg (micrograms) of activity.

This relationship may be used to determine either the number of units of activity or the weight or volume containing a specified number of units, as shown below:

$$\frac{\text{Units of activity (given)}}{\text{Weight or volume (given)}} = \frac{\text{Units of activity (given or desired)}}{\text{Weight or volume (given or desired)}}$$

Example

Calculate the volume of insulin U-100 to be taken to inject 50 units dose. (U-100 insulin contains 100 units per mL)

Solution

$$\frac{\text{Units of activity (given)}}{\text{Weight or volume (given)}} = \frac{\text{Units of activity (given or desired)}}{\text{Weight or volume (given or desired)}}$$

Or, $\frac{\text{100 units}}{\text{1 mL}} = \frac{\text{40 units}}{\text{x mL}}$

$x = \frac{\text{40 units}}{\text{100 units}}\ \text{mL}$

Ans. 0.4 mL

Example

Sterile penicillin G sodium powder contains 1600 units per mg. How many milligrams of the sterile powder are to be taken to administer 500000 units?

Solution

$$\frac{\text{Units of activity (given)}}{\text{Weight or volume (given)}} = \frac{\text{Units of activity (given or desired)}}{\text{Weight or volume (given or desired)}}$$

$$\text{or, } \frac{1600 \text{ units}}{1 \text{ mg}} = \frac{500000 \text{ units}}{\text{x mg}}$$

$$\text{or, } x = \frac{500000 \text{ units}}{1600 \text{ mg}}$$

Ans. 312.5 mg

Example

A diabetic patient receives 20 units of insulin twice daily. The vial contains 10 mL of insulin U-100, in how many days the vial will be exhausted?

Solution

In a day the patient receives 2 × 20 units = 40 units.

10 ml of U-100 insulin contains = 10 × 100 units = 1000 units of insulin

$$\frac{\text{Units of activity (given)}}{\text{Weight or volume (given)}} = \frac{\text{Units of activity (given or desired)}}{\text{Weight or volume (given or desired)}}$$

$$\text{or, } \frac{40 \text{ units}}{1 \text{ day}} = \frac{1000 \text{ units}}{x \text{ days}}$$

$$\text{or, } x = \frac{1000 \text{ units} \times \text{days}}{40 \text{ units}}$$

Ans. 25 days

The units and micrograms of potency of some official drugs and their respective weight equivalents are given in Table 1.1

Table 1.1 Potency (Activity units) of some important drug substances

Drug substance	Potency as per the USP
Ampicillin Sodium	Not less than 845 μg and not more than 988 μg of
Antihemophilic Factor	Ampicillin per mg
Bacitracin	Not less than 100 Antihemophilic Factor Units per g of
Bacitracin Zinc	protein
Cephalothin Sodium	Not less than 40 Bacitracin Units per mg
Chymotrypsin	Not less than 40 Bacitracin Units per mg
Clindamycin HCl	Not less than 850 μg of Cephalothin per mg
Colistimethate Sodium	Not less than 1000 USP Chymotrypsin Units per mg
Digitalis	Not less than 800μg of Clindamycin per mg

Table 1.1 ***contd...***

Erythromycin Estolate	390 μg Colistin per mg
Gentamycin Sulfate	Not less than 1 USP Digitalis Unit per 100 mg
Heparin Calcium	Not less than 600 μg of erythromycin per mg
Heparin Sodium	Not less than 590μg of Gentamycin per mg
Insulin	Not less than 140 USP Heparin Units per mg
Insulin Human	Not less than 140 USP Heparin Units per mg
Kanamycin Sulfate	Not less than 26.5 USP Insulin Units per mg
Mitomycin	Not less than 27.5 USP Insulin Human Units per mg
Neomycin Sulfate	Not less than 750 μg of Kanamycin per mg
Nystatin	Not less than 970μg Mitomycin per mg
Pancreatin	Not less than 600 μg of neomycin per mg
	Not less than 4400 USP Nystatin Units per mg
Penicillin G Benzathine Penicillin G Potassium	Not less than 25 USP Units of amylase activity, not less than 2 USP Units of lipase activity, and Not less than 25 USP Units of protease activity per mg
Penicillin G Sodium Penicillin V	Not less than 1090 and not more than 1272 Penicillin G Units per mg
Penicillin V Potassium Polymyxin B Sulfate	Not less than 1440 and not more than 1680 Penicillin G Units per mg
Streptomycin Sulfate Tobramycin	Not less than 1500 and not more than 1750 Penicillin G Units per mg
Trypsin, crystallized Vancomycin	Not less than 1525 and not more than 1780 Penicillin V Units per mg
Vasopressin Vitamin A	Not less than 1380 and not more than 1610 Penicillin V Units per mg
	Not less than 6000 Polymyxin B Units per mg
	Not less than 650 μg and Not more than 850 μg of streptomycin per mg
	Not less than 900 μg of Tobramycin per mg
	Not less than 2500 USP Trypsin Units per mg
	Not less than 950 μg Vancomycin per mg
	Not less than 300 Vasopressin Units per mg
	1 USP Vitamin A Unit equals the biologic activity of 0.3 μg of the all-*trans* isomer of retinol

Example

The monograph of I.P. for Concentrated vitamin A oil states that it contains not less than 500000 Units of vitamin A per g and not less than 95% and not more than 110% of the stated number of Units per g. What would be the purity expression in terms of percent for a sample containing 475000 Units of vitamin A per g?

Solution

As per I.P. the lowest limit in terms of Units is 500000 which is equivalent to 95%.

$$\frac{500000\text{ Units}}{95\%} = \frac{475000\text{ Units}}{x\%}$$

or, $$x = \frac{475000 \times 95}{500000}$$

Ans. 90.25%

Example

Streptomycin sulphate 75 kg has been bought and analyzed. The potency of the drug is found to be 710 μg per mg. According to Master Formula 70 kg of 100% potency is required for a lot. Find out how much of the drug is to be issued by the store.

Solution

The limits of potency of the drug being from 650 to 850μg/mg; the potency of 750 [(650+850)/2] μg/mg represents 100%.

Thus, the potency, 710 μg/mg represents $\frac{710 \times 100}{750} = 94.67\%$

Say, x kg of 94.67% is equivalent to 70 kg of 100%

The amount of drug to be issued = $\frac{70 \times 100}{94.67}$

Ans. 73.94 kg

Exercise

1. The weights have been recorded differently by different students. Add 12 kg 85 mg, 95 kg 349 g, 1kg 986 g 446 mg, 764.9 g, 3.6437 kg, 6.643 g and write the result in the form of mixed units.

   Ans: 113 kg 750 g 81 mg

2. Add 0.0025 kg, 1750 mg, 2.25 g, and 825,000 μg, and express the answer in grams.

   Ans: 7.325 g

3. A capsule contains the following amounts of medicinal substances: 0.075 g, 20 mg, 0.0005 g, 4 mg, and 500 μg. What is the total weight of the substances in the capsule?

   Ans: 100 mg

4. Each ml of a solution contains 1.04 g, 45 mg, 0.8 mg, 520 mcg of various ingredients. Calculate total quantity of ingredients per ml?

Ans: 1 g 86.32 mg

5. Add 51 L, 0.85 L and 395 mL. Express the total volume in milliliters.

Ans: 52245 ml

6. From a stock of 2.55 g Cyanocobalamine 770 mg is taken. How much is left?

Ans: 1780 mg or 1 g 780 mg

7. A cloth piece of length 4 meter was cut into pieces. Length of each is 1 foot 6 inches. Calculate the length of balance cloth.

Ans: 13.48 inch or 34.24 cm

8. There are five bottles of Almond oil; two bottles of 1 quart, one bottle of 1 pint, one bottle of 500 ml, and one bottle of 1L. Find out the total quantity of almond oil.

Ans: 3865 ml or 3 L 865 ml

9. A thermometer records 98 °C. Convert this temperature to Fahrenheit scale.

Ans: 208.4 °F

10. If the normal body temperature is 98.6 °F. What would it be in Centigrade scale?

Ans: 37 °C

11. A sample is found to contain 590 units of drug per mg. A dosage form containing 200000 units is prepared. How many milligram of the drug shall remain per unit dosage form?

Ans: 338.98 mg per dosage form

12. The monograph of I.P. for Concentrated vitamin A oil states that it contains not less than 500000 Units of vitamin A per g and not less than 95% and not more than 110% of the stated number of Units per g. What would be the purity expression in terms of units for a sample containing 98.5% of vitamin A?

Ans: 518421 units per g

12. Each Paracetamol tablet contains 650 mg of paracetamol. How many such tablets can be prepared from 15 kg of paracetamol?

Ans: 23076.9

13. An injectable solution contains 50 µg of a drug substance in each 0.5 mL, find out the volume to be injected so that a patient receives 0.25 mg of the drug substance.

Ans: 2.5 ml

14. A prefilled syringe contains 25 mg of drug in 2 mL of solution. How many micrograms of drug would be administered if 0.5 mL of the solution is injected?

Ans: 6250 µg

15. Each tablet contains the following ingredients:

Aspirin 325 mg

Calcium Carbonate 27.5 mg

Citric Acid 90.5 mg

Potassium Bicarbonate 29.5 mg

Sodium Bicarbonate 46.0 mg

Magnesium stearate 5 mg

Starch 25 mg

Talcum 5 mg

PVP 27.5 mg

(a) Calculate the total weight, in grams, of the ingredients in each tablet.

(b) How many tablets could be made with a supply of 5 kg of aspirin?

Ans: (a) 561, (b) 15384.6

16. The dimensions of a microscopic slide are 10.8 cm by 2.6 cm. Express these dimensions in corresponding inches and area in sq in. (1 inch = to 2.54 cm)

Ans: 4.25 in, 1.02 in, 4.34 sq in

17. An inhaler contains 20 mg of drug, how many inhalation doses can be delivered if each inhalation-dose contains 80 µg?

Ans: 250 doses

18. A formulation contains 0.3 mg of drug in each milliliter. Which of the following would be the equivalent expression of concentration?

(a) 0.03 mg/0.1 dL

(b) 300 mcg/0.01 dL

(c) 3 mcg/0.01 cL

(d) 300 mcg/10 cL

Ans: (b) 300 µg/0.01dL

19. An intravenous solution contains 520µg of drug substance per 5 ml. How many milligrams of the drug would be administered if 540ml of the solution is infused?

Ans: 280.8 mg

20. An analytical instrument can measure quantities of a chemical substance up to nanogram/ml. How many times more capable is this instrument than one that can measure microgram/ml?

Ans: 1000 times

21. A solution for IV injection contains 125 mg of drug in each 15 mL of injection. What would be the concentration of drug in terms of µg/µL?

Ans: 8.33 µg/µL

22. According to the label claim each milliliters of Ampicillin sodium injection contains 125 mg of Ampicillin100%. If the Ampicillin sodium used contains 900 µg of Ampicillin per mg, calculate the amount of Ampicillin present in two milliliters of injection. The potency limits of Ampicillin sodium is 845 to 988µg/mg.

Ans: 254.6 mg

23. A tube is 2ft 5 inches long and 7 inches wide. Convert the dimensions in terms of centimeter.

Ans: 73.66cm long and 17.78 cm wide

24. A mixing tank is 1.6 meter in height and its width is 0.98meter. Convert the dimensions in foot and inches.

Ans: 5 ft 2.99 inches long and 3ft 2.58 inches

25. The prophylactic dose of riboflavin is 2 mg. How many grams of riboflavin would be required to prepare 50000 tablets with 10% overage?

Ans: 110 mg

2

Measurements of Mass and Volume

Pharmaceutical measurement is an important activity, it is necessary for all sorts activities related to manufacture, analysis, and in pharmacy practice. It includes equipments and methods used. Accurate weighing and measuring the materials is a skill which is acquired through professional education and training.

This chapter focuses on:

- Instruments required for volumetric measurement and characterization of their differences in application and accuracy.
- Knowledge about sensitivity and its application in calculations.
- Calculations using the aliquot method.
- Understanding of percentage of error in pharmaceutical measurement.

Measurement of Weight

Wide range of weights, balances, and scales are available - sensitive electronic analytic balances, prescription balances, and large-capacity industrial scales which are used in manufacturing and analysis of pharmaceutical products.

The selection of an appropriate balance and weights depends on the type of measurement to be done. Each instrument used must meet established standards for sensitivity, accuracy, and capacity.

Class A prescription balances are designed for weighing of medicinal or pharmaceutical substances required in small-scale compounding. Some prescription balances have a weigh beam and rider, and others a dial, to add up to 1 gram of weight. The weights are put on the right hand pan of the balance and the material to be weighed is placed on the left-hand pan.

This type of balance is sensitive to 6 mg or less without load and with a load of 10 grams in each pan. Usually most of the commercially available Class A balances have a maximum capacity of weighing 120 g and not less than 120 mg should be weighed to avoid errors of greater than 5%.

The term *sensitivity* is defined as the load that will cause a change of one division on the index plate of the balance. It may be determined by the following procedure:

1. The balance is leveled.
2. The rest point of the balance is determined.
3. Sensitivity shall be the smallest weight that can shift the rest point to one division on the index plate.

There are high-precision electronic analytical balances with greater accuracy than a Class A prescription balance. Such balances can be used to weigh very small quantities. Many of these balances can be used to weigh accurately 0.1 milligram.

Every balance has two limits for its capacity - the minimum amount and maximum amount of a material that can be weighed. There is a relation among sensitivity, error and minimum weigh table quantity.

$$\text{Minimum weigh table quantity} = \frac{\text{Sensitivity} \times 100}{\text{Error (\%)}}$$

Measurement of Volume

Volume is a derived property of an object. It is derived from length. Hence, its unit is a derived one. Pipette, micropipettes, burettes and volumetric flasks are the instruments used for measurement of volume. These are used mainly in analytical procedures. Calibrated vessels are also used to measure the volume in commercial manufacturing. On the basis of degree of precision required, the measuring instruments should be selected. In general, the most common instruments for measuring volume of liquid up to 1000 ml are cylinders; while for the measurement of small volumes, a calibrated syringe or a pipette is used. Measuring cylinders are graduated and calibrated in SI or metric units. These are made of both glass and plastic. These are available in a number of capacities, ranging from 5 to 1000 milliliters and greater.

Some rules to avoid greater error in measurement are:

- Use a measuring cylinder whose capacity is either equal to or just more than the volume to be measured.
- Small volumes should not be measured in large cylinders, the error may increase.
- The cylinder with narrow bore or chamber should be used; the error will be less while reading the meniscus.

According to the *United States Pharmacopeia*, a deviation of ± 1 mm in the meniscus reading causes an error of approximately 0.5 milliliter, when a 100 ml cylinder is used; while an error of 1.8 ml tales place if a comparable graduated conical cylinder is used.

Aliquot Method of Weighing and Measuring

If the degree of required precision in measurement is beyond the capacity of the instrument available, the desired precision can be achieved by calculating and measuring by aliquot method. Aliquot means a fraction, or portion, or a part of an exact number.

Weighing by the Aliquot Method

This method is used when the material to be weighed is less than the minimum weighing capacity of the balance.

In this method an amount larger than the required is weighed first with the desired degree of accuracy. The material weighed is diluted with a known amount (weighed amount) of an inert material, and then a portion (aliquot) of the mixture that contains the desired amount of the needed substance is weighed. The method involves three steps and is described as follows:

Say, 6 mg of a drug is to be weighed and the balance available cannot weigh 6 mg; it can weigh minimum100 mg and maximum up to 160 g.

- **Step I:** Multiply 6 with 20; that is, 120 mg of the drug is weighed first.
- **Step II:** Weigh accurately 2.280 g of an inert material; say lactose. Mix the drug with lactose thoroughly. The total weight of mixture becomes 120 mg + 2280 mg = 2400 mg (20 times of 240 mg). Thus, 2400 mg of powder contain 120 mg of the drug.

- **Step III:** Now weigh 120 mg (2400 mg $\times \frac{1}{20}$) of the powder accurately.

Thus, the aliquot of the powder mix, **120 mg** contains 6 mg of the drug. (Answer)

Arithmetic verification:

2400 mg of powder contains 120 mg of the drug,

Or, 120mg of the drug is present in 2400mg of the powder

Hence, 6 mg of the drug will be contained by $\frac{2400 \times 6}{120}$ = 120 mg of the powder.

Example

A balance is having sensitivity of 10 mg with an error of 5%. Calculate the minimum weighhtable quantity.

Solution

Given that the sensitivity of balance = 10 mg and error = 5%

Then, minimum weightable quantity = $\frac{10 \times 100}{5}$

Ans. 200 mg

Example

A balance has sensitivity of 5 mg with an error of 2%. It can weigh maximum amount of 150 g. How can you weigh 125 mg of a drug using lactose as the inert material?

Solution

The minimum weighhtable quantity = $\frac{5 \times 100}{2}$ = 250 mg

Thus, any amount less than 250 mg cannot be weighed with desired accuracy.

Hence, aliquot method is to be used.

Step I: The quantity of drug to be weighed = 125 mg.

The multiple of this quantity is weighed

= 125 mg × 2 = 250 mg

Step II: The maximum quantity can be weighed is 150 g. The inert material to be mixed should be multiple of 125.

Say, 6.25 g or 6250 mg would be the weight of lactose and drug. Then, the amount of lactose to be weighed and mixed thoroughly = 6250 mg – 250 mg = 6000 mg.

Step III: 6250 mg is 25 times of 250 mg (6250 ÷ 250 = 25).

Thus, 6250 mg × $\frac{1}{2}$ = 3125 mg of the powder mix is weighed which will contain 125 mg of the drug.

Ans: Thus, **3125 mg** of the powder mix will contain 125 mg of the drug.

Arithmetic verification

$$\frac{62500 \text{ mg (Dilution)}}{250 \text{ mg (Dilution)}} = \frac{3125 \text{ mg}}{x \text{ mg}}$$

or, $$x = \frac{3125 \times 250}{62500} = 125 \text{ mg}$$

Example

Calculate the minimum amount of an inert material to be required to weigh 5 mg of a drug using a balance having sensitivity of 6 mg with 5% error. The balance can weigh maximum of 120 g.

Solution

The minimum quantity the balance can weigh = $\frac{6 \times 100}{5}$ = 120 mg and maximum 120 g.

Step I: The quantity of drug to be weighed = 5 mg. The quantity of the drug is weighed = 120 mg which is 24 times of 5 mg.

Step II: The minimum amount of inert material to be mixed would be calculated as;

Let x mg is minimum amount of inert material to be mixed;

Then, (x + 120) mg should be multiple of 120 whose $\frac{1}{24}$ th would be 120 mg, the minimum weighhtable quantity.

or, $$\frac{x}{24} + \frac{120}{24} = 120$$

$$(x + 120) = 120 \times 24 = 2880 \text{ mg}$$

$$x = 2880 - 120 = 2760 \text{ mg}$$

Ans. So, minimum 2760 mg of inert material would be required.

Percentage of Error in Weighing

Various scales and balances are used for pharmaceutical weighing for various purposes. Each of these has a particular degree of precision. A balance may be used to weigh small quantity of material for analytical purpose or large quantity of material for manufacturing purpose. In each case the degree of accuracy would be specific. Hence, the knowledge of the *sensitivity requirement* of the balance being used is most important in weighing to ensure a specified degree of accuracy. The sensitivity of a balance can be used to determine the percentage of error in a given weighing.

Example

When the maximum potential error is ± 5 milligrams in a total of 100 milligrams, what is the percentage of error?

Solution

Error is ± 5 mg out of 100 mg; that is, the measured weight would be either less than 100 mg or more than 100 mg

Ans. Percentage of error $= \frac{5 \text{ mg} \times 100\%}{100 \text{ mg}} = 5\%$

Example

A balance before calibration measures 500 mg which is desired also, when the material is re-measured in a calibrated balance shows 495 mg. Find out the error in the first balance?

Solution

Desired weight = 500 mg,

Actual weight = 495 mg

Difference between the weights = 500 mg – 495 mg = 5 mg

Ans. Percentage of error $= \frac{5 \text{ mg} \times 100\%}{500 \text{ mg}} = 1\%$

Percentage of Error in Measuring Length

Similar to the measurement of volume and weight, measurement of length is necessary to calculate area, volume, etc. Hence, there are different scales used for different purposes. For example, simple scale is used to measure the diameter of a heap of powders in determination of angle of repose of powders or simply to measure the height of a liquid filled in bottle; while slide caliper is used to measure thickness or diameter of a tablet. Hence, each device will have specific accuracy. Ordinary metric scales can measure the smallest length of 1 mm, sometimes up to 0.5 mm; while the slide caliper can measure up to 0.01 mm due to the vernier attached to the main scale. Therefore, a scale is selected depending on the purpose.

A scale may have error; while accuracy and precision in measuring length are equally important. Accordingly the error in measurement of length should also be determined. In fact, each scale being used needs to be calibrated and validated also as is done in case of balance and volume measuring devices.

$$\text{Percentage of Error} = \frac{\text{Error} \times 100\%}{\text{Length desired}}$$

Example

The diameter of a circle is measured using an ordinary scale and found to be 15.5 cm. When it is measured by a certified scale, it measures 15.45 cm. Find out the percentage of error.

Solution

The desired length = 15.5 cm, actual length = 15.45 cm

Difference between desired and actual (error) = 15.50 cm – 15.45 cm = 0.05 cm

$$\textbf{Ans. } \text{Percentage of error} = \frac{0.05 \text{ cm} \times 100\%}{15.5 \text{ cm}} = 0.32$$

Example

The diameter of a tablet is measured using a scale and found to be 11.9 mm. When the same is measured using a slide caliper it is found to be 11.95 mm. Calculate the error in first determination.

Solution

The correct value (diameter) = 11.95 mm,

Difference in two measurements = 11.95 mm – 11.9 mm = 0.05 mm

Percentage of error = $\frac{0.05 \text{ cm} \times 100\%}{11.95 \text{ cm}}$

Ans. 0.42

Example

The average thickness and diameter of a tablet were measured and found 3.0 mm and 10.0 mm respectively. The thickness and diameter were re-measured using a certified instrument and found to be 3.12 mm and 10.4 mm respectively. Find out the % error in the first instrument and % variation in the values of surface area.

Solution

1. the correct thickness of the tablet = 3.12 mm

   Difference in measurement = 3.12 mm – 3.0 mm = 0.12 mm

   Thus, percent error in first measurement = $\frac{0.12 \times 100}{3.12} = 3.85$

   The correct diameter of the tablet = 10.4 mm

   Difference in measurement = 10.4 mm – 10.0 mm = 0.4 mm

   Thus, percent error in first measurement = $\frac{0.4 \times 100}{10.4}$

   Ans. 3.85

2. The surface area of the tablet = $2\,\pi r \times h$

   (where, r = radius and h = thickness of the tablet)

   According to the first measurement, the surface area of the tablet

   = 2 × 3.14 × 5 × 3 = 94.2 sq mm

   According to the second measurement, the surface area of the tablet = 2 × 3.14 × 5.2 × 3.12 = 101.88 sq mm

   The percent variation in surface area = $\frac{(101.88 - 94.2) \times 100}{101.88}$

   Ans. 7.54

Measurement of Area

The area of a rectangle is the product of its length and breadth. If the length is L and breadth is B, then the area, $A = L \times B$.

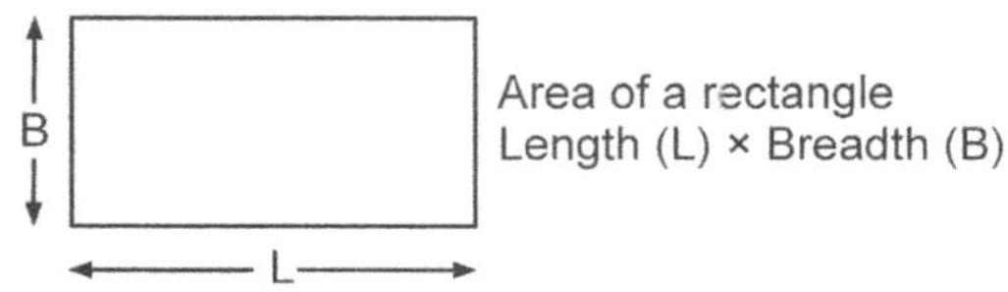

The unit of area is derived from length unit. It is very simple; the square of length units is generated by multiplying the two length units. Since very long the popular units are square feet, square yards, square miles and acre, etc.

There is a Pharmaceutical relevence in learning how to measure the area. For example, to calculate the area of manufacturing premises or AUC in biopharmaceutical assessment of drug.

British System

The area of land has been expressed in terms of acres, rods and in case of relatively smaller area the unit used is square feet. These units are of the British system and still we use these units. Hence, these are mentioned here.

Acre

This unit had been traditionally used and is still in use to express the area of agricultural land. In England *one acre is the area bounded by one furlong long by one chain wide.*

Thus, 1 acre = 1 furlong × 1 chain

= 220 yards × 22 yards

= 4840 square yards

= 43560 square feet

Rood

The term rood came from the term rod. One rood is one forth of an acre. The area of one furlong by one rod is called one rood.

Thus, 1 rood = 1 furlong × 1 rod

$= 220 \text{ yards} \times 5\frac{1}{2} \text{ yards}$

= 1210 square yards

$= \frac{1}{4} \text{ acre}$

The values of units for area used in the British system are given in the table below:

Units	Value	Units	Value
1 sq thou	0.000001 sq in	1 sq chain	16 sq rod = 484 sq yd
1 sq ft	144 sq in	1 rood	2.5 sq chain = 40 sq rod = 1210 sq yd
1 sq yd	9 sq ft = 1296 sq in	1 acre	10 sq chain = 160 sq rod = 4840 sq yd
1 sq rod	30.25 sq yd = 272.25 sq ft	1 sq mile	640 acre

Metric System

The units of metric system used in measuring the length are used by squaring them. For example, square millimeter (sq mm), square centimeter (sq cm), square meter (sq m), etc.

Example

The length of a room is 1.4 m and breadth is 1.0 m. Find out the area of the room.

Solution

Given that the length, A = 1.4 m

Breadth, B = 1.0 m

Then, area $\frac{AB}{A \times B}$ = 1.4 m × 1.0 m

Ans. 1.4 sqm

Example

A rectangular floor is 22 ft long and 12 ft wide. Find out its area and express the in sq m also. (1 m = 39.37 in).

Solution

$1\text{ m} = 39.37\text{ in} = \frac{39.37}{12}\text{ ft} = 3.28\text{ ft}$

or, $1\text{ ft} = \frac{1}{3.28}\text{ m} = 0.305\text{ m}$

Area of the floor = 22 ft × 12 ft = 264 sq ft. (Answer)

= 22 × 0.305 m × 12 × 0.305 m

Ans. 24.56 sq m

Example

The length of a rectangular glass plate, A is 25.5 ft and breadth is15 ft. The length of another rectangular plate, B is 29.9 ft and its breadth is 9.9 ft. Calculate.

1. the areas of two plates,
2. which plate is bigger in area, and
3. how many times?

Solution

1. Area of the plate A = 25.5 ft × 15 ft = 382.5 sq ft (Answer)

   Area of the plate B = 29.9 ft × 9.9 ft = 296.01 sq ft (Answer)
2. The area of plate A is bigger. (Answer)
3. The area of A is bigger than that of B in times = $\frac{382.5 \text{ sq ft}}{296.01 \text{ sq ft}}$

Ans. $0.279 \approx 0.3$

Example

The areas of two rectangular plots, A and B are 1900 sq ft and 200 sq m respectively. Which one is bigger and how much? (1 m = 3.28 ft)

Solution

1 m = 3.28 ft,

1 sq m = 3.28 ft × 3.28 ft = 10.76 sq ft

The area of plot A = 1900 sq ft

The area of plot B = 200 sq m = 200 × 10.76 sq ft = 2152 sq ft

Hence, (1) the plot B is bigger than plot A. (Answer)

Difference in area = 2152 sq ft – 1900 sq ft = 252 sq ft.

Hence, (2) the area of plot B is **252 sq ft** more than that of A. (Answer)

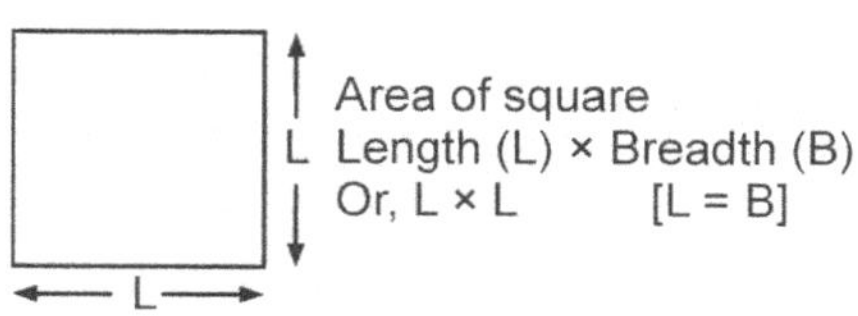

A square is a rectangle whose four sides are equal in length. Thus its area, $A = L \times L = L^2$.

Example

A plate is of square shape. The length of its side is 12 m; find out the area and express in sq ft.

(1 m = 3.28 ft)

Solution

The length of each side of the plate is 12 m; its area = 12 m × 12 m = **144 sq m** (Answer)

1 m = 3.28 ft

1 sq m = 3.28 ft × 3.28 ft = 10.76 sq ft

144 sq m = 144 × 10.76 sq ft

Ans. 1549.44 sq ft

Example

A piece of land is rectangular in shape. If it is cut into two pieces, each plot becomes square. The area of square plot is 1540 sq ft. Find out the length of the original rectangular plot.

Solution

Area of the square plot = 1540 sq ft

Area of a square = L^2 = 1540 sq ft. (L is the length of any side of the square)

$L = \sqrt{1540} = 39.24$ ft

The area of original plot = 2 × area of the square plot

The area of rectangular plot = 2 × 1540 sq ft = 3080 sq ft

The breadth of rectangular plot = length of the square = 39.24 ft

Length of rectangular plot = 2 × 39.24 ft

Ans. 78.48 ft

There is confusion over the definition of trapezium and trapezoid, in USA and UK. Trapezium is a quadrilateral; that is having four sides. In USA it is defined as a quadrilateral with no parallel sides; while in UK it is defined as a quadrilateral with two sides parallel.

According to the British system the area of trapezium $= \frac{1}{2}$(sum of lengths of two parallel sides × vertical height)

If the lengths of two parallel sides are a and b, and the vertical height (perpendicular distance between two parallel sides) is h; then the area $= \frac{1}{2}(a + b) \times h$

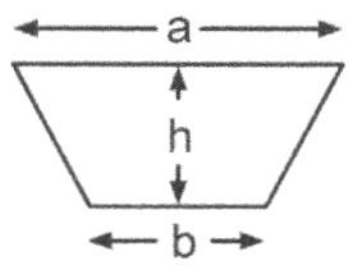

Area of trapezium

$\frac{1}{2}(a + b) \times h$

h = vertical height

Example

The lengths of two parallel sides of a trapezium are 45 cm and 15 cm, and these are separated by a perpendicular distance of 5 cm. Calculate the area of the trapezium.

Solution

Area of a trapezium $= \frac{1}{2}$ [sum of lengths of two parallel sides × vertical height]

$= \frac{1}{2}(45\text{cm} + 15\text{ cm}) \times 5\text{ cm}$

Ans. 300 sq cm

Example

Prove that the area of a trapezium is $\frac{1}{2}$ [sum of lengths of two parallel sides × vertical height]

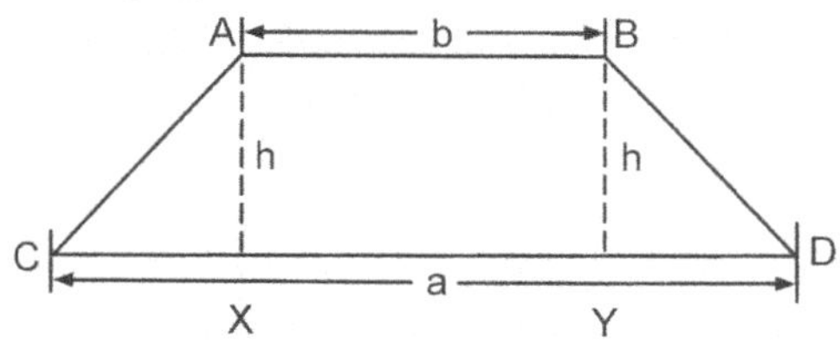

Solution

Let us assume that ABDC is a trapezium, and

AB = XY = b, CD = a, and the vertical distance between them, AX or BY = h. It contains one rectangle, AXYB and two right angled triangles, ACX and BYD.

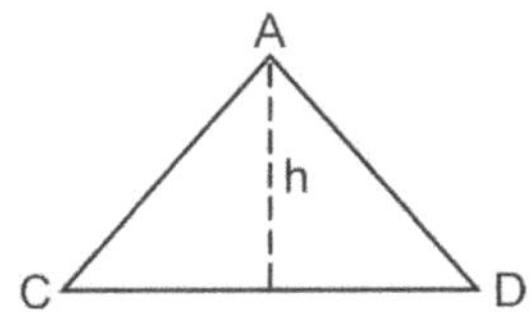

When the triangles are separated out and joined together, they form the triangle, A'C'D'.

So, the area of ABDC = area of AXYB + area of A'C'D' (area of ACX + area of BYD).

$$= bh + \frac{1}{2}(a - b)h \quad [CD = CX + XY + YD = CX + AB + YD]$$

$$C'D' = CD - AB = a - b$$

$$= bh + \frac{1}{2}ah - \frac{1}{2}bh$$

$$= \frac{1}{2}ah + \frac{1}{2}bh$$

$$= \frac{1}{2}(a + b)h$$

$= \frac{1}{2}$ (length of one parallel side + length of other parallel side) × vertical height.

Thus, the area of a trapezium is $\frac{1}{2}$ [sum of lengths of two parallel sides × vertical height] [Proved]

Example

Calculate the area of a trapezium whose parallel sides are 17.8 ft and 10.3 ft long, and the vertical height is 5.4 ft.

Solution

The lengths of the parallel sides are 17.8 ft and 10.3 ft, and the vertical height is 5.4 ft.

Area of trapezium = $\frac{1}{2}$ (length of one parallel side + length of other parallel side) × vertical height.

$$= \frac{1}{2}(17.8 \text{ ft} + 10.3 \text{ ft}) \times 5.4 \text{ ft}$$

$$= \frac{1}{2}(27.3 \text{ ft}) \times 5.4 \text{ ft}$$

Ans. 73.71 sq ft

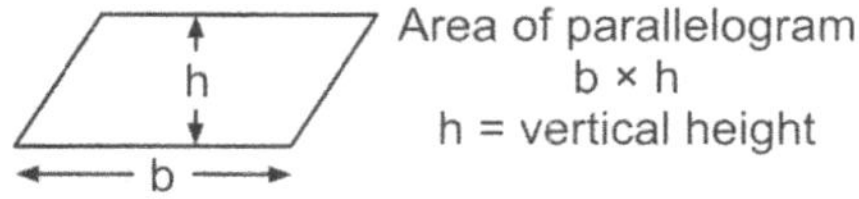

A **parallelogram** is a quadrilateral with opposite sides are parallel; hence, opposite angles are equal. A quadrilateral with equal sides is called rhombus. In a parallelogram opposite sides are equal in length and opposite angles are equal in measure.

The area of a parallelogram = base × vertical height.

Example

The lengths of base and vertical height of a parallelogram are 14.6 m and 6.2 m respectively. Find out the area of the parallelogram.

Solution

Length of the base, b = 14.6 m

Vertical height, h = 6.2 m

Area of the parallelogram = b × h = 14.6 m × 6.2 m

Ans. 90.52 sq m

Example

The base of a parallelogram is 7.8 cm and vertical height is 3.4 cm at one position. When the parallelogram is rotated to 90° the length of the base becomes 5.3 cm. Find out the vertical height at this position.

Solution

When the length of the base = 7.8 cm and vertical height = 3.4 cm

Area of the parallelogram = 7.8 cm × 3.4 cm = 26.52 sq cm.

After 90° rotation the length of the base = 5.3 cm; but the area remains same.

Vertical height = ? (Say, it is b cm)

Then, 5.3 cm × b cm = 26.52 sq cm

$$\text{Hence, b} = \frac{26.52 \text{ sq cm}}{5.3 \text{ cm}} = 5.00 \text{ cm. (Answer)}$$

The length of the vertical height is 5.00 cm. (Answer)

A rhombus is an equilateral quadrilateral whose any two opposite sides are parallel; all the four sides are of same length. There are three methods to calculate the area of a rhombus.

Method I: Base Times Height method; Area of a rhombus = Base × Vertical height

---

Example

The side of a rhombus is 20 cm long and the vertical height is 14 cm. Find out the area of the rhombus.

Solution

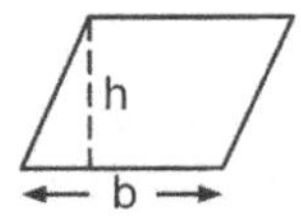

Length of one side, b = 20 cm

Vertical height, h = 14 cm

Area of the rhombus = Base × vertical height

= 20 cm × 14 cm

= 280 sq cm (Answer)

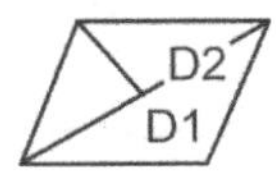

Method II: Diagonal method; Area of a rhombus = $\frac{1}{2}$ × first-diagonal × second-diagonal

According to the definition, the diagonals of a rhombus connect the opposite corners (vertices) in the centre of the shape. The diagonals of a rhombus are perpendicular to each other and form four right angles at the point of intersection.

Example

The diagonals of a rhombus are 12 cm and 16 cm respectively. Calculate the area of the rhombus.

Solution

Area of the rhombus = $\frac{1}{2}$ × first-diagonal × second-diagonal

= $\frac{1}{2}$ × 12 cm × 16 cm

Ans. 96 sq cm

Example

The diagonals of a kite are 11 cm and 40 cm. What would be the area of the kite?

Solution

$$\text{Area of the rhombus} = \frac{1}{2} \times \text{first-diagonal} \times \text{second-diagonal}$$
$$= \frac{1}{2} \times 11 \text{ cm} \times 40 \text{ cm}$$

Ans. 220 sq cm

Method III: Trigonometry method; Area of a rhombus = (any side)^2 × Sin A. The opposite angles of a rhombus are equal and any one of the two pairs of angles can be taken for calculation.

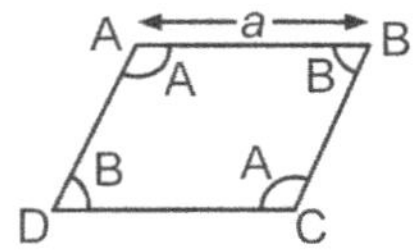

Example

The length of a side of a rhombus is 5 cm and an internal angle measure 50°. Find out the area of the rhombus.

Solution

$$\text{Area of a rhombus} = (\text{any side})^2 \times \text{Sin A} \; [\, a = 5 \text{ cm and angle B} = 50^\circ]$$
$$= 5^2 \times 0.766$$
$$= 25 \times 0.766$$

Ans. 19.15 sq cm

A **triangle** is three sided polygon. Triangles are of three types on the basis of measure of angles.

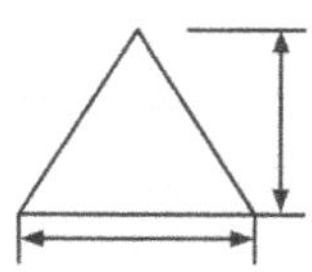

- Acute triangle (each of three angles is less than 90°),
- Right angle triangle (one angle is 90°) and
- Obtuse triangle (one angle is more than 90°).

Again triangles may be of three types based on the length of the sides:

- Equilateral triangle (all three sides are equal),
- Isosceles triangle (any two sides are equal) and
- Scalene triangle (none of the sides are equal).

As the area of a parallelogram is $a \times$ h, the area of a triangle would be $\frac{1}{2} \times a \times$h; where a is the base and h is the vertical height.

Example

The base of a triangle is 15 cm and its height is 25 cm. Find out the area.

Solution

The area of a triangle = $\frac{1}{2} \times a \times \text{h}$

[a = 15 cm and h = 25 cm]

$= \frac{1}{2} \times 15 \text{ cm} \times 25 \text{ cm}$

Ans. 187.5 sq cm

Example

The area of a triangular carpet is 5 sq ft and its base is 25 ft; calculate the height of the carpet.

Solution

The area of a triangle = $\frac{1}{2} \times a \times \text{h}$ [a = 5 ft, h = ?]

The area of a triangular carpet = 25 sq ft = $\frac{1}{2} \times 5 \text{ ft} \times \text{h}$

$\text{h} = \frac{25 \text{ sq ft}}{5 \text{ ft}}$

Ans. 5 ft (Answer)

The area of an **ellipse** is $\pi \times a \times$ b; where a is minor axis and b is major axis.

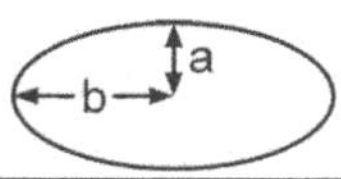

Area of ellipse πab

Example

A piece of elliptical cloth whose major axis is 10 cm and minor axis is 4 cm. Find out the area of the cloth.

Solution

Area of an ellipse = $\pi \times a \times$ b [a = 4 cm and b = 10 cm]

The area of elliptical cloth = 3.14 × 4 × 10

Ans. 125.6 sq cm

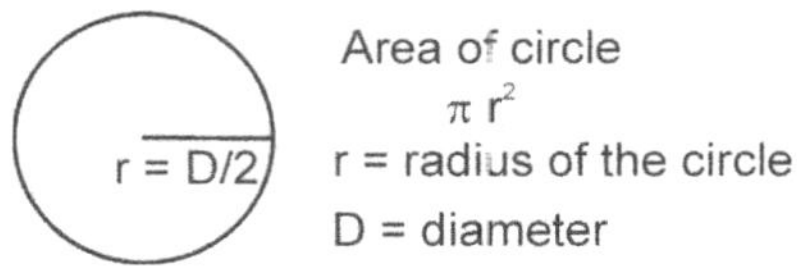

The distance around a **circle** is its circumference; distance across a circle through its centre is diameter. The ratio of the circumference of a circle to its diameter is represented by π (pi). The diameter, D of a circle is twice of its radius, r. The circumference is $2\pi r$ and area of the circle is πr^2; when r is its radius.

Example

The diameter of a circle is 28 cm, calculate its area.

Solution

Area of a circle = πr^2. $\quad$ [$r = \frac{1}{2} \times$ diameter and $\pi = 3.14$]

$$\text{Area of the given circle} = \pi \left(\frac{D}{2}\right)^2 = 3.14 \times \left(\frac{28}{2}\right)^2$$

$$= 3.14 \times 14 \times 14$$

$$= 615.44 \text{ sq cm (Answer)}$$

When calculating the area of a **sector**, actually a fractional part of the area of the entire circle is being calculated. The fraction is determined by the ratio of the central angle of the sector to the "entire central angle" of 360°.

Example

The central angle of a circle is 180° and its radius is 28 cm. What would be area of the sector?

Solution

The central angle, θ = 180° and r = 25 cm

$$\text{The area of the circle} = \frac{\theta}{360} \pi r^2$$

$$= \frac{180^o}{360^o} \times 3.14 \times 25 \text{ cm} \times 25 \text{ cm}$$

$$= \frac{1}{2} \times 1962.5$$

Ans. 981.25 sq cm

Example

If the value of θ is 45° and the diameter of the circle is 3 cm, calculate the area of the sector.

Solution

The central angle, $\theta = 45^\circ$ and r = 3 cm

The area of the circle $= \frac{\theta}{360}\pi r^2$

$$= \frac{45^\circ}{360^\circ} \times 3.14 \times 3\text{cm} \times 3\text{cm}$$

$$= 0.125 \times 28.26 = 3.53 \text{ sq cm (Answer)}$$

The area of **sector** of a circle can be calculated as;

The area of sector of a circle $= \frac{L}{2\pi r}\pi r^2$; where r is the radius and L is the length of arc of the circle. The circumference of a circle is $2\pi r$.

Example

The radius of a circular field is 24 ft and length of a arc is 15 ft. Find out the area of the sector.

Solution

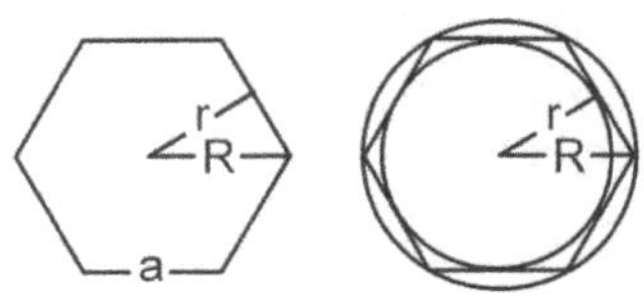

r = apothem (radius of the inscribed circle)
R = radius of the circum circle
a = length of a side
n = number of sides

Area of a sector $= \frac{\theta}{360}\pi r^2$

Where θ is the angle of the sector.

The radius, r = 24 ft and the length of the arc, L = 15 ft.

Then, area of the sector $= \frac{L}{2\pi r}\pi r^2 = \frac{15}{2\times3.14\times24} 3.14 \times 24 \times 24$

$$= \frac{27129.6}{150.72} = \textbf{180 sq ft.} \text{ (Answer)}$$

The area of a **regular polygon** can be calculated by using various formulas:

1. Area $= \frac{1}{2}$ r 2πR
2. Area $= \frac{1}{2}$ n × *a* × r (n = number of sides of the polygon)
3. Area $= \frac{1}{2} n \times R^2 \times \sin \frac{360^o}{n}$

   $= n \times r^2 \times \tan \frac{180^o}{n}$

Surface Area

The surface area of a solid material is the total area of all the surfaces of the material. In other words, surface area is the total area of surface of a three-dimensional object.

It can be explained in terms of a three-dimensional shape of a solid that has length, breadth and depth. For example, a sphere and a cube have three dimensions; while a circle and square are two dimensional. A cube does not have any curved surface; while a sphere has. The unit of surface area is square of length unit, such as sq cm, sq ft, etc.

Surface area of a **cube** is the area of six squares which cover it. The area of each square is a^2; where a is the length of any side. Thus, surface area of the cube is $6a^2$.

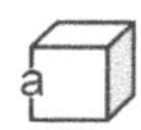

The surface area of a **rectangular prism** is the area of the six rectangles that cover it. Out of six sides the top and bottom are of same dimensions or area, the front and back have same dimensions or area, and the left and right sides are of same area. If the length and breadth of top or bottom side are a and b, then the area would be $a \times$ b. Similarly, if the depth is c, then the area of front or back side is $a \times$ c; and the area of right or left side would be b × c.

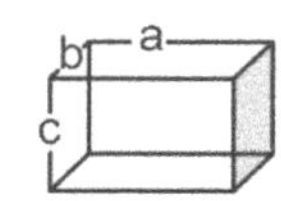

Rectangular prism

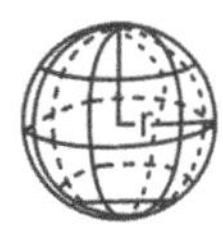

Sphere

Thus, the surface area of the prism = 2ab + 2bc +2ac.

Example

The length, breadth and depth of a rectangular prism are 4, 2, and 1 m respectively. Find out its surface area.

Solution

Given that, the length, $a = 4$m

Breadth, b = 2m, and the depth, c = 1m

Then, c

$$= 2(4\times2 + 2\times1 + 1\times4)$$

$$= 2\times14$$

Ans. 28 sq m

Example

The depth of a rectangular prism is half of its breadth which is half of its length. If the depth of the rectangular prism is 2m, calculate the surface area of the prism.

Solution

Given that the breadth of the prism, b = 2c, or 2 × depth of the prism;

The length of the prism, a = 2b, or 2 × breadth of the prism.

The depth of the prism, c = 2m.

The surface area of the prism = $2ab + 2bc + 2ac$.

$$= 2(2\times2c\times2c + 2c\times c + 2\times2c\times c)$$

$$= 2(8c^2 + 2c^2 + 4c^2)$$

$$= 28c^2$$

$$= 28\times2^2 \text{ sq m}$$

$$= 112 \text{ sq m (Answer)}$$

Surface area of a **sphere** is $4\pi r^2$; where r is the radius.

Example

If the diameter of a sphere is 6 cm, calculate the surface area of the sphere.

Solution

Given that the diameter of the sphere = 6 cm

The surface area of the sphere is $4\pi r^2$

The radius, $r = \frac{1}{2} \times \text{diameter} = \frac{1}{2} \times 6 \text{ cm} = 3 \text{ cm}$

Then, the surface area of the sphere = $4 \times 3.14 \times 3^2$ sq cm

= 113.04 sq cm (Answer)

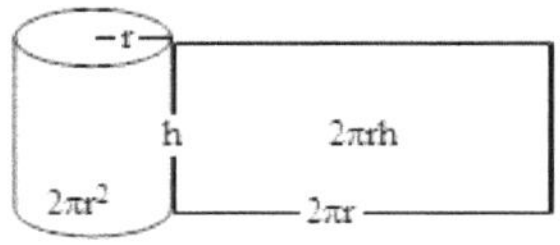

Surface area of symmetrical **cylinder** is the sum of the area of the top, bottom and side. The area of top and bottom are same; which is equal to the area of a circle. The side portion if peeled off look like a rectangular sheet whose length would be the circumference of the circle and breadth would be height of the cylinder.

The area of top and bottom surface = $\pi r^2 + \pi r^2$ and that of the side = $2\pi r \times h$.

Thus, the surface area of the cylinder = $2\pi r^2 + 2\pi rh$.

Example

One mild steel pipe 190 cm wide and 3.25 m long needs to be painted externally. If 0.1 ml of paint is required per sq cm, how many liters of paint would be required?

Solution

Given that the diameter of the cylinder, d = 190 cm

The radius, $r = \frac{d}{2} = \frac{190}{2} = 95$ cm, and

Height of the cylinder, h = 3.25 m = 3.25 × 100 cm = 325 cm

The external surface area of the cylinder = $2\pi rh$

= 2 × 3.14 × 95 × 325 sq cm

= 193895 sq cm

Per sq cm 0.1 ml paint is required.

Hence, paint required for 193895 sq cm = $\frac{0.1\text{ml} \times 193895 \text{ sq cm}}{1 \text{sq cm}}$ = 19389.5 ml

$= \frac{19389.5 \text{ ml}}{1000}$

Ans. 19.389 lts

Example

A hollow pipe is prepared with a 14mm metal sheet. The length of the pipe 1.4 m and outer diameter is 0.9 m. Find out the inner surface area.

Solution

The inner diameter of the pipe = 0.9 m – 14 mm = 0.9 m – 0.014 m = 0.886 m

The length of the pipe = 1.4 m

Surface area of the pipe = $2\pi r \times h$

$$= 2 \times 3.14 \times \frac{0.886}{2} \text{ m} \times 1.4 \text{ m}$$

$$= 2 \times 3.14 \times 0.443 \times 1.4 \text{ sq m}$$

Ans. 3.895 sq m

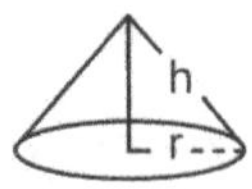

Surface area of a **right circular cone** is $\pi r (r + \sqrt{r^2 + h^2})$; where r is the radius and h is the height of the cone.

Example

A cone like tent is to be made covered with canvas cloth. The tent is 2.10 m high and 2.25 m wide. Calculate how many sq m of cloth would be required.

Solution

Given that, the height of the cone, h = 2.10 m

The diameter, d = 2.25 m; the radius, $r = \frac{2.25}{2}$ m = 1.125 m

The surface area of the cone = $\pi r (r + \sqrt{r^2 + h^2})$

$$= 3.14 \times 1.125\ (1.125 + \sqrt{1.125^2 + 2.1^2})$$

$$= 3.5325\ (1.125 + \sqrt{1.2656 + 4.41})$$

$$= 3.5325\ (1.125 + 2.3823)$$

$$= 12.3895 \text{ sq m}$$

Ans. 12.39 sq m

Measuring Volume by the Aliquot Method

The principle of measuring volume by aliquot method is same as that of weight. When small volume of a liquid is to be measured with great precision, this method is used. The steps involved are:

- Select a multiple of the desired volume of a liquid and measure with the required precision.
- Dilute the multiple quantity of the liquid with a solvent miscible with the liquid to be measured. The volume of the solvent is a multiple of the liquid.
- Divide the mixture by the same factor and measure the aliquot of the diluted liquid that contains the desired quantity.

Example

There is a 10 ml cylinder graduated from 2 to 10 ml, each small division represents 1ml. How you would measure 0.4 ml of sulphuric acid by the aliquot method?

Solution

Say, 2 milliliters is set as the volume of the aliquot and 5 is selected as the multiple,

Then;

Step I: Measure 5×0.4 mL = 2 mL of the acid

Step II: Dilute 2 ml of the acid with 8 mL of water to make10 mL.

Step III: Measure $\frac{1}{5}$ th of 10 ml diluted acid, or 2 mL of diluted acid. Thus, **2 ml** of diluted acid contain

Ans. 0.4 mL of sulphuric acid

Example

Using a 5 mL graduated cylinder whose smallest division represents 0.5 mL. How would you measure 0.2 ml of peppermint oil by the aliquot method? Alcohol is the diluent.

Solution

Say, 5 is chosen as the multiple, then:

Step I: Measure 5×0.2 ml = 1 mL of peppermint oil.

Step II: Dilute 1 ml of peppermint oil with 4 mL of alcohol and mix. 5 mL of diluted oil is obtained.

Step III: Measure $\frac{1}{5}^{th}$ of 5 ml of diluted oil; that is 1 mL.

Thus, **1 ml** of diluted oil contains 0.2 mL of peppermint oil. (Answer)

Percentage Error

Measurements are never *absolutely* accurate. It is important to know the limitations of the instruments used and the magnitude of the errors that may be incurred excluding the personnel error. During measurement of a volume of liquid or weight of a material, two quantities are important to ascertain:

1. The *apparent* weight or volume measured, and
2. The percent age of error in the volume or weight measured.

Percentage of error may be defined as *the maximum potential error multiplied by 100 and divided by the quantity desired.* The mathematical expression is as follows:

$$\text{Percentage of Error} = \frac{\text{Error} \times 100\%}{\text{Quantity desired}}$$

Percentage of Error in Volumetric Measurement

It has been mentioned earlier that the precision obtained in a given measurement depends on several factors such as;

- The selection of the measuring device,
- The volume of liquid to be measured, and
- The skill and care of the personnel involved in measuring or weighing.

The percentage of error in a measurement of volume may be calculated from the equation given above. The extent of error may be determined through devices of greater precision in comparison to the volume measured.

Example

A liquid was measured 72 ml using a graduated cylinder; subsequently on examination, using a narrow-gauge burette, it was found to be 73 ml. What was the percentage of error in the original measurement?

Solution

73 ml – 72 ml = 1 ml was the error in measurement of 72 ml

$$\text{Percentage of error} = \frac{1\text{ ml} \times 100\%}{72\text{ ml}}$$

Ans. 1.39%

Example

Using an ordinary pipette 2 ml of a solution is measured and thereafter a certified pipette is used to measure 2 ml of the same solution. The certified pipette indicates that 2.075 ml has been measured by the ordinary pipette in place of 2 ml. Find out the percentage of error?

Solution

Error = Actual – Desired

= 2.075 ml – 2 ml = 0.075 ml

$$\text{Percentage of error} = \frac{0.075\text{ ml} \times 100\%}{2\text{ ml}}$$

Ans. 3.75%

Example

A burette has been found to have +3% of error in its graduation. How many milliliters it will measure if 7.5 ml is to be measured?

Solution

Desired volume = 7.5 ml and Error is +3%. It means that the measured volume > 7.5 ml

Assume that the measured volume = x ml; then the difference would be $(x - 7.5)$ ml

$$\text{So, } 3 = \frac{(x-7.5)\text{ ml} \times 100\%}{7.5\text{ ml}}$$

or, $3 \times 7.5 = 100x - 7.5 \times 100$ or, $100x = 750 + 22.5 = 772.5$

or, $x = \frac{772.5}{100} = 7.7725$ ml or 7.8 ml

Hence, the burette will measure

Ans. 7.8 ml

Example

A burette has been found to have (-) 3% of error in its graduation. How many milliliters it will measure if 7.5 ml is to be measured?

Solution

Desired volume = 7.5 ml and Error is (-) 3%. It means that the measured volume < 7.5 ml

Assume that the measured volume = x ml; then the difference would be $(7.5 - x)$ ml

So, $3 = \frac{(7.5 - x) \text{ ml} \times 100\%}{x \text{ ml}}$

or, $3x = 7.5 \times 100 - 100x$

or, $100x + 3x = 750$

or, $103\,x = 750$; $x = \frac{750}{103} = 7.28$ ml or 7.3 ml

Hence, the burette will measure

Ans. 7.3 ml

Volume of Different Shapes

Shapes	Volume
Cube	a^3; [a is the length of any side.]
Rectangular Prism	$a \times b \times c$; [a, b, and c are three sides of the prism.]
Sphere	$\frac{4}{3}\pi \times r^3$; [r is the radius of the sphere.]
Ellipsoid	$\frac{4}{3}\pi \times r_1 \times r_2 \times r_3$; [$r_1$, r_2, and r_3 are the radii of the ellipsoid on three axes, x, y and z.]
Cylinder	$\pi r^2 h$; [r is the radius of circle and h is the height of the cylinder.]
Cone	$\frac{1}{3}\pi r^2 h$; [r is the radius of the circle and h is lateral height of the cone.]

Example

The diameter of cylindrical vessel is 1 m and height is 2.4 m, calculate the capacity of the vessel to hold liquid.

Solution

The capacity to hold liquid refers to the volume.

Diameter of the vessel = 1 m; then the radius, r = 0.5 m = 5 dm [1 m = 10 dm]

Height of the vessel, h = 2.4 m = 24 dm

Volume of the vessel = $\pi r^2 h$ = 3.14 × 5 dm × 5 dm× 24 dm

= 1884 cubic decimeter

Ans. 1884 liter

Example

A rectangular packet measures 5 ft long, 3.2 ft wide and 1.6 ft in breadth. How many meters of paper would be required to wrap the packet?

Solution

Paper required to wrap the packet = surface area of the packet

Surface area of a rectangle = 2 (a × b + b × c + c × a); where a, b, and c are measures of length, breadth and width.

Given that a = 5 ft, b = 3.2 ft, and c = 1.6 ft

Surface area of the packet

= 2(5 ft × 3.2 ft + 3.2 ft × 1.6 ft + 1.6 ft × 5 ft)

= 2(16 + 4.8 + 8)

= 57.6 sq ft

= 57.6 × 0.0903 sq m

[1 m = 3.28 ft; so, 1 sq ft = 0.093 sq m]

Ans. 5.2 sq m paper would be required

Example

To fill 12 bottles of 5.6 cm height and 3.8 cm wide in a corrugated box with 3mm ply partition between two bottles what should be the inner dimensions of the box? The arrangement of bottles would be 4 × 3.

Solution

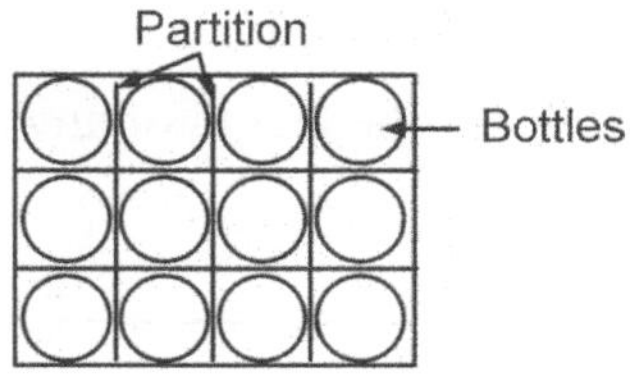

The height of the bottle shall be inner height of the box.

Diameter of bottle = 3.8 cm

Height of bottle = 5.6 cm

Thickness of the partition ply = 3mm

The pattern of arrangement would 4×3; (shown in figure)

That is, the length inside the box = 3.8 cm × 4 + 3× 3 mm

= 15.2 cm + 0.9 cm

= 16.10 cm

The inside breadth of the box = 3.8 cm × 3 + 2 × 3 mm

= 11.4 cm + 0.6 cm

= 12.00 cm

Thus, inner dimensions of the box would be 16.10 cm in length, 12.00 cm in breadth and 5.6 cm in height. (Answer)

Example

Using liquid displacement method the volume of a cube has been found equal to that of a sphere. If the diameter of sphere is 4mm, find out the side-length of the cube. The volume of the sphere is 25 cubic mm.

Solution:

The volume of a cube = a^3; where a is the length of any side.

The volume of a sphere = $\frac{4}{3}\pi \times r^3$; where r is the radius of the circle.

Given that the diameter of the sphere (circle) = 2r = 4 mm; r = 2 mm

Volume of the sphere = 25 cubic mm

That is, $\frac{4}{3}\pi \times r^3$ = 25 cubic mm = a^3

or, $a^3 = \frac{4}{3} \times 3.14 \times 2^3 = 33.49$ cu mm

or, $a^3 = 33.49$ cu mm

or, $a = 3.2235$ mm

Thus, the length of any side of the cube is

Ans. 3.225 mm

Exercise

1. 75 mg of metronidazole benzoate is to be weighed using a prescription balance with a sensitivity requirement of 6 mg, how this can be weighed with an error not greater than 5% using aliquot method?

Ans: Metronidazole benzoate 150 mg + 250 mg of diluent, 200 mg of the mixture is to be taken.

2. A prescription balance has sensitivity requirement of 6 mg. How can you weigh 10 mg of salbutamol sulphate with an error not exceeding 5% using lactose as the diluent?

Ans: Salbutamol sulphate 100 mg + 1300 mg of lactose, 140 mg of the mixture is to be taken.

3. A prescription balance has sensitivity requirement of 4 mg. How can you weigh 8 mg of a drug with an error not exceeding 5% using lactose as the diluent?

Ans: Drug 80 mg + 1920 mg of lactose, 200 mg of the mixture is to be taken.

4. A torsion prescription balance has a sensitivity requirement of 5 milligrams. Explain how you would weigh 10 milligrams of atropine sulfate with an accuracy of ± 5%, using lactose as the diluent.

Ans: Atropine sulfate 100 mg + 900 mg of lactose, 100 mg of the mixture containing 10 mg of atropine sulfate is to be taken.

5. Using a 5 mL graduated cylinder in units of 0.5 mL, how would you obtain the required amount of clove oil (0.2 mL) using the aliquot method and alcohol as the diluent?

Ans: Clove oil 1 ml + 4 ml of alcohol, 1 ml of the mixture containing 0.2 ml of Clove oil is to be taken.

6. According to a formula 0.5 milliliter of hydrochloric acid is required. How can it be measured using a 10-milliliter cylinder graduated from 2 to 10 milliliters and 1-milliliter division?

Ans: Hydrochloric acid 2ml + 6 ml of water, 2ml of the mixture containing 0.5 ml of hydrochloric acid is to be taken.

7. Using a graduated cylinder, a pharmacist measured 30 milliliters of a liquid. On subsequent examination, using a narrow-gauge burette, it was measured and found to be 31 milliliters. What was the percentage of error in the first measurement?

Ans: 3.33%

8. When the maximum potential error is ± 2 milligrams in a total of 100 milligrams, what is the percentage of error?

Ans: 2%

9. In a 10 ml cylinder 5 ml of distilled water is put and weighed. The weight of the cylinder changes from 32.8052 g to 37.7984 g; assuming the density of water unity calculate the percentage error in the measurement.

Ans: 0.2%

10. The average thickness of a tablet were measured and found 3.4 mm. The thickness was re-measured using a certified instrument and found to be 3.45 mm. Find out the error in the first instrument and express in percent.

Ans: 1.45%

11. During performing test for angle of repose the diameter and height of the powder hip were measured using an ordinary scale. The measurement was repeated using a certified scale. The figures are given below. Calculate the percentage error in the first measurement.

Ordinary scale		**Certified scale**	
Diameter	Height	Diameter	Height
5.75 cm	7.25 cm	5.55 cm	7.00 cm

Ans: 3.6%

12. The volume of a cylindrical vessel was calculated by measuring its depth and internal diameter using an ordinary tape. The results were verified by measuring the vessel using a certified tape. The

measurements are given in table below. Calculate the percentage error in the first measurement and the effect on measurement of volume of the vessel.

Ordinary scale		**Certified scale**	
Diameter	Depth	Diameter	Depth
1.47 m	2.10 m	1.40 m	2.00 m

Ans: Error in first tape is **5%** and it caused **15.6%** error in volume

13. The sensitivity of a balance is 0.1 mg and error is 5%. What would be minimum amount that can be weighed?

Ans: 2 mg

14. A balance can weigh a minimum amount of 1 mg with an acceptable error of 2%. Find out the sensitivity of the balance.

Ans: 0.02 mg

15. A pipette measures 7.65 ml in place 7.55 ml. What would be the error in the pipette?

Ans: +1.31%

16. A burette has (–) 2% error. If someone wish to measure 40.05 ml of a solution how much should be measured?

Ans: 39.26 ml

17. The dimensions of paper board cartoon are 12 cm × 5 cm × 3 cm. To pack 48 of such cartoons what should be the available space on the box? Assume that packing arrangement would be 4×3×4.

Ans: 36 cm × 20 cm × 12 cm

18. A liquid mixing tank has full volume of 3000 lt; as per norm 70% of the volume can be used for mixing. If the height of allowable level is 6 ft, calculate the total height of the tank.

Ans: 2.76 m

19. A sheet of aluminium measuring 8 ft by 4 ft is used to prepare a cylindrical container having 3.2 ft height and 2.0 ft diameter with top and bottom lid. Calculate the area of the sheet wasted.

Ans: 5.62 sq ft

20. A solid metal tube displaces 125 ml of water. Calculate the diameter of tube if its length is 3 cm.

Ans: 3.64 cm

21. An piece of land measures 5 chains by 41 chains. Find out the area of the land. (1 chain = 22 yards)

Ans: 99220 sq yd

22. Divide 4 acres of land into 8 equal parts. What would be the area of each piece of land in square feet?

Ans: 21780 sq ft

23. A bottle is 9 in high with cap and 4 in outer diameter. To pack the bottle in a paper made box what should be the inner dimension of the box in terms of millimeter?

Ans: 228.6mm in height and 101.6mm wide (plus adequate clearance)

24. A spherical solid body is immersed completely in water. If the radius of the sphere is 6in, then calculate how many milliliters of water would be displaced.

Ans: 4719.47 ml

25. The values of three radii of 4cm, 2.8cm, and 2.81cm of an egg are there. What would be its volume?

Ans: 41.96 ml

3

FUNDAMENTAL CALCULATIONS

Pharmaceutical calculations refer to the study of the basic principles of mathematics that are necessary for correct preparation, safety and for effective use of pharmaceuticals. This chapter reminds the students about some previously learned mathematics.

The chapter illustrates:

- How the common fractions, decimal fractions, and percentages can be converted to their corresponding equivalent expressions and the application of each in further calculations.
- Utilization of exponential notations.
- How the method of ratio and proportion can be applied for solving the problems.
- How the method of dimensional analysis can be applied for solving problem.
- About significant figures.

Fractions

A fraction is the portion of a whole; such as $\frac{1}{3}$, $\frac{7}{8}$, etc. These are used in pharmaceutical calculations.

- For addition or subtraction of the fractions, a *common denominator* is used.

Examples

Addition of $\frac{1}{3}$ and $\frac{1}{4}$

Solution

The denominators of the two fractions are made same by taking lowest common multiple (LCM)

$$\frac{1}{3} = \frac{1\times4}{3\times4} = \frac{4}{12} \text{ and } \frac{1}{4} = \frac{1\times3}{4\times3} = \frac{3}{12}$$

So, $$\frac{1}{3} + \frac{1}{4} = \frac{4}{12} + \frac{3}{12} = \frac{4+3}{12}$$

Ans. $\frac{7}{12}$ (Ans)

Example

Subtraction of $\frac{1}{4}$ from $\frac{1}{3}$

Solution

The denominators of the two fractions are made same by taking lowest common multiple (LCM)

$$\frac{1}{3} = \frac{1\times4}{3\times4} = \frac{4}{12} \text{ and } \frac{1}{4} = \frac{1\times3}{4\times3} = \frac{3}{12}$$

So, $$\frac{1}{3} - \frac{1}{4} = \frac{4}{12} - \frac{3}{12} = \frac{4-3}{12} = \frac{1}{12} \text{ (Ans)}$$

- The multiplication and division of the fractions are explained by the following examples.

Examples

Multiply $\frac{1}{3}$ by $\frac{7}{8}$

Solution

$$\frac{1}{3} \times \frac{7}{8} = \frac{1\times7}{3\times8} = \frac{7}{24} \text{ (Ans)}$$

Examples

What would be $\frac{1}{5}^{th}$ of 150.

Solution

$\frac{1}{5} \times 150 = 30$ (Answer)

Examples

Divide $\frac{3}{5}$ by $\frac{1}{5}$

Solution

$\frac{3}{5} \div \frac{1}{5} = \frac{3}{5} \times \frac{5}{1} = \frac{15}{5} = 3$ (Answer)

A *fraction* with a denominator of 10 or multiple of 10 is called decimal fraction. It is usually expressed decimally instead of common fraction. For example, $\frac{3}{10}$ is expressed as 0.3 or $\frac{35}{10}$ is expressed as 3.5. When there is no integer before the decimal point, zero is used.

Example

Express $\frac{3}{5}$ in terms of decimal.

Solution

$\frac{3}{5} = \frac{3\times2}{5\times2} = \frac{6}{10} = 0.6$ (Answer)

Example

Express 0.125, 1.25 and 12.5 in terms of fractions

Solution

$$0.125 = \frac{125}{1000} = \frac{25\times5}{25\times5\times8} = \frac{1}{8}$$

$$1.25 = \frac{125}{100} = \frac{25\times5}{25\times4} = \frac{5}{4} = 1 + \frac{1}{4} = 1\frac{1}{4}$$

$$12.5 = \frac{125}{10} = \frac{5\times25}{5\times2} = \frac{25}{2} = 12 + \frac{1}{2} = 12\frac{1}{2}$$

Percent

The term *percent* means per cent; that is per hundred. The symbol used to express the term is %. For example, 20% means 20 per 100 or $\frac{20}{100}$ or $\frac{1}{5}$.

Conversion of fraction into percent is explained as:

Example

Express the fraction, $\frac{2}{5}$ in terms of percent

Solution

$$\frac{2}{5} = \frac{2\times20}{5\times20} = \frac{20}{100} = 20\% \quad \text{or,} \quad \frac{2}{5} \times 100 = 20\%$$

Example

Convert 0.25 to percent

Solution

$$0.25 \times 100 = \mathbf{25\%} \quad \text{or,} \quad 0.25 \times 100 = \frac{25}{100} \times 100 = 25\%$$

25%

Example

Convert 15% to fraction

Solution

$$15\% = \frac{15}{100} = \frac{3\times5}{20\times5} = \frac{3}{20}$$

Example

Convert 0.15% to fraction

Solution

$$0.15\% = \frac{0.15}{100} = \frac{15}{100\times100} = \frac{3\times5}{20\times5\times100} = \frac{3}{2000}$$

Exponential Notation

There are some large numbers of high magnitudes which are very difficult to express as such. Thus, exponential notation or powers of 10 is used to express. For example, 1000000000000000 = 10^{15}. 10^{15} is the exponential notation of 1000000000000000.

This is explained as follows:

Example

Express the number 2534 and 0.00056 in terms of exponential notation

Solution

$$2534 = \frac{2534}{1000} \times 1000 = 2.534 \times 10 \times 10 \times 10 = 2.534\times10^3$$

$$0.00056 = \frac{56}{100000} = 56 \times10^{-1}\times10^{-1}\times10^{-1}\times10^{-1}\times10^{-1} = 56\times10^{-5}$$

$$0.00056 = \frac{5.6}{10000} = 5.6 \times10^{-1}\times10^{-1}\times10^{-1}\times10^{-1} = 5.6\times10^{-4}$$

In this manner when the numbers are written, the first part, e.g., 5.6 is called the *coefficient.* One figure is written to the left of the decimal point. The second part, e.g., - 4 is the *exponential factor* or *power of 10.* For example, 21000 can be converted to 2.1×10^4; the decimal point is moved to 4 places to the left. Hence 4 is the exponent and 2.1 is coefficient. Similarly, 0.0000021 can be converted to 2.1×10^{-6}; the decimal point is moved to 6 places to the right with the *negative* sign. Hence, the exponent is –6 and 2.1 is the coefficient.

- *Multiplication* of exponentials:
  1. In multiplication of exponential number the exponents are *added.*

     For example, $10^5 \times 10^6 = 10^{5+6} = 10^{11}$ $[a^n \times a^m = a^{m+n}]$,
  2. The coefficients are multiplied as usual.

     For example, $2.37\times10^5 \times 4.21\times10^9 = (2.37 \times 4.21) \times10^{9+5} = 9.9777\times10^{14}$.

     $7.32\times10^6 \times 3.57\times10^{-3} = 7.32 \times 3.57\times10^{6+(-3)} = 26.1324\times10^{6\ -3} = 26.1324\times10^3$

- Division of exponents: in division of exponential number the exponents are *subtracted.*

  For example, $10^9 \div 10^5 = 10^{9-5} = 10^4$ [$a^m \div a^n = a^{m-n}$].

  $10^9 \div 10^{-5} = 10^{9-(-5)} = 10^{9+5} = 10^{\mathbf{14}}$ [$a^m \div a^{-n} = a^{m+n}$].

  2. The coefficients of the numbers are divided as per arithmetic principle.

     For example, $7\times10^9 \div 3.5\times10^5 = 7\div3.5\times10^9\div10^5 = 2\times10^{9-5} = 2\times10^4$.

- In case of *addition* and *subtraction* of exponentials, the expressions are to be converted (by moving the decimal points) to the forms having any common power of 10; then the coefficients are to be added or subtracted. The result should be rounded off to the number of *decimal places* contained in the *least* precise component, and it should be expressed with only one figure to the left of the decimal point.

Example

$2.9\times10^5 + 3.1\times10^3$

Solution

$$2.9 \times10^5 = 2.9\times10^2 \times 10^3$$
$$= 290\times10^3 + 3.1 \times 10^3$$
$$= (290 + 3.1) \times 10^3$$
$$= 293.1 \times 10^3$$

Similarly, $3.1 \times 10^3 = \frac{3.1}{100} \times 100 \times 10^3 = 0.031 \times 10^5 + 2.9 \times10^5$

$$= (0.031 + 2.9) \times 10^5 = 2.931 \times 10^5$$

Example

$2.9 \times 10^5 - 3.1 \times 10^3$

Solution

$2.9 \times 10^5 = 2.9 \times 10^2 \times 10^3 = 290 \times 10^3$

$-\underline{3.1 \times 10^3}$

286.9×10^3

Similarly, 2.9×10^5

$$-3.1 \times 10^3 = -\frac{3.1}{100} \times 100 \times 10^3 = \underline{-0.031 \times 10^5}$$

$$2.869 \times 10^5$$

Ratio and Proportion

Ratio

The relative magnitude of two quantities is called their ***ratio***. Since a ratio relates the relative value of two numbers, it can be reduced to a common fraction. For example, a ratio, 3:4 can be expressed as 3/4. It is read as '3 is to 4'; not as 'three fourth'. The rules applicable to fractions are applicable to ratios also;

- *If the two terms of a ratio are multiplied or divided by the same number, the value remains unchanged.*

  For example, $\frac{3}{7} \times \frac{2}{2} = \frac{6}{14}$; similarly, $\frac{8}{20} \div \frac{4}{4} = \frac{8/4}{20/4} = \frac{2}{5}$

- The terms of a ratio must be of the same kind, for the *value* of a ratio is an abstract number expressing how many *times* greater or smaller the first term (or numerator) is than the second term (or denominator).

  For example, a ratio of 30:6 or 30/6 may be 30cm/6cm, or 30lts/6lts, etc.

- If the value of two ratios are same, they become *equivalent.* If two ratios are equivalent, the *product of the numerator of the one and the denominator of the other shall be equal to the product of the denominator of the one and the numerator of the other.*

  For example, $\frac{1}{3}$ is equivalent to $\frac{3}{9}$; or $\frac{1}{3} = \frac{3}{9}$; then $3 \times 3 = 1 \times 9$

  This is applicable to the reciprocals of the original fractions; that is for $\frac{3}{1}$ and $\frac{9}{3}$. Thus, in these ratios also the cross products are equal ($3 \times 3 = 1 \times 9$).

- The *numerator of the one fraction would be equal to the product of its denominator and the other fraction.*

For example, in case of $\frac{2}{5}$ and $\frac{4}{10}$, the numerator of $\frac{2}{5}$ is $2 = 5 \times \frac{4}{10} = 2$;

Similarly with other fraction, $\frac{4}{10}$, the numerator $4 = 10 \times \frac{2}{5} = 4$

- *If the numerator of one fraction is divided by the other fraction the quotient of the division would be equal to the numerator of the first fraction.*

For example, the fractions are $\frac{2}{7}$ and $\frac{4}{14}$

Then, $7 = 2 \div \frac{4}{14} = 2 \times \frac{14}{4} = 7$ and $14 = 4 \div \frac{2}{7} = 4 \times \frac{7}{2} = 14$

Proportion

The equality of two ratios is expressed in the form of ***proportion***. In any of the three standard forms a proportion can be written. For example,

(i) a : b = c : d

(ii) a : b :: c : d

(iii) $\frac{a}{b} = \frac{c}{d}$

Each of the three expressions is read as; '*a is to b as c is to d*', and *a* and *d* are called the *extremes* (outer members) and *b* and *c* are called *means* (middle members).

In any proportion, *the product of the extremes is equal to the product of the means.* With the help of this rule a missing term of any proportion can be determined when the other three terms are known.

For example, the proportion is $\frac{a}{b} = \frac{c}{d}$

Then, $a = \frac{bc}{d}$, $b = \frac{ad}{c}$, $c = \frac{ad}{b}$ and $d = \frac{bc}{a}$

All the terms of the proportion should carry same unit, such as g, kg, m*l*, *l*t, cm, km, etc. or no unit (numbers only) to know proper relationship between the ratios of a proportion.

Example

5 tablets contain 1.5 g of paracetamol, how many milligrams of the drug should be present in 15 tablets?

Solution

1 g = 1000 mg

1.5 g = 1.5 × 1000 =1500 mg

Let us assume that 15 tablets contain x mg of paracetamol

Then, $\frac{5 \text{ tabs}}{15 \text{ tabs}} = \frac{1500 \text{ mg}}{x \text{ mg}}$

So, $x = \frac{15 \text{ tabs}}{5 \text{ tabs}} \times 1500 \text{ mg} = 4500 \text{ mg}$

Example

If 15 tablets contain 4500mg of paracetamol, how many milligrams of paracetamol shall be present in 5 tablets?

Solution

$\frac{15 \text{ tabs}}{5 \text{ tabs}} = \frac{4500 \text{ mg}}{x \text{ mg}}$

Let us assume 5 tabs contain x mg of paracetamol

So, $x = \frac{5 \text{ tabs}}{15 \text{ tabs}} \times 4500 \text{ mg} = 1500 \text{ mg}$

Example

If 65 ml represent the $2/3^{rd}$ of a volume, how many milliliters would represent $3/7^{th}$ of the volume?

Solution

$2/3^{rd}$ of 1 ml = $1 \times \frac{2}{3} = 0.67$ ml

$3/7^{th}$ of 1 ml = $1 \times \frac{3}{7} = 0.43$ ml

Let us assume that $3/7^{th}$ of the volume = x ml

Now $$\frac{0.67\text{ ml}}{0.43\text{ ml}} = \frac{65\text{ ml}}{x\text{ ml}}$$

So, $$x = \frac{65\text{ml} \times 0.43\text{ ml}}{0,67\text{ml}} = 41.72\text{ ml}$$

Variation

The previous examples explain the direct relationship or proportional relationship between cause and effect. For example, if 5% (cause) is 5 in 100 then 10% would be 10 (effect) in 100. But, there may be inverse relationship between cause and effect. That is, twice the cause may result half the effect. For example, the concentration of a solution will decrease, if its volume is increased by dilution.

Let us explain with an example.

Example

If 10 ml of a 10% solution is diluted to 50ml, what would be the concentration of the diluted solution?

Solution

Let us assume that the concentration of diluted solution is x%.

According to the law of proportion

$$\frac{10\text{ ml}}{50\text{ ml}} = \frac{x\%}{10\%}$$

or, $$x = \frac{10\text{ ml} \times 10\%}{50\text{ ml}} = 2\%$$

Example

According to the formula 75 kg of drug having 100% of potency is to be added. If the actual potency of drug is 98.8%, how much drug should be taken?

Solution

Let us assume that x kg of drug is required.

According to the law of proportion

$$\frac{100\%}{98.8\%} = \frac{x\text{ kg}}{75\text{ kg}}$$

or, $$x = \frac{100\% \times 75\text{ kg}}{98.8\%} = 75.91\%$$

Logarithm

The concept of logarithm was first introduced by the British Mathematician John Napier in 1550. As such multiplication, division, indices and roots of large numbers are time consuming process and are prone to error. By using the technique of logarithm such huge calculations can be made easy.

Due to limitation of the scope we shall not go into detail, shall use the laws that are used in calculations. The laws of algorithm are:

- $\log_a \left(\frac{m}{n}\right) = \log_a m - \log_a n$
- $\log_a (mn) = \log_a m + \log_a n$
- $\log_a (m^n) = \text{n} \log_a m$
- $\log_a 1 = 0$ (since, $a^0 = 1$)
- $\log_a a = 1$ (since, $a^1 = a$)
- $\log_a m = \frac{\log_b m}{\log_b a}$ (where, $a \neq 0$, $\text{b} \neq 0$ and are real number)

If $\log_a y = x$

Then, $\text{y} = \text{antilog}_{10}\, x$

Usually, in common logarithm the base is 10 and it is mentioned in the logarithmic equation; for example, 'log 547' is expressed as $\log_{10} 547$. Logarithm of a positive number, $(\text{m}\times 10^x)$ is written as $\log(\text{m} \times 10^{\text{p}})$ has two parts – characteristic ('p' stands for characteristic) and mantissa ('log m' is the mantissa).

Characteristic of a Common Logarithm

Characteristic of a common logarithm is a positive integer and is one less than the number of digits in integral part of that number.

Number	0.3452	0.03452	0.003452	0.0003452	3.452	34.52	345.2	3452
Number of digits in integral part of the number	-	-	-	-	1	2	3	4
Number of zeros after decimal point in the number	-	1	2	3	-	-	-	-
Characteristic	–1	–2	–3	–4	0	1	2	3

Mantissa

To determine the mantissa of a common logarithm the logarithm table is to be used and the following steps are to be followed;

1. The decimal point has no effect in finding mantissa. If the number of digits are more than four, round it up to four. For example, 12.9745 is rounded to 1297 or 12.9475 is rounded to 1295.

***Note*:** The *decimal point is ignored to find out the characteristic.*

2. The first two digits are used to determine the row of the logarithm table. If there is only one digit number, then zero should be added to it. For example, 12 are the first two digits of the number 1297 or 1295.
3. The third digit is used to determine the column in the log table and the value of third digit is noted from the column.
4. The fourth digit is used to determine the column in mean difference log table.
5. Add the two figures with respect to third and fourth digits (step 3 and 4) to calculate the required mantissa.

No.	Four-Place Logarithm										Proportional Parts								
	0	1	2	3	4	5	6	7	8	9	1	2	3	4	5	6	7	8	9
10	.0000	.0043	0086	.0128	.0170	.0212	.0253	.0294	.0334	.0374	4	8	12	17	21	25	29	33	37
11	.0414	.0453	.0492	.0531	.0569	.0607	.0645	.0682	.0719	.0755	4	8	11	15	19	23	27	30	34
12	.0792	.0828	.0864	.0899	.0934	.0969	.1004	.1038	.1072	.1106	3	7	10	14	17	21	24	28	31
13	.1139	.1173	.1206	.1239	.1271	.1303	.1335	.1367	.1399	.1430	3	6	10	13	16	19	23	26	29

Illustration:

1. The number 12. 9475 is rounded up to 1295.
2. From log table the value of 12 in column headed by 9 is 0.1106
3. The value of 12 in mean difference column headed by 5 is 0.0017

Total 0.1106 + 0.0017 = 0.1123

Thus, log 12.9475 is 0. 1123

Antilogarithm

If $\log_a y = x$; the positive number y is called the antilogarithm of the number x.

Hence, $y = \text{antilog}_{10} x$

No.	Four-Place Logarithm										Proportional Parts								
	0	1	2	3	4	5	s 6	7	8	9	1	2	3	4	5	6	7	8	9
52	.7160	.7168	.7177	.7185	.7193	.7202	.7210	.7218	.7226	.7235	1	2	2	3	4	5	6	7	7
53	.7243	.7251	.7259	.7267	.7275	.7284	.7292	.7300	.7308	.7316	1	2	2	3	4	5	6	6	7
54	.7324	.7332	.7340	.7348	.7356	.7364	.7372	.7380	.7388	.7396	1	2	2	3	4	5	6	6	7

No.	Four-Place Antilogarithm										Proportional Parts								
	0	1	2	3	4	5	6	7	8	9	1	2	3	4	5	6	7	8	9
.72	5248	5260	5272	5284	5297	5309	5321	5333	5346	5358	1	2	4	5	6	7	9	10	11
.73	5370	5383	5395	5408	5420	5433	5445	5458	5470	5483	1	3	4	5	6	8	9	10	11
.74	5495	5508	5521	5534	5546	5559	5572	5585	5598	5610	1	3	4	5	6	8	9	10	12

Illustration:

(i) log 10 = 1, antilog 1 = 10

(ii) log 539.2 = 0.7316 + 2 = 0.7318, antilog 2.7318 = 539.3

(iii) log 0.54 = –1.7324, antilog –1.7324 = 0.5395 + 5 = 0.540

(iv) log 0.054 = –2.7324, antilog –2.7324 = 0.5395 + 5 = 0.054

Example

Find the values of the following using logarithm.

(a) 0.0076×1.5342 (b) $97.645 \div 2.9867$

(c) $\dfrac{5.5432 \times \sqrt{75.4531}}{2.2341}$ (d) $\sqrt{\dfrac{56.3231}{9.8657}}$

(e) $\sqrt{\dfrac{0.0148 \times 0.274}{0.8735}}$ (f) $(0.8931)^{-4}$

Solution

(a) Let $x = 0.0076 \times 1.5342$

Taking log on both sides; $\log x = \log (0.0076 \times 1.5342)$

$= \log 0.0076 + \log 1.5342$

$= -3.8808 + 0.1858$

$= -2.0666$

$x = \text{antilog} -2.0667$

Ans. 0.01166

(b) Let $x = 97.645 \div 2.9867$

Taking log on both sides; $\log x = \log (97.645 \div 2.9867)$

$= \log 97.645 - \log 2.9867$

$= 1.9896 - 0.4752$

$= 1.5144$

$x = \text{antilog } 1.5144$

Ans. 32.69

(c) Let $x = \dfrac{5.5432 \times \sqrt{75.4531}}{2.2341}$

Taking log on both sides; $\log x = \dfrac{5.5432 \times \sqrt{75.4531}}{2.2341}$

$= \log (5.5432 \times \sqrt{75.4531}) - \log 2.2341$

$= \log 5.5432 + \log \sqrt{75.4531} - \log 2.2341$

$= \log 5.5432 + \log (75.4531)^{1/2} - \log 2.2341$

$= \log 5.5432 + \frac{1}{2} \log 75.4531 - \log 2.2341$

$= 0.7437 + \frac{1}{2} \times 1.8777 - 0.3491$

$= 0.7437 + 0.9388 - 0.3491$

$= 1.3334$

$x = \text{antilog } 1.3334 = 21.57$

Ans. 21.57

(d) Let $x = \sqrt{\dfrac{56.3231}{9.8657}}$

Taking log on both sides; $\log x = \log \sqrt{\dfrac{56.3231}{9.8657}}$

$= \log \left(\dfrac{56.3231}{9.8657}\right)^{\frac{1}{2}}$

$= \dfrac{1}{2} (\log 56.3231 - \log 9.8657)$

$$= \frac{1}{2}(1.7507 - 0.9942)$$

$$= 0.3782$$

$$x = \text{antilog } 0.3782$$

Ans. 2.390

(e) Let $x = \sqrt{\frac{0.0148 \times 0.274}{0.8735}}$

$$\log x = \log \sqrt{\frac{0.0148 \times 0.274}{0.8735}} = \log \left(\frac{0.0148 \times 0.274}{0.8735}\right)^{\frac{1}{2}}$$

$$= \frac{1}{2} \log \frac{0.0148 \times 0.274}{0.8735}$$

$$= \frac{1}{2} [\ \log 0.0148 + \log 0.274 - \log 0.8735)$$

$$= \frac{1}{2} [\log 1.48 \times 10^{-2} + \log 2.74 \times 10^{-1} - \log 8.735 \times 10^{-1}]$$

$$= \frac{1}{2} [0.1703 - 2 + 0.4378 - 1 - (0.9412 - 1)]$$

$$= \frac{1}{2} [0.1703 + 0.4378 - 0.9412 - 2 - 1 + 1]$$

$$= \frac{1}{2} [- 2 - 0.3331]$$

$$= - 1.1666$$

$$= -1 + 1 - 1 - 0.1666$$

$$= -2 + 0.8334$$

$$= -2.8334$$

$$x = \text{antilog } -2.8334 = 6.814 \times 10^{-2}$$

Ans. 0.06814

(f) Let $x = (0.8931)^{-4}$

$$\log x = \log (0.8931)^{-4}$$

$$= - 4 \log 0.8931$$

$$= - 4(\log 8.931 \times 10^{-1})$$

$$= - 4(- 1 + 0.9509)$$

$= -4 \times (-0.0491)$

$= 0.1964$

$x = \text{antilog } 0.1964$

Ans. 1.571

Example

If $a^3 = 2197$; find the value of a using logarithm.

Solution

Given that, $a^3 = 2197$

So, $\log a^3 = \log 2197$

$3 \log a = 3.3418$

$$\log a = \frac{3.3418}{3} = 1.1139$$

so, $a = \text{antilog of } 1.1139$

Ans. 13.00

Example

If $x^5 = 759375$; find the value of x using logarithm.

Solution

Given that, $x^5 = 759375$

So, $\log x^5 = \log 759375$

So, $5 \log x = 5.8804$

$$\log x = \frac{5.8804}{5} = 1.1761$$

so, $x = \text{antilog of } 1.1761$

Ans. 15.00

Alligation

This is an arithmetic method used to solve the problems related to mixture of components of different strengths. There are two types of alligation – alligation medial and alligation alternate.

- *Alligation medial* method is used to calculate the strength of a component present in all the two or three preparations. For example, two or three alcohol solutions of known volumes containing known amount of alcohol are mixed. The content of alcohol in the final mixture can be determined by alligation medial method.

Example

Find out the % age concentration of alcohol in a mixture prepared by mixing 150ml of 40% alcohol, 275ml of 38% alcohol and 75ml of 90% of alcohol.

Solution

150 ml solution × 40% = 60 ml

275 ml solution × 38% = 104.5 ml

75 ml solution × 90% = 67.5 ml

500 ml solution × x% = 232 ml

Thus, 500 ml of solution contains 232 ml of alcohol

Then, the concentration of alcohol (x) in the mixture = $\frac{232}{500} \times 100\%$

Ans. 46.4%

Example

A reprocessed batch of aspirin tablet contains 75kg of granules of 73.05% aspirin, 46 kg of 72.85% aspirin, 52.4kg of 72.39% of aspirin and 39kg of 71.98% of aspirin. Calculate the aspirin content of the mixture in percent.

Solution

75 kg × 73.05% = 54.79 kg

46 kg × 72.85% = 33.51 kg

52.4 kg × 72.39% = 37.93 kg

39 kg × 71.98% = 28.07 kg

Thus, 212.4 kg of granules × x % = 157.3 kg

Then the average drug content of the mixture = $\frac{157.3\text{kg}}{212.4\text{kg}} \times 100$

Ans. 74.06%

Example

Extracts obtained from three lots were mixed with 2.07kg of an inert substance. The mixture contains 12.09kg having 0.95% active constituent, 14.60kg having 0.895% active constituent, and 11.75kg having 1.03% active constituent. Find out the content of active constituent in the final mixture.

Solution

$0.00\% \times 2.07 \text{ kg} = 0 \text{ kg}$

$0.95\% \times 12.09 \text{ kg} = 0.115 \text{ kg}$

$0.895\% \times 4.60 \text{ kg} = 0.131 \text{ kg}$

$1.03\% \times 11.75 \text{ kg} = 0.121 \text{ kg}$

Thus, $x\% \times 40.51\text{kg} = 0.367 \text{ kg}$

Then, the content of active constituent in the final mixture $(x) = \dfrac{0.367\text{kg}}{40.51\text{kg}} \times 100$

Ans. 0.906%

- *Alligation alternate* is used to find out at what proportions or quantities two or more preparations are to be mixed to get a mixture of a desired concentration of a common ingredient. For example, a solution of a specified concentration is to be prepared by mixing two or more solutions of different known concentrations of the same ingredient. The proportion or volumes of each solution to be mixed may be calculated by alligation alternate. The strength of the mixture should be within the strengths of the preparations being mixed.

Example

In what proportion 95% alcohol and 50% alcohol are to be mixed to prepare 70% alcohol?

Solution

The required strength of the alcohol is lower than the alcohol of higher strength and 20% higher than the alcohol of lower strength.

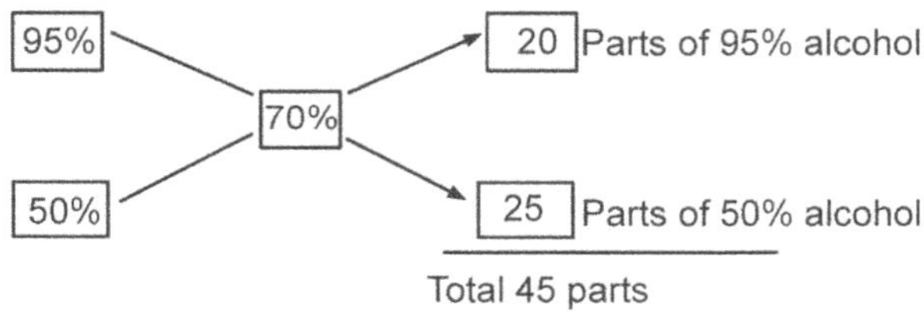

The proportion of mixing is as follows:

Thus, each 45 volume of alcohol of 50% strength can be prepared by mixing 20 parts of 95% alcohol and 25 parts of 50% alcohol. Then, the ratio of mixing is 20:25 or 4:5. (Answer)

The validity of this relationship can be verified mathematically as follows:

Percent given	Percent desired	Proportional parts required
a		x
b		y

The ratio of x to y can be derived as:	$ax + by = c(x + y)$
	$= cx + cy$
or,	$ax - cx = cy - by$
or,	$x(a - c) = y(c - b)$
So,	$\frac{x}{y} = \frac{c-b}{a-c}$

Putting the values of a, b, c, x and y (a = 95%, b = 50%, c = 70%, $x = 20$, and y = 25) in the above equation;

$$\frac{x}{y} = \frac{70-50}{95-70} = \frac{20}{25} = \frac{4}{5}.$$

Hence, the ratio determined by alligation method is verified.

Example

In what proportion 20% framycetin sulphate ointment is to be mixed with a suitable ointment base to make 1% framycetin sulphate ointment?

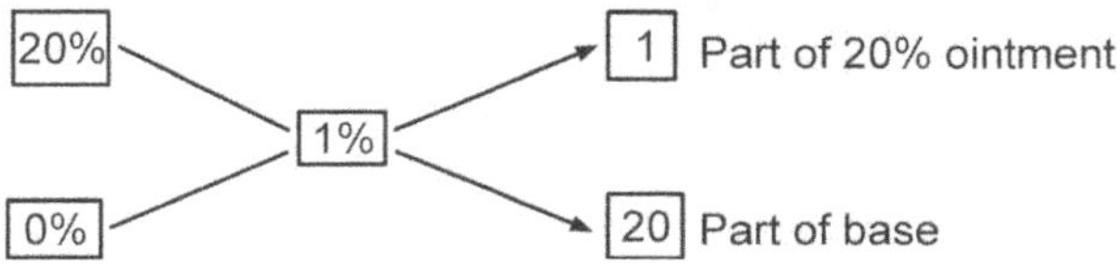

Solution

Thus, 1 part of 20% framycetin sulphate ointment is to be mixed with 20 parts of base. The ratio of mixing shall be 1:20.

Example

How many parts of 98% sulphuric acid are to be added to water to prepare 10% of sulphuric acid?

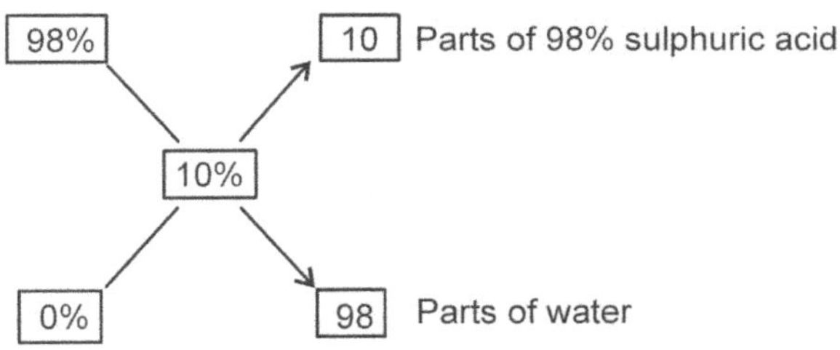

Solution

Thus, 10 ml of 98% sulphuric acid is to be mixed with 98 ml of water to prepare 10% solution of sulphuric acid. (Answer)

Example

A mixture of 15% alcohol is prepared by mixing 5%, 25%, and 60% alcohol. In which proportion these have been mixed?

Solution

Since, the concentration of alcohol in two lots (25% and 60%) are more than required concentration, these should be linked to the required concentration (5%) separately.

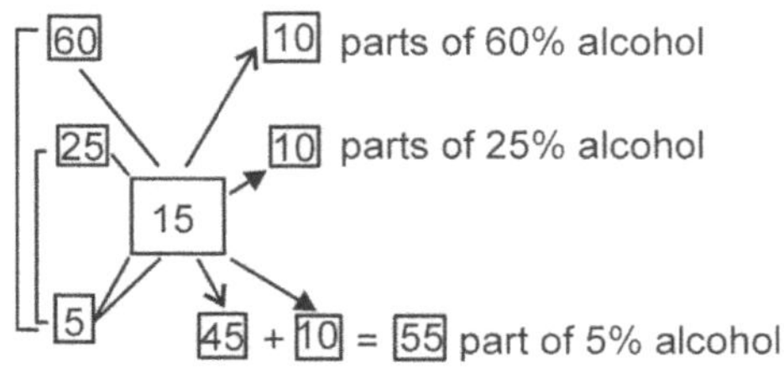

The proportion of mixing of dilute alcohols (60%:25%:5%) would be 10:10:55 = 2:2:11 (Answer)

Arithmetic verification: $60 \times 2 = 120$

$25 \times 2 = 50$

$5 \times \underline{11} = \underline{55}$

Total $15 = 225$

$225 \div 15 = 15\%$

Example

In what proportions 22%, 13%, 7%, and 2% zinc oxide ointments are to be mixed to produce a 10% ointment?

Solution

Ointments having concentrations (13% and 7%) nearer to desired concentration are paired and two ointments having concentrations (22% and 2%) away from the desired concentration are paired separately.

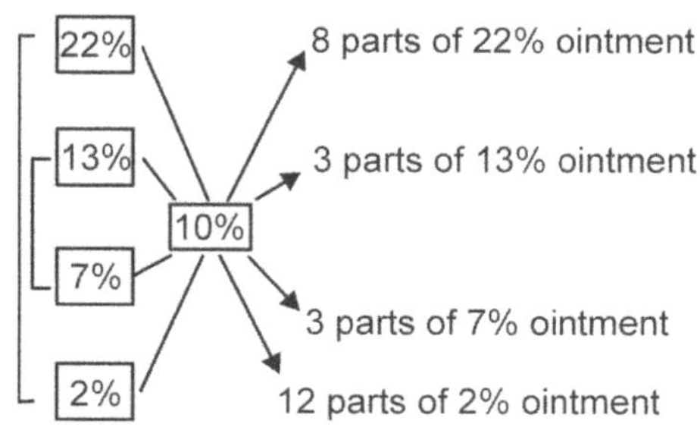

Thus, the proportion of mixing of the ointments 22%, 13%, 7% and 2% are 8 parts, 3 parts, 3parts, and 12 parts respectively.

The proportion is 8 : 3 : 3 : 12 (Answer)

Arithmetic verification:

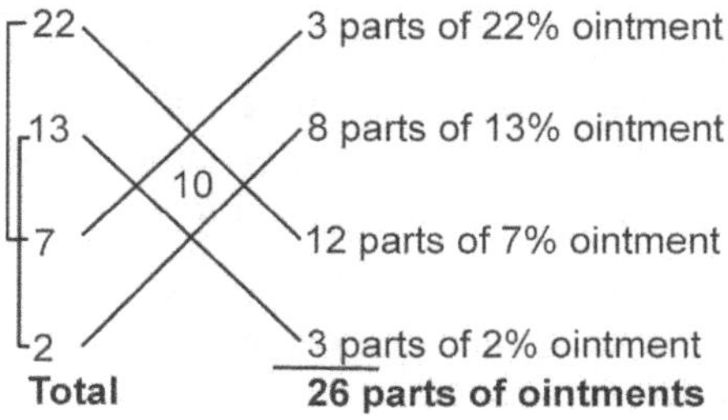

$22 \times 8 = 176$

$13 \times 3 = 39$

$7 \times 3 = 21$

$2 \times \underline{12} = \underline{24}$

Total 26 260

$260 \div 26 = 10\%$

The result is verified.

This may be done in another way as shown;

The proportion may be 3:8:12:3 (Answer)

Arithmetic verification:

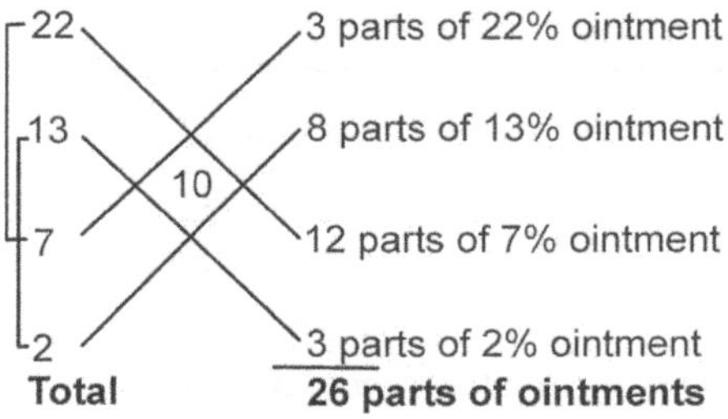

$22 \times 3 = 66$

$13 \times 8 = 104$

$7 \times 12 = 84$

$2 \underline{\times 3} = \underline{6}$

26 260

$260 \div 26 = 10\%$

The result is verified.

Significant Figures

When the objects are counted accurately, the answer is expressed in the form of a numerical figure and the total number of objects is taken at its face value. Such figures are said to be *absolute.* During measurement the last figure to the right is considered to be an approximate depending on the accuracy and limit of precision of the measurement.

For example, the volume of a liquid is measured and expressed as 321 ml. The number may be interpreted as follows: 300 ml + 20 ml + 1 ml.

Third figure 1 may be an approximate figure. That is 1 ± a fraction, depending on how accurately the measurement has been done and how much it is precise. There may be a negligible variation in measuring this 1 ml. In fact, this usually happens during any measurement, whether volume, weight, or length. Thus, the right figure may not be significant depending on the precision of the measuring device used and accuracy of the measurement. It would not be correct to measure 9.57 ml of a liquid using a graduated cylinder calibrated in units of 1ml or to weigh 51.268 grams using a balance having sensitivity of 0.01 gram. Thus, 10ml in place of 9.57ml or 51g in place of 51.268g is taken.

Significant figures are defined as the consecutive figures that can express accurately enough the value of a denominate number for a particular purpose.

The *accuracy* depends on the number of significant figures present in a denominate, except the right figure. Any digit in a given denominate number must be considered as significant, even a zero depending on its position in the denominate. For example, in a denominate number 3057, zero is significant; but in a denominate number 0357, the left zero is not significant. The significance of zero in a denominate may be summarized as follows:

- *Zero between any two digits is significant.*

  For example, the number 1052 consist of four significant figures, and 1004 consists of four significant figures.

- *Zero to the left of the first digit is not significant; it indicates only the location of decimal point in case of decimal number.*

  For example, 035 have only two significant figures; 0.35 has only two significant figures. The zero in the second number indicates how many tenths and hundredths are in the number. Similarly, 0.005 has only one significant figure, 5. Zero before the decimal and two zeros after the decimal indicate that the value of 5 is one thousand.

- *However, zero to the right of the decimal point sometimes may be considered as significant.*

  For example, 0.505 has three significant figures-5, 0, and 5.

Rounding of Figures and Rules for Rounding

Frequently we record a value correct to a 'certain' decimal places. For example, a number 3.54689 may be rounded to *four decimal places* - 3.5469 having *five significant figures*. Thus, rounding of a number should be done logically. The rules for rounding are given below:

Rules for Rounding

- Keep the figures that can provide practical value of the measurement. Leave the figure which is found to be uncertain.

For example, a scale, calibrated in centimeter and one small division is 1mm, is used to measure a length and reported as 7.255 cm or 72.55 mm. Since the smallest division is 1mm, measuring a length less than 1mm needs approximation. Hence, 72mm can be measured correctly. 0.5mm is an approximate figure. Measuring 0.005 mm is impossible. Thus, 72.55 mm should be rounded to 72.5 mm.

- Eliminate the extra or superfluous figures. Add 1 to the last figure retained, if the first figure being eliminated is 5 or greater than 5. If the first figure being eliminated is less than 5, there shall be no change in the figures retained. If the first figure being eliminated is more than 5, there shall be next higher figures.

  For example, 9.4562 can be rounded to second decimal as 9.46 and can be rounded to third decimal as 9.456.

- Before addition or subtraction rounding should be avoided, the result should only be rounded to desired decimal points.

  For example, 52.0054, 4.2356, and 76.98 are to be added. The addition is done as usual and the result becomes 133.221 which are rounded to 133.2 or 133.22. Similarly, 32.5412 are subtracted from 76.9005. The result 44.3593 is then rounded to 44.359 or 44.36.

- Before multiplication or division rounding of figures are not done to get correct result. After division or multiplication the result is rounded to required decimal point.

  For example, 58.00747 ÷ 4.278 = 13.559537 rounded to 13. 56 (rounded to second decimal) or 13.559 (rounded to third decimal).

- If an approximate number is divided or multiplied by an absolute number, the result should be rounded to the same of significant figures as in the approximate number.

  For example, 5.7804 (significant figure is 5) is multiplied by 23, the product is 132.9492 which is rounded to 132.95 having 5 significant figures.

Estimation

Rationality of a numeric computation is an estimation of the answer. If the method used is wrong, a wrong answer would be obtained. By using a mechanical repetition of the calculation the error would not be detected.

The estimating process is simple and performed as follows:

- The numbers given in a problem are *mentally* rounded off to slightly larger or smaller numbers containing fewer significant figures. For example, 78 would be rounded off to 80, and 832 to 800.
- The computations are performed, as far as possible mentally. The result obtained would to be somewhat greater or smaller than the correct answer, but would be close enough to serve as an estimate.

In case of addition:

- The figures in the leftmost column are added.
- Add the remaining figures of each number, more or less than one-half of the value of the figures just added.
- The sum of the leftmost column and half for every number in the column becomes the estimate.

Example

Add 4579, 6578, 7823, 5509, and 9452

Solution

The figures in the thousands column are added; the result is 31000.

On addition of each number on average contributing 500 the result is 2500.

Then, the estimate becomes 31000 + 2500 = 33500 (Answer)

The actual answer is 33941.

In case of multiplication,

- Two leftmost numbers are first multiplied.
- To the right of the product put zeros. The number of zeros should be equal to the number of digits neglected.
- The number becomes a fair estimate of the multiplication.

Example

Multiply 628 and 4597.

Solution

Multiply 6 and 4. The product is 24. $[6 \times 4 = 24]$

The number of figures not multiplied is 5 [2, 8, 5, 9 and 7]

Then, the estimated product becomes 2400000. (Answer)

The actual product is 2886916

In case of division:

- The given numbers are rounded off to get practical approximate.
- Divide, and put zeros equal to the number of figures left out.

Example

Divide 4255 by 6.5

Solution

The number 4255 is rounded off to 4200 and 6.5 is rounded off to 7.

Then 42 is divided by 7 mentally, the result becomes 6. Two zeros were not considered during division.

Hence the estimated result becomes 600. (Answer) The actual result is 654.61

Exercise

1. Add $\frac{3}{7}, \frac{5}{2}, \frac{5}{9}$ and $\frac{7}{12}$

   Ans: $4\frac{17}{252}$

2. Simplify $\frac{2}{5}+\frac{4}{10}+\frac{3}{5}+\frac{7}{10}$

   Ans: $2\frac{1}{10}$

3. Subtract $\frac{17}{35}$ from $\frac{2}{7}$

   Ans: $\frac{7}{35}$

4. Simplify $\frac{2}{7}+\frac{3}{7}-\frac{1}{7}$

   Ans: $\frac{4}{7}$

5. Multiply $\frac{8}{42}$ by $\frac{7}{16}$

Ans: $\frac{1}{12}$

6. Divide $\frac{8}{42}$ by $\frac{7}{16}$

Ans: $\frac{64}{147}$

7. Express 0.245, 0.0025 and 2.5 in terms of fraction.

Ans: $\frac{49}{200}$, $\frac{1}{400}$ and $\frac{5}{2}$

8. Express $\frac{13}{100}$ and $\frac{27}{1000}$ in terms of decimals.

Ans: 0.13 and 0.027

9. Find out the Estimate value and actual value of the following

(a) 768 × 5521 — **Ans: 4000000** (4240128)

(b) 8975 × 689834 — **Ans: 6300000000** (5922010150)

(c) 66589×2431178 — **Ans: 140000000000** (161889711842)

(d) 77.05×75.132 — **Ans: 5600.00** (5788.92)

(e) 0.06523 × 8745 — **Ans: 540** (570.43)

10. Express the fraction, $\frac{3}{5}$ in terms of percent and decimal.

Ans: 60% and 0.6

11. Express the number 5432 and 0.00087 in terms of exponential notation.

Ans: 5.432×10^3 and 8.7×10^4

12. Add $22.7453 \times 10^7 + 1.045 \times 10^7 + 8.9873 \times 10^7$

Ans: 32.7776×10^7

13. Multiply 7.328×10^7 by 4.81×10^{14}

Ans: 35.25×10^{21}

14. Divide 8.361×10^{15} by 3.28×10^7

Ans: 2.55×10^8

15. Thirteen pots contain 19.5g of a material, how many grams of the material should be present in twenty pots?

Ans: 30 g

16. Find the value of the following

(a) log 0.006754 **Ans: 3.8296**

(b) log 0.04675 **Ans: 2.6698**

(c) log 0.3476 **Ans: 1.5411**

17. Find the value of the following

(d) log 6.982 **Ans: 0.8440**

(e) log 89.24 **Ans: 1.9506**

(f) log 1.437×10^{-5} **Ans: -5.1564**

(g) log 7.753×10^{5} **Ans: 5.8895**

18. Solve the following using logarithm

(a) 67.86×87.54 **Ans: 5940**

(b) $30.07 \div 5.436$ **Ans: 5.53**

19. Multiply 3367214 by 78962, and write down the estimated and actual values.

Ans: 210000000000 (265881951868)

20. Divide 9677246 by 86904, and write down the estimated and actual values.

Ans: 120 (111.355)

21. The assay value of a material received is 98.99%. As per formula for 100kg lot size 70 kg of this material with 100% potency is required. Calculate the amount of the material to be used for a lot size of 150 k.

Ans: 106.1kg

22. A reprocessed batch of tablet contains 78 kg of granules of 74.65% of drug and 45 kg of 70.05% of drug, Calculate the drug content of the mixture in percent.

Ans: 72.96%

23. In what proportion 20.0% of alcohol and 15.0% of alcohol are to be mixed with water to make 17.5% alcohol? Use the method of alligation.

Ans: 8 pts of 20%, 1 pt of 15% and 1 pts of water

24. In what proportion 10% Gentamycin sulphate ointment is to be mixed with a suitable ointment base to make 1% Gentamycin sulphate ointment?

Ans: 1 pt of 10% and 10 pts of base

25. A mixture of 20% hydrochloric acid is prepared by mixing 7.5%, 22.5%, and 50% hydrochloric acid solutions. In which proportion these have to be mixed?

Ans: 32.5 pts of 7.5%, 12.5 pts of 22.5% and 12.5 pts of 50% of HCl

4

DENSITY, SPECIFIC GRAVITY AND SPECIFIC VOLUME

The density of a substance is a concrete number; for example, 1.16 g/mL (Hydrochloric acid). The specific gravity is a ratio of two densities. It is an abstract number; for example, 1.165 (Hydrochloric acid). The density depends on temperature and varies with the units of measure used. The specific gravity has no unit and is therefore a constant value for any substance, if measured under same conditions. It is important to note that specific gravity is a *factor* that provides the information about the heaviness or lightness of a substance than water. For example, a liquid with a specific gravity of 1.45 indicates that it is 1.45 times heavier than water; similarly a liquid having specific gravity of 0.975 indicates that the liquid is 0.85 times lighter than water.

The chapter provides the information about:

- Definition of the terms, density, specific gravity, and specific volume, method of determination of each and related calculations.
- Correct application of the term specific gravity in converting weight to volume and volume to weight.

Density

The term *density (ρ or d)* is defined as *the mass per unit volume of a substance at a particular temperature.* It is usually expressed as *grams* per *cubic centimeter (g/cc)* or *grams* per *milliliter (g/mL).* One gram is considered as the mass of 1 mL of water at 4°C; hence, the density of water is 1 g/cc at 4°C. According to the *United States Pharmacopeia* 1 mL should be considered as the equivalent of 1 cc and the density of water may be expressed as 1 g/mL; while one milliliter of mercury weighs 13.6 g; hence, the density of mercury is 13.6 g/mL.

Thus, density may be calculated as:

$$\text{Density} = \frac{\text{Mass}}{\text{Volume}}$$

Example

If 100 mL of concentrated hydrochloric acid weigh 116 g, what would be its density?

Solution

$$\text{Density} = \frac{\text{Mass}}{\text{Volume}}$$

$$= \frac{116\text{ g}}{100\text{ mL}} = 1.16\text{ g/mL}$$

Example

At 25°C, the weight of 25 mL of Sorbitol solution (70%) is 32.1252 g. Find out its density.

Solution

Density of Sorbitol solution (70%) at 25°C = $\frac{32.1252\text{ g}}{25\text{ mL}}$

Ans. 1.285 g/mL

Use of Density to Determine Alcohol Content

Many pharmaceutical liquid preparations contain alcohol. Thus, it is necessary to determine alcohol content in the preparation. The preparation is distilled by specified method and the distillate is collected in a 100 ml volumetric flask. Hence a diluted solution of alcohol is obtained. Density of this solution is measured at 20 °C and using the table, content of alcohol present in the distillate solution is determined. There after the content of alcohol is calculated as follows;

For example, a 25 ml of actual preparation is taken for distillation. After distillation 100ml of distillate is collected for determination of density. Say, the specific gravity of the distillate is 0.98187 at 20°C. Form the table it represents alcohol content of 10%v/v. That is, 10ml of alcohol is present in 100ml of distillate.

Thus, 25 ml of the preparation contains 10 ml of alcohol;

100 ml of preparation contains $\frac{10 \times 100}{25}$ = 40%v/v of alcohol.

Ethanol w/v%	Specific gravity at		Ethanol w/v%	Specific gravity at		Ethanol w/v%	Specific gravity at	
	20°C	25°C		20°C	25°C		20°C	25°C
0	0.99823	0.99708	35	0.94494	0.94146	70	0.86766	0.86340
0.1	0.99804		35.1	0.94475		70.1	0.86742	
0.2	0.99785		35.2	0.94456		70.2	0.86718	
0.3	0.99766		35.3	0.94438		70.3	0.86694	
0.4	0.99748		35.4	0.94419		70.4	0.86671	
0.5	0.99729		35.5	0.94400		70.5	0.86647	
0.6	0.99710		35.6	0.94382		70.6	0.86623	
0.7	0.99692		35.7	0.94363		70.7	0.86599	
0.8	0.99673		35.8	0.94344		70.8	0.86575	
0.9	0.99655		35.9	0.94325		70.9	0.86551	
1	0.99636	0.9952	36	0.94306	0.93952	71	0.86527	0.86100
1.1	0.99618		36.1	0.94287		71.1	0.86503	
1.2	0.99599		36.2	0.94268		71.2	0.86479	
1.3	0.99581		36.3	0.94249		71.3	0.86455	
1.4	0.99562		36.4	0.94230		71.4	0.86431	
1.5	0.99544		36.5	0.94211		71.5	0.86407	
1.6	0.99525		36.6	0.94192		71.6	0.86383	
1.7	0.99507		36.7	0.94172		71.7	0.86339	
1.8	0.99489		36.8	0.94153		71.8	0.86335	
1.9	0.99471		36.9	0.94134		71.9	0.86311	
2	0.99453	0.99336	37	0.94114	0.93756	72	0.86287	0.85859
2.1	0.99435		37.1	0.94095		72.1	0.86263	
2.2	0.99417		37.2	0.94075		72.2	0.86239	
2.3	0.99399		37.3	0.94056		72.3	0.86215	
2.4	0.99381		37.4	0.94036		72.4	0.86191	
2.5	0.99363		37.5	0.94017		72.5	0.86167	
2.6	0.99345		37.6	0.93997		72.6	0.86143	
2.7	0.99327		37.7	0.93978		72.7	0.86119	
2.8	0.99310		37.8	0.93958		72.8	0.86095	
2.9	0.99292		37.9	0.93939		72.9	0.86071	

Table *contd...*

Ethanol w/v%	Specific gravity at		Ethanol w/v%	Specific gravity at		Ethanol w/v%	Specific gravity at	
	20°C	25°C		20°C	25°C		20°C	25°C
3.1	0.99257		38.1	0.93899		73.1	0.86022	
3.2	0.99240		38.2	0.93879		73.2	0.85998	
3.3	0.99222		38.3	0.93859		73.3	0.85974	
3.4	0.99205		38.4	0.93840		73.4	0.85950	
3.5	0.99188		38.5	0.93820		73.5	0.85926	
3.6	0.99171		38.6	0.93800		73.6	0.85902	
3.7	0.99154		38.7	0.93780		73.7	0.85878	
3.8	0.99137		38.8	0.93760		73.8	0.85854	
3.9	0.99120		38.9	0.93740		73.9	0.85830	
4	0.99103	0.98984	39	0.93720	0.93353	74	0.85806	0.85376
4.1	0.99087		39.1	0.93700		74.1	0.85781	
4.2	0.99070		39.2	0.93680		74.2	0.85757	
4.3	0.99053		39.3	0.93660		74.3	0.85733	
4.4	0.99037		39.4	0.93640		74.4	0.85709	
4.5	0.99020		39.5	0.93620		74.5	0.85685	
4.6	0.99003		39.6	0.93599		74.6	0.85661	
4.7	0.98987		39.7	0.93579		74.7	0.85636	
4.8	0.98971		39.8	0.93559		74.8	0.85612	
4.9	0.98954		39.9	0.93539		74.9	0.85588	
5	0.98938	0.98817	40	0.93518	0.93148	75	0.85564	0.85134
5.1	0.98922		40.1	0.93498		75.1	0.85540	
5.2	0.98906		40.2	0.93478		75.2	0.85515	
5.3	0.98890		40.3	0.93458		75.3	0.85491	
5.4	0.98874		40.4	0.93437		75.4	0.85467	
5.5	0.98859		40.5	0.93417		75.5	0.85443	
5.6	0.98843		40.6	0.93396		75.6	0.85419	
5.7	0.98827		40.7	0.93376		75.7	0.85394	
5.8	0.98811		408	0.93356		75.8	0.85370	
5.9	0.98796		40.9	0.93335		75.9	0.85346	
6	0.98780	0.98656	41	0.93314	0.92940	76	0.85322	0.84891
6.1	0.98765		41.1	0.93294		76.1	0.85297	
6.2	0.98749		41.2	0.93273		76.2	0.85273	
6.3	0.98734		41.3	0.93253		76.3	0.85249	

Table *contd...*

Ethanol w/v%	Specific gravity at		Ethanol w/v%	Specific gravity at		Ethanol w/v%	Specific gravity at	
	20°C	25°C		20°C	25°C		20°C	25°C
6.4	0.98718		41.4	0.93232		76.4	0.85225	
6.5	0.98703		41.5	0.93212		76.5	0.85200	
6.6	0.98688		41.6	0.93191		76.6	0.85176	
6.7	0.98673		41.7	0.93170		76.7	0.85152	
6.8	0.98658		41.8	0.93149		76.8	0.85128	
6.9	0.98642		41.9	0.93129		76.9	0.85103	
7	0.98627	0.98500	42	0.93107	0.92729	77	0.85079	0.84647
7.1	0.98612		42.1	0.93086		77.1	0.85055	
7.2	0.98597		42.2	0.93065		77.2	0.85031	
7.3	0.98582		42.3	0.93044		77.3	0.85006	
7.4	0.98567		42.4	0.93023		77.4	0.84982	
7.5	0.98553		42.5	0.93002		77.5	0.84958	
7.6	0.98538		42.6	0.92981		77.6	0.84933	
7.7	0.98523		42.7	0.92960		77.7	0.84909	
7.8	0.98508		42.8	0.92939		77.8	0.84884	
7.9	0.98493		42.9	0.92918		77.9	0.84860	
8	0.98478	0.98346	43	0.92897	0.92516	78	0.84835	0.84403
8.1	0.98463		43.1	0.92876		78.1	0.84811	
8.2	0.98449		43.2	0.92855		78.2	0.84787	
8.3	0.98434		43.3	0.92834		78.3	0.84762	
8.4	0.98419		43.4	0.92812		78.4	0.84738	
8.5	0.98404		43.5	0.92791		78.5	0.84713	
8.6	0.98389		43.6	0.92770		78.6	0.84689	
8.7	0.98374		43.7	0.92749		78.7	0.84664	
8.8	0.98360		43.8	0.92728		78.8	0.84640	
8.9	0.98345		43.9	0.92707		78.9	0.84615	
9	0.98331	0.98193	44	0.92685	0.92301	79	0.84590	0.84158
9.1	0.98316		44.1	0.92664		79.1	0.84566	
9.2	0.98301		44.2	0.92642		79.2	0.84541	
9.3	0.98287		44.3	0.92621		79.3	0.84517	
9.4	.98273		44.4	0.92600		79.4	0.84492	
9.5	0.98258		44.5	0.92579		79.5	0.84467	
9.6	0.98244		44.6	0.92557		79.6	0.84443	

Table *contd...*

Ethanol w/v%	Specific gravity at		Ethanol w/v%	Specific gravity at		Ethanol w/v%	Specific gravity at	
	20°C	25°C		20°C	25°C		20°C	25°C
9.7	0.98229		44.7	0.92536		79.7	0.84418	
9.8	0.98215		44.8	0.92515		79.8	0.84393	
9.9	0.98201		44.9	0.92493		79.9	0.84369	
10	0.98187	0.98043	45	0.92472	0.92085	80	0.84344	0.83911
10.1	0.98172		45.1	0.92450		80.1	0.84319	
10.2	0.98158		45.2	0.92429		80.2	0.84294	
10.3	0.98144		45.3	0.92408		80.3	0.84270	
10.4	0.98130		45.4	0.92386		80.4	0.84245	
10.5	0.98117		45.5	0.92365		80.5	0.84220	
10.6	0.98103		45.6	0.92343		80.6	0.84196	
10.7	0.98089		45.7	0.92322		80.7	0.84171	
10.8	0.98075		45.8	0.92300		80.8	0.84146	
10.9	0.98061		45.9	0.92279		80.9	0.84121	
11	0.98047	0.97897	46	0.92257	0.91868	81	0.84096	0.83664
11.1	0.98033		46.1	0.92236		81.1	0.84072	
11.2	0.98019		46.2	0.92214		81.2	0.84047	
11.3	0.98006		46.3	0.92193		81.3	0.84022	
11.4	0.97992		46.4	0.92171		81.4	0.83997	
11.5	0.97978		46.5	0.92150		81.5	0.83972	
11.6	0.97964		46.6	0.92128		81.6	0.83947	
11.7	0.97951		46.7	0.92106		81.7	0.83923	
11.8	0.97937		46.8	0.92085		81.8	0.83898	
11.9	0.97923		46.9	0.92063		81.9	0.83873	
12	0.97910	0.97753	47	0.92041	0.91649	82	0.83848	0.83415
12.1	0.97896		47.1	0.92019		82.1	0.83823	
12.2	0.97883		47.2	0.91997		82.2	0.83798	
12.3	0.97869		47.3	0.91976		82.3	0.83773	
12.4	0.97855		47.4	0.91954		82.4	0.83748	
12.5	0.97842		47.5	0.91932		82.5	0.83723	
12.6	0.97828		47.6	0.91910		82.6	0.83698	
12.7	0.97815		47.7	0.91889		82.7	0.83674	
12.8	0.97801		47.8	0.91867		82.8	0.83649	
12.9	0.97788		47.9	0.91845		82.9	0.83624	

Table *contd...*

Ethanol w/v%	Specific gravity at		Ethanol w/v%	Specific gravity at		Ethanol w/v%	Specific gravity at	
	20°C	25°C		20°C	25°C		20°C	25°C
13	0.97775	0.97661	48	0.91823	0.91426	83	0.83599	0.83164
13.1	0.97761		48.1	0.91801		83.1	0.83574	
13.2	0.97748		48.2	0.91780		83.2	0.83549	
13.3	0.97735		48.3	0.91758		83.3	0.83523	
13.4	0.97722		48.4	0.91736		83.4	0.83498	
13.5	0.97709		48.5	0.91714		83.5	0.83473	
13.6	0.97696		48.6	0.91692		83.6	0.83448	
13.7	0.97683		48.7	0.91670		83.7	0.83423	
13.8	0.97670		48.8	0.91648		83.8	0.83398	
13.9	0.97657		48.9	0.91626		83.9	0.83373	
14	0.97643	0.97472	49	0.91604	0.91208	84	0.83348	0.82913
14.1	0.97630		49.1	0.91582		84.1	0.83323	
14.2	0.97617		49.2	0.91560		84.2	0.83297	
14.3	0.97604		49.3	0.91538		84.3	0.83272	
14.4	0.97591		49.4	0.91516		84.4	0.83247	
14.5	0.97578		49.5	0.91494		84.5	0.83222	
14.6	0.97565		49.6	0.91472		84.6	0.83196	
14.7	0.97552		49.7	0.91450		84.7	0.83171	
14.8	0.97539		49.8	0.91428		84.8	0.83146	
14.9	0.97526		49.9	0.91406		84.9	0.83120	
15	0.97514	0.97334	50	0.91384	0.90985	85	0.83095	0.82660
15.1	0.97501		50.1	0.91361		85.1	0.83070	
15.2	0.97488		50.2	0.91339		85.2	0.83044	
15.3	0.97475		50.3	0.91317		85.3	0.83019	
15.4	0.97462		50.4	0.91295		85.4	0.82994	
15.5	0.97450		50.5	0.91272		85.5	0.82968	
15.6	0.97438		50.6	0.91250		85.6	0.82943	
15.7	0.97425		50.7	0.91228		85.7	0.82917	
15.8	0.97412		50.8	0.91206		85.8	0.82892	
15.9	0.97400		50.9	0.91183		85.9	0.82866	
16	0.97387	0.97199	51	0.91160	0.90760	86	0.82840	0.82405
16.1	0.97374		51.1	0.91138		86.1	0.82815	
16.2	0.97361		51..2	0.91116		86.2	0.82789	

Table *contd...*

Ethanol w/v%	Specific gravity at		Ethanol w/v%	Specific gravity at		Ethanol w/v%	Specific gravity at	
	20°C	25°C		20°C	25°C		20°C	25°C
16.3	0.97349		51.3	0.91093		86.3	0.82763	
16.4	0.97336		51.4	0.91071		86.4	0.82738	
16.5	0.97323		51.5	0.91049		86.5	0.82712	
16.6	0.97310		51.6	0.91026		86.6	0.82686	
16.7	0.97297		51.7	0.91004		86.7	0.82660	
16.8	0.97284		51.8	0.90981		86.8	0.82635	
16.9	0.97272		51.9	0.90959		86.9	0.82609	
17	0.97259	0.97062	52	0.90936	0.90534	87	0.82583	0.82148
17.1	0.97246		52.1	0.90914		87.1	0.82557	
17.2	0.97233		52.2	0.90891		87.2	0.82531	
17.3	0.97220		52.3	0.90869		87.3	0.82505	
17.4	0.97207		52.4	0.90846		87.4	0.82479	
17.5	0.97194		52.5	0.90824		87.5	0.82453	
17.6	0.97181		52.6	0.90801		87.6	0.82427	
17.7	0.97168		52.7	0.90779		87.7	0.82401	
17.8	0.97155		52.8	0.90756		87.8	0.82375	
17.9	0.97142		52.9	0.90734		87.9	0.82349	
18	0.97129	0.96923	53	0.90711	0.90307	88	0.82323	0.81888
18.1	0.97116		53.1	0.90689		88.1	0.82297	
18.2	0.97103		53.2	0.90666		88.2	0.82271	
18.3	0.97089		53.3	0.90644		88.3	0.82245	
18.4	0.97076		53.4	0.90621		88.4	0.82219	
18.5	0.97063		53.5	0.90598		88.5	0.82193	
18.6	0.97050		53.6	0.90576		88.6	0.82167	
18.7	0.97037		53.7	0.90553		88.7	0.82140	
18.8	0.97024		53.8	0.90531		88.8	0.82114	
18.9	0.97010		53.9	0.90508		88.9	0.82088	
19	0.96997	0.96782	54	0.90485	0.90079	89	0.82062	0.81626
19.1	0.96984		54.1	0.90463		89.11	0.82035	
19.2	0.96971		54.2	0.90440		89.2	0.82009	
19.3	0.96957		54.3	0.90417		89.3	0.81983	
19.4	0.96944		54.4	0.90395		89.4	0.81956	
19.5	0.96931		54.5	0.90372		89.5	0.81930	

Table *contd...*

Ethanol w/v%	Specific gravity at		Ethanol w/v%	Specific gravity at		Ethanol w/v%	Specific gravity at	
	20°C	25°C		20°C	25°C		20°C	25°C
19.6	0.96917		54.6	0.90349		89.6	0.81903	
19.7	0.96904		54.7	0.90327		89.77	0.81877	
19.8	0.96891		54.8	0.90304		89.8	0.81850	
19.9	0.96877		54.9	0.90281		89.9	0.81824	
20	0.96864	0.96639	55	0.90258	0.89850	90	0.81797	0.81362
20.1	0.96850		55.1	0.90236		90.1	0.81770	
20.2	0.96837		55.2	0.90213		90.2	0.81744	
20.3	0.96823		55.3	0.90190		90.3	0.81717	
20.4	0.96810		55.4	0.90167		90.4	0.81690	
20.5	0.96796		55.5	0.90145		90.55	0.81664	
20.6	0.96783		55.6	0.90122		90.6	0.81637	
20.7	0.96769		55.7	0.90099		90.7	0.81610	
20.8	0.96756		55.8	0.90076		90.8	0.81583	
20.9	0.96742		55.9	0.90054		90.9	0.81556	
21	0.96729	0.96495	56	0.90031	0.89621	91	0.81529	0.81094
21.1	0.96716		56.1	0.90008		91.1	0.81502	
21.2	0.96702		56.2	0.89985		91.2	0.81475	
21.3	0.96688		56.3	0.89962		91.3	0.81448	
21.4	0.96675		56.4	0.89939		91.44	0.81421	
21.5	0.96661		56.5	0.89917		91.55	0.81394	
21.6	0.96647		56.6	0.89894		91.6	0.81366	
21.7	0.96634		56.7	0.89871		91.7	0.81339	
21.8	0.96620		56.8	0.89848		91.8	0.81312	
21.9	0.96606		56.9	0.89825		91.9	0.81285	
22	0.96592	0.96348	57	0.89803	0.89392	92	0.81257	0.80823
22.1	0.96578		57.1	0.89780		92.1	0.81230	
22.2	0.96564		57.2	0.89757		92.2	0.81203	
22.3	0.96551		57.3	0.89734		92.3	0.81175	
22.4	0.96537		57.4	0.89711		92.4	0.81148	
22.5	0.96523		57.5	0.89688		92.5	0.81120	
22.6	0.96509		57.6	0.89665		92.6	0.81093	
22.7	0.96495		57.7	0.89643		92.7	0.81066	
22.8	0.96481		57.8	0.89620		92.8	0.81038	

Table *contd...*

Ethanol w/v%	Specific gravity at		Ethanol w/v%	Specific gravity at		Ethanol w/v%	Specific gravity at	
	20°C	25°C		20°C	25°C		20°C	25°C
22.9	0.96467		57.9	0.89597		92.9	0.81010	
23	0.96453	0.96199	58	0.89574	0.89162	93	0.80983	0.80549
23.1	0.96439		58.1	0.89551		93.1	0.80955	
23.2	0.96425		58.2	0.89528		93.2	0.80928	
23.3	0.96411		58.3	0.89505		93.3	0.80900	
23.4	0.96396		58.4	0.89482		93.4	0.80872	
23.5	0.96382		58.5	0.89459		93.5	0.80844	
23.6	0.96368		58.6	0.89436		93.6	0.80817	
23.7	0.96354		58.7	0.89413		93.7	0.80789	
23.8	0.96340		58.8	0.89390		93.8	0.80761	
23.9	0.96326		58.9	0.89367		93.9	0.80733	
24	0.96312	0.96048	59	0.89344	0.88931	94	0.80705	0.80272
24.1	0.96297		59.1	0.89321		94.1	0.80677	
24.2	0.96283		59.2	0.89298		94.2	0.80649	
24.3	0.96269		59.3	0.89275		94.3	0.80621	
24.4	0.96254		59.4	0.89252		94.44	0.80593	
24.5	0.96240		59.5	0.89229		94.5	0.80565	
24.6	0.96225		59.6	0.89206		94.6	0.80537	
24.7	0.96211		59.7	0.89183		94.7	0.80509	
24.8	0.96196		59.8	0.89160		94.8	0.80480	
24.9	0.96182		59.9	0.89137		94.9	0.80452	
25	0.96168	0.95895	60	0.89113	0.88699	95	0.80424	0.79991
25.1	0.96153		60.1	0.89090		95.1	0.80395	
25.2	0.96139		60.2	0.89067		95.2	0.80367	
25.3	0.96124		60.3	0.89044		95.3	0.80338	
25.4	0.96109		60.4	0.89021		95.4	0.80310	
25.5	0.96094		60.5	0.88998		95.5	0.80281	
25.6	0.96080		60.6	0.88975		95.6	0.80253	
25.7	0.96065		60.7	0.88951		95.7	0.80224	
25.8	0.96050		60.8	0.88928		95.8	0.80195	
25.9	0.96035		60.9	0.88905		95.9	0.80166	
26	0.96020	0.95738	61	0.88882	0.88446	96	0.80138	0.79706
26.1	0.96005		61.1	0.88859		96.1	0.80109	

Table *contd...*

Ethanol w/v%	Specific gravity at		Ethanol w/v%	Specific gravity at		Ethanol w/v%	Specific gravity at	
	20°C	25°C		20°C	25°C		20°C	25°C
26.2	0.95990		61.2	0.88836		96.2	0.80080	
26.3	0.95975		61.3	0.88812		96.3	0.80051	
26.4	0.95959		61.4	0.88789		96.4	0.80022	
26.5	0.95944		61.5	0.88766		96.5	0.79993	
26.6	0.95929		61.6	0.88743		96.6	0.79963	
26.7	0.95914		61.7	0.88720		96.7	0.79934	
26.8	0.95898		61.8	0.88696		96.8	0.79905	
26.9	0.95883		61.9	0.88673		96.9	0.79875	
27	0.95867	0.95576	62	0.88650	0.88233	97	0.79846	0.79415
27.1	0.95851		62.1	0.88626		97.1	0.79816	
27.2	0.95836		62.2	0.88603		97.2	0.79787	
27.3	0.95820		62.3	0.88580		97.3	0.79757	
27.4	0.95805		62.4	0.88557		97.4	0.79727	
27.5	0.95789		62.5	0.88533		97.5	0.79698	
27.6	0.95773		62.6	0.88510		97.6	0.79668	
27.7	0.95757		62.7	0.88487		97.7	0.79638	
27.8	0.95742		62.8	0.88463		97.8	0.79608	
27.9	0.95726		62.9	0.88440		97.9	0.79578	
28	0.95710	0.95410	63	0.88417	0.87998	98	0.79547	0.79117
28.1	0.95694		63.1	0.88393		98.1	0.79517	
28.2	0.95678		63.2	0.88370		98.2	0.79487	
28.3	0.95662		63.3	0.88347		98.3	0.79456	
28.4	0.95646		63.4	0.88323		98.4	0.79426	
28.5	0.95630		63.5	0.88300		98.5	0.79396	
28.6	0.95613		63.6	0.88277		98.6	0.79365	
28.7	0.95597		63.7	0.88253		98.7	0.79335	
28.8	0.95581		63.8	0.88230		98.8	0.79305	
28.9	0.95565		63.9	0.88206		98.9	0.79274	
29	0.95548	0.95241	64	0.88183	0.87763	99	0.79543	0.78814
29.1	0.95532		64.1	0.88160		99.11	0.79213	
29.2	0.95516		64.2	0.88136		99.2	0.79182	
29.3	0.95499		64.3	0.88113		99.33	0.79151	
29.4	0.95483		64.4	0.88089		99.4	0.79120	

Table *contd...*

Ethanol w/v%	Specific gravity at		Ethanol w/v%	Specific gravity at		Ethanol w/v%	Specific gravity at	
	20°C	25°C		20°C	25°C		20°C	25°C
29.5	0.95466		64.5	0.88066		99.55	0.79089	
29.6	0.95450		64.6	0.88042		99.6	0.79059	
29.7	0.95433		64.7	0.88019		99.7	0.79028	
29.8	0.95416		64.8	0.87995		99.8	0.78997	
29.9	0.95400		64.9	0.87972		99.9	0.78966	
30	0.95382	0.95067	65	0.87948	0.87527	100	0.78934	0.78506
30.1	0.95365		65.1	0.87925				
30.2	0.95349		65.2	0.87901				
30.3	0.95332		65.3	0.87878				
30.4	0.95315		65.4	0.87854				
30.5	0.95298		65.5	0.87831				
30.6	0.95281		65.6	0.87807				
30.7	0.95264		65.7	0.87784				
30.8	0.95247		65.8	0.87760				
30.9	0.95230		65.9	0.87737				
31	0.95212	0.94890	66	0.87713	0.87291			
31.1	0.95195		66.1	0.87689				
31.2	0.95178		66.2	0.87666				
31.3	0.95161		66.3	0.87642				
31.4	0.95143		66.4	0.87619				
31.5	0.95126		66.5	0.87595				
31.6	0.95108		66.6	0.87572				
31.7	0.95091		66.7	0.87548				
31.8	0.95074		66.8	0.87524				
31.9	0.95056		66.9	0.87501				
32	0.95038	0.94709	67	0.87477	0.87054			
32.1	0.95020		67.1	0.87454				
32.2	0.95003		67.2	0.87430				
32.3	0.94985		67.3	0.87406				
32.4	0.94967		67.4	0.87383				
32.5	0.94950		67.5	0.87359				
32.6	0.94932		67.6	0.87336				
32.7	0.94914		67.7	0.87312				

Table *contd...*

Ethanol w/v%	Specific gravity at		Ethanol w/v%	Specific gravity at		Ethanol w/v%	Specific gravity at	
	20°C	25°C		20°C	25°C		20°C	25°C
32.8	0.94896		67.8	0.87288				
32.9	0.94878		67.9	0.87265				
33	0.94860	0.94525	68	0.87241	0.86817			
33.1	0.94842		68.1	.87218				
33.2	0.94824		68.2	0.87194				
33.3	0.94806		68.3	0.87170				
33.4	0.94788		68.4	0.87147				
33.5	0.94770		68.5	0.87123				
33.6	0.94752		68.6	0.87099				
33.7	0.94734		68.7	0.87075				
33.8	0.94715		68.8	0.87052				
33.9	0.94697		68.9	0.87028				
34	0.94679	0.94337	69	0.87004	0.86579			
34.1	0.94660		69.1	0.86981				
34.2	0.94642		69.2	0.86957				
34.3	0.94624		69.3	0.86933				
34.4	0.94605		69.4	0.86909				
34.5	0.94587		69.5	0.86885				
34.6	0.94568		69.6	0.86862				
34.7	0.94550		69.7	0.86838				
34.8	0.94531		69.8	0.86814				
34.9	0.94512		69.9	0.86790				

Specific Gravity

Specific gravity (sp gr) is a ratio of the density of a substance to that of water at a particular temperature. It is expressed decimally and it does not have any unit. Water is used as the reference for the specific gravities determination of both liquids and solids; while for gases hydrogen is used as reference.

Specific gravity may be calculated by dividing the weight of a given substance by the weight of an equal volume of water at the same temperature.

$$\text{Specific gravity} = \frac{\text{Weight of substance}}{\text{Weight of equal volume of water at same temperature}}$$

$$= \frac{\text{Density of substance}}{\text{Density of water at the same temperature}}$$

Example

The weight of 10 mL of water is 9.9602 g and that of Sorbitol solution (70%) is 12.85 g at 25°C. What would be the specific gravity of sorbitol solution?

Solution

Specific gravity of sorbitol solution at 25°C

$$= \frac{\text{Weight of 10 ml of sorbitol solution}}{\text{Weight 10 ml of water at the } 25^{\circ}\text{C}}$$

$$= \frac{12.85 \text{ g}}{9.9602 \text{ g}}$$

$$= 1.29013 \text{ (Answer)}$$

Or, Specific gravity of sorbitol solution at 25°C

$$= \frac{\text{Density of sorbitol solution}}{\text{Density of water at the } 25^{\circ}\text{C}}$$

$$= \frac{1.285 \text{ g/ml}}{0.99602 \text{ g/ml}} = 1.2901 \text{ (Answer)}$$

Example

If 96.05 ml of a liquid weighs 94.897 g at 25°C, what would its specific gravity?

Solution

The weight of 96.05 ml of water at 25°C = 96.05 ml× 0.99602 g/ml = 95.67 g

[Density of water at 25°C = 0.99602 g/ml]

Then, the specific gravity of the liquid $= \frac{94.897 \text{ g}}{95.67 \text{ g}} = 0.9919$ (Answer)

The specific gravity of some common liquids are given in Table 4.1

Table 4.1 Specific gravity of some common liquids at 25°C

Substance	Specific gravity	Substance	Specific gravity
Ether (at 20°C)	0.71	Propylene glycol	1.03
Isopropyl alcohol	0.78	Clove oil	1.04
Acetone	0.79	Liquefied phenol	1.07
Alcohol	0.81	Polysorbate 80	1.08
Liquid petrolatum	0.87	Polyethylene glycol 400	1.13
Benzene	0.88	Hydrochloric acid	1.16
Peppermint oil	0.90	Glycerin	1.25
Olive oil	0.91	Syrup	1.31
Arachis oil	0.92	Nitric acid	1.42
Peanut oil	0.92	Chloroform	1.47
Cod liver oil	0.92	Nitroglycerin	1.59
Castor oil	0.92	Phosphoric acid	1.70
Sesame oil	0.96	Sulphuric Acid	1.84
Water	1.00	Mercury	13.6

Note:

1. *Substances having specific gravity less than 1 are lighter than water*
2. *Substances having specific gravity more than 1 are heavier than water*

Determination of Specific Gravity of Liquid

Materials required:

1. One clean pycnometer
2. Distilled water
3. Hot-air oven
4. Sample liquid

Pycnometer is a special glass bottle used to determine specific gravity. Pycnometer is generally available for laboratory use, its volume ranges from 1 mL to 50 mL. Glass stopper with a capillary opening is fitted to the Pycnometer. The stopper when inserted into the mouth of the pycnometer allows trapped air and excess fluid to come out.

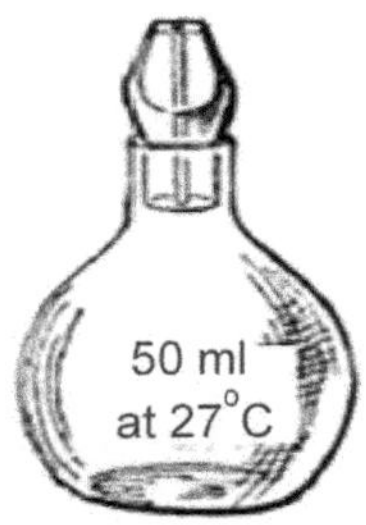

Pycnometer

For determining specific gravity, temperature is a factor which needs to be maintained. For this reason some pycnometers have thermometers attached. The clean, dry and empty pycnometer is first weighed (W_g) and then filled with water and weighed (W_1). The difference in weights (W_1 – W) g is the weight of the water. During determination a specific temperature is maintained. The water is removed and the pycnometer is dried. The sample liquid is placed in the pycnometer, kept at same temperature for at least 10 min. It is then weighed (W_2). The difference in weight (W_2 – W) g is the weight of the liquid. The specific gravity of the liquid $= \frac{W_2 - W}{W_1 - W}$

The calculation of specific gravity is demonstrated in the following example.

Example

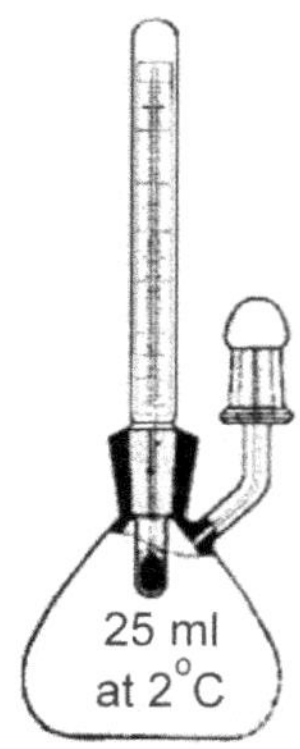

Pycnometer fitted with a thermometer

The volume of pycnometer

= 50 ml

The weight of empty pycnometer

= 121.7635 g at 25°C

The weight of pycnometer + water

= 171.5660 g at 25°C

The weight of pycnometer + liquid

= 172.9768 g at 25°C

Calculate the specific gravity of the liquid.

Weight of 50 ml of water at 25°C

= 171.5660 g – 121.7635 g

= 49.8025 g

Weight of 50 ml of liquid at 25°C

= 172.9768 g – 121.7635 g

= 51.2133 g

Thus, the specific gravity of the liquid at 25°C $= \frac{51.2133\text{ g}}{49.8025\text{ g}}$

s = 1.0283 (Answer)

or

$$\text{The density of water at } 25^{\circ}\text{C} = \frac{49.8025 \text{ g}}{50 \text{ ml}} = 0.99605 \text{ g/ml}$$

$$\text{The density of the liquid at } 25^{\circ}\text{C} = \frac{51.2133 \text{ g}}{50 \text{ ml}} = 1.0243 \text{ g/ml}$$

$$\text{So, the specific gravity of the liquid at } 25^{\circ}\text{C} = \frac{1.0243 \text{ g/ml}}{0.99605 \text{ g/ml}}$$

Ans. 1.0284

Displacement or Plummet Method

The specific gravity of a solid or insoluble liquid can be determined by the displacement or plummet method. This method is based on the *Archimedes' principle,* which states that when a body is immersed in a liquid, it displaces an amount of the liquid equal to its own volume. As a result an apparent loss in weight, equal to the weight of the displaced liquid is observed. This method is commonly used to determine the density of a solid.

The body is suspended in water and weighed. Then it is suspended in the liquid of which the specific gravity is to be determined and weighed. These weights are subtracted from the weight of the body in air. Thus, the weights of equal volumes of water and the liquid are obtained and used to calculate the specific gravity of the body.

Example

The weights of a glass paper weight are as follows; (1) 15.4932 g in air, (2) 10.8915 g when immersed in water, and (3) 11.9127 g when immersed in oil. Calculate the specific gravity of the oil.

Solution

The weight of the oil displaced (the volume equal to the paper weight) = 15.4932 g – 11.0127g

= 4.4805 g

The weight of the water displaced (the volume equal to the paper weight) = 15.4932g–10.8915 g = 4.6017 g

$$\text{Then the specific gravity of the oil} = \frac{4.4805 \text{ g}}{4.6017 \text{ g}}$$

Ans. 0.9736

Example

A piece of metal weighs 39.0854g in air and weighs 34.9871g when fully immersed in water at 25°C, the density of water is 0.99607g/ml. Find out the density of the metal.

Solution

As per Archimedes' principle the metal piece displaces water equal to its own volume and the weight of water displaced = loss of weight of metal piece in water.

Loss of weight of metal piece in water = 39.0854 g – 34.9871 g

$$= 4.0983\text{g}$$

Volume of displaced water = volume of metal piece

$$= \frac{4.0983\text{g}}{0.99697\ \text{g/ml}} \text{ (Density of water at 25°C = 0.99607g/ml)}$$

$$= 4.114\ \text{ml}$$

$$\text{Density of the metal} = \frac{\text{Weight in air}}{\text{volume}} = \frac{39.0854\text{g}}{4.114\ \text{ml}}$$

$$= 9.687\text{g/ml (Answer)}$$

Density of Solid

As defined earlier density is the weight of unit volume of a substance. For a nonporous substance the density can be determined by measuring its weight and volume directly or indirectly. If an insoluble solid material is immersed in a liquid of known density the solid material displaces the liquid equal to its volume. By measuring the volume of the displaced liquid the volume of known weight of the solid can be determined.

Example

A solid metal when immersed in water 20 ml of water is displaced. The weight of the metal is 43.9764g. Find out the density.

Solution

The volume of the solid = volume of water displaced = 20 ml

The weight of the solid = 43.9764g

$$\text{Density of the metal} = \frac{43.9764\ \text{g}}{20\ \text{ml}} = 2.1988\ \text{g/ml} \approx 2.20\ \text{g/ml}$$

Example

A rectangular solid slab made of metal is 4.5 ft long, 0.75 ft thick and 2 ft wide. The weight of the slab is 414.75 kg. Calculate the density (g/cm^3) of the metal used.

Solution

1 ft = 30.48 cm = 0.3048 m

Length = 4.5 ft = 4.5 × 0.3048 m = 1.37 m

Breadth = 2 ft = 2 × 0.3048 m = 0.6096 m

Thickness = 0.75 ft = 0.75 × 0.3048 m = 0.228 m

Volume of the slab = 1.37 m × 0.6096 m × 0.228 m = 0.1904 m^3

$= 0.1904 \times 100 \times 100 \times 100\ cm^3 = 190400\ cm^3$

$$\text{Density of the metal} = \frac{\text{weight}}{\text{volume}} = \frac{414.75 \times 1000}{190400}\ g/ml$$

Ans. 2.178g/cm^3

Density of Powder

Determination of density of powders should be done carefully. Because solid particles are of different natures;

- Hard and smooth
- Rough and spongy
- Porous, and
- Nonporous.

Density is calculated by determining the weight of unit volume of a substance. In fact, determination of volume of powders is difficult. Most powders have microscopic cracks, internal poses and capillary spaces.

Density of powders may be categorized into three types:

- **True density** is the actual density. In case of porous material, voids or internal pores may be more than molecular or atomic dimensions in the crystal lattice. In such case, best method is gas displacement method such as helium displacement method. Helium can penetrate into the smallest pores and is not adsorbed by the powders.
- **Granule density** is the density of the granules measured by liquid displacement method. Liquid may be mercury, benzene or water.

Mercury is most suitable because it neither dissolves any solid, nor enters into the pores smaller than 10μm. If the powders are nonporous, true density and granule density become equal and can be successfully measured by liquid displacement method.

- **Bulk density** is the weight of powders of unit bulk volume. It is measured using a measuring cylinder.
- **Tapped density** is the density of powders measured by tapping powders of known weight filled in a cylinder. The volume after tapping is measured for calculating the density.

Determination of Density of Powder

In general the density is determined in the laboratory by using standard pycnometer. The method is illustrated with the help of an example.

Assume, the weight of a 50 ml clean and dry pycnometer = a g

The pycnometer is filled with water and the weight of a 50 ml pycnometer + 50 ml water = b g

Thus, weight of 50 ml of water = (b – a) g

The pycnometer is dried again and then some amount of dry powders is carefully filled in.

The weight of powder + pycnometer = x g

The weight of powder inside the pycnometer = (x – a) g

Then water is poured into the pycnometer to fill its $3/4^{th}$ volume carefully, so that no powder comes out.

The pycnometer is closed and shaken, so that the entrapped air, if any, can be removed. After careful shaking for few times, the pycnometer is filled with water and weighed.

The weight of powders + water + pycnometer = y g

Then the weight of water less than 50 ml-volume occupied by powders in the pycnometer = (y – x) g

Now, the volume of (x – a) g of powders = [50 - (y – x)] ml [if, density of water is 1.0g/ml]

$$\text{Hence, density of powder} = \frac{(x - a)}{[50-(y - x)]} \text{ g/ml}$$

Example

The weight of 50 ml empty pycnometer is 38.7342 g. The density of water is 1.00 g/ml at 25 °C. An amount of 13.0455 g of powder was filled in pycnometer; total weight becomes 91.2267 g. Find out the density of the powder. Assume that the experimental temperature is 25°C.

Solution

Weight of powder + water + pycnometer = 91.2267g

Weight of powder + water = 91.2267g – 38.7342 g = 52.4925g

Weight of powder present in the pycnometer = 13.0455g

Then, weight of water present in the pycnometer = 52.4925g – 13.0455g = 39.4470g

That is the volume of water present with 13.0455g of powder = 39.4470 ml

The volume of 13.0455g of powder = 50.0 ml – 39.4470 ml = 10.553 ml

$$\text{Hence, density of powder} = \frac{13.0455\text{g}}{10.553\text{ ml}}$$

Ans. 1.236 g/ml

Computation of Weight Using Specific Gravity and Volume

In some calculations specific gravity can be used to calculate weight and volume. In such calculations, specific gravity is used as a factor and the result should contain significant figures not more than the number in the factor. The weight of a substance can be calculated if its specific gravity or density and volume are known. The formula used for this purpose is;

$$\text{Density} = \frac{\text{Mass}}{\text{Volume}}$$

$$\text{or, Mass} = \text{Density} \times \text{Volume}$$

Note: In fact, multiplication of milliliters by specific gravity does not yield grams. Using density (g/ml) in place of specific gravity produces gram. However, the equation becomes feasible by assuming that the volume of the liquid in question is equal to the volume of water. This is explained through the following example.

Example

Calculate the weight of 2500 ml of castor oil having specific gravity of 0.92.

Assuming that the weight of 1 ml of water is 1.0 g

Solution

Weight of 2500 ml of water = 2500 ×1.0 g = 2500 g

Then the weight of 2500 ml of castor oil = 2500 × 0.92 g = 2300 g (Answer)

Weight of a liquid = weight of water of same volume × specific gravity of the liquid

Computation of Volume using Specific Gravity and Weight

The volume of a liquid can be calculated if its weight and specific gravity are known. The computation is done using the following equation:

$$\text{Volume (ml)} = \frac{\text{Weight (grams)}}{\text{Specific gravity}}$$

Example

Calculate the volume of 598 g of glycerin having specific gravity of 1.25.

Solution

Assuming that 598 g of water occupy a volume of 598 ml

$$\text{The volume of 598 g of glycerin} = \frac{598 \text{ ml}}{1.25}$$

Ans. 478.4 ml

Example

Calculate the volume of 595 lb of nitric acid having specific gravity of 1.42.

Solution

1 lb = 454 g

595 lb = 454×595 g = 270130 g

The volume of 270130 g = 270130 ml

So, the volume of 270130 g of nitric acid = $\frac{270130 \text{ ml}}{1.42}$ = 190232.4 ml

$= \frac{190232.4 \text{ ml}}{1000}$

Ans. 190.2324 L

Applications of Specific Gravity in Pharmacy

- To convert the weight of an ingredient or preparation to volume or vice versa. Suppose, in a formula the amount of a liquid ingredient is given in weight and it is convenient to measure in volume or vice versa. In such cases specific gravity of the liquid is used for conversion.
- For calculation of equivalent strength of a preparation in terms of either weight or volume, specific gravity is used.
- To prepare Total Parenteral Nutrition (TPN) admixtures using automated compounder. The required amounts of components of large volume parenterals such as dextrose, amino acids, water, etc. can be mixed in correct proportion on the basis of their specific gravity. The weights of components are automatically calculated, based on the specific gravity, volume, and percentage concentration of the solutions used, such as 70% dextrose injection, in the admixture.
- Specific gravity helps to diagnose disease also. The specific gravity of urine in normal persons remains within 1.010 to 1.025 when fluid intake is normal. It indicates both the concentration of particles in the urine and degree of hydration. The specific gravity of urine increases due to – (1) excess of waste products or electrolytes in urine; for example, glucosurea (presence of glucose in urine) or proteinurea (presence of protein in urine). (2) Excessive water loss, (3) low fluid intake, or for other reasons. The specific gravity of the urine may decrease due to – (1) diabetes insipidus, (2) malfunction of kidney, (3) increased fluid intake, (4) intravenous hydration, or other factors.

Specific Volume

The term *specific volume* is usually defined as a ratio of the volume of a substance to the volume of an equal weight of another substance taken as a reference standard at the same temperature. Water is normally used as the standard.

Specific gravity is a ratio of two weights of equal volumes; while specific volume is a ratio of two volumes of equal weights. Therefore, specific gravity and specific volume are *reciprocals*; that is, if they are multiplied together, the product is 1.

Specific volume may be calculated by dividing the volume of a given mass by the volume of an equal weight of water. Thus, it indicates how much greater (or smaller) in volume of a mass of a substance in comparison to the volume of same weight of water at a definite temperature. Let us explain it with the help of an example.

$$\text{Volume of substance} = \frac{\text{Weight of the substance}}{\text{Specific gravity}}$$

$$\text{Weight of a substance} = \text{Specific gravity} \times \text{volume of substance}$$

$$\text{Specific volume} = \frac{1}{\text{Specific gravity}}$$

Example

The volume of 25 g of glycerin is 20 mL and the volume of 25 g of water is 25 mL under the same conditions. Find out the specific volume of the glycerin.

Solution

According to the definition specific volume of glycerin

$$= \frac{\text{Volume of 25 g of glycerin}}{\text{Volume of 25 g of water}}$$

$$= \frac{20 \text{ ml}}{25 \text{ ml}}$$

Ans. 0.8

Example

Calculate the specific volume of sulphuric acid which has specific gravity of 1.84.

Solution

The specific volume of sulphuric acid $= \frac{1}{1.84}$

Ans. 0.543

Example

Calculate the specific gravity of propylene glycol which has specific volume of 0.97.

Solution

The specific gravity of propylene glycol $= \frac{1}{0.97}$

Ans. 1.03

Exercise

1. A piece of metal weighs 12.7481 g and its volume is 1.62ml. Find out its density.

   Ans: 7.869g/ml

2. 300 L of Glycerol weighs 375 kg. Calculate its specific gravity.

   Ans: 1.25

3. At a particular temperature 500 ml of water weighs 498.08 g and 250 L of Isopropyl alcohol weighs 195 kg. Calculate the specific gravity of isopropyl alcohol.

   Ans: 0.783

4. The weight of 350 L of sesame oil is 369 kg. Calculate the specific gravity of the oil.

   Ans: 1.054

5. The weight of empty pycnometer is 34.8735 g, it weighs 60.3476 g when filled with water, and 59.5592 g when filled with another liquid. Find out the specific gravity.

   Ans: 969

6. The composition of a modified Ringer's solution is as follows:

Potassium chloride	0.15 g
Sodium chloride	4.3 g
Calcium chloride	0.165 g
PEG 3350	30 g
Water of injection	490 ml

The final volume of this solution would be 500 ml. Calculate the specific gravity of the solution.

Ans: 1.049

7. The volume of 125 g of a liquid is 158 ml. Calculate the specific volume of the liquid.

Ans: 1.264

8. At room temperature theobroma oil is solid and melts at 34°C. It has specific gravity of 0.86. What would be the weight of 45 ml of theobroma oil required for making suppositories?

Ans: 38.7 g

9. The composition of a gel base is as follows:

Gelatin	21.7 g
Glycerol	77.5 ml
Purified water	10.8 ml

Calculate the total weight of the formula. (Specific gravity of glycerol is 1.25)

Ans: 129.38 g

10. Composition of 40 suppositories is given below;

Glycerin	72.8 g
Sodium stearate	7.2 g
Purified water	4 ml

The specific gravity of glycerin is 1.25. Calculate the volume of glycerin required for 75 numbers of suppositories.

Ans: 109.2 ml

11. If the density of a liquid is 1.034g/ml and that of water is 0.99607 g/ml at 25°C, what would be specific gravity of the liquid?

Ans: 1.038

12. The weight of 50 ml empty pycnometer is 38.9982 g. The density of water is 1.00 g/ml at 25°C. An amount of 10.1685 g of powder was filled in pycnometer; total weight becomes 90.6087 g. Find out the density of the powder. Assume that the experimental temperature is 25°C.

Ans: 1.188g/ml

13. The weights of a piece of metal are as follows; (1) 25.0913 g in air, (2) 21.3955 g when immersed in water, and (3) 21.8912 g when immersed in oil. Calculate the specific gravity of the oil.

Ans: 0.8658

14. What would be the weight of 3.5 fl. oz. of a liquid (in grams), having a density of 1.008g/ml? (1 fl. oz. equals to 29.57ml)

Ans: 104.32g

15. What would be the cost of 1000 L of glycerin, specific gravity 1.25, bought at Rs.104.50 per kg?

Ans: Rs. 130625

16. A pycnometer weighs 27.8235 g. When filled with water, it weighs 77.6571 g and weighs 76.7628 g when filled with another liquid. Calculate the specific gravity of the liquid.

Ans: 0.982

17. The length of solid tube is 15 cm and its diameter is 4 cm. it weighs 500 g at 25°C. Find out the density of the material of construction.

Ans: 2.654g/cc

18. The dimensions of two cubes, A and B are same, but materials of construction are different. If the weight of cube A is 607.5g and that of B is 289.2g, what would be the ratio of their densities?

Ans: A: B :: 5:2.4

19. Two bodies have same weights but their volumes are 270 cubic cm and 180 cubic cm. find out the relation between their densities.

Ans: 2 : 3

20. Half of a body when immersed in water, the water level increases by 55.2ml. If the density of the material is 7.87g/cc, what would be the weight of the body?

Ans: 868.85g

21. 50g of powders were filled in a cylinder and tapped using bulk density apparatus. The volume of the powders was 38ml after tapping. Find out the bulk density of the powders.

Ans: 1.316g/ml

22. To make 1 liter of 1N solution 98g of concentrated sulphuric acid is to be diluted with water up to 1 liter. if the density of concentrated sulphuric acid is 1.84g/ml, how many milliliters of the acid are to be taken?

Ans: 53.3ml

23. Calculate the volume of 600 g of glycerin having specific gravity of 1.25.

Ans: 480ml

24. According to the manufacturing formula the preparation should contain 10%v/v of alcohol (96.5%). If the density of 96.5% alcohol is 0.7999g/ml at 20°C; what should be alcohol content in terms of %w/v?

Ans: 7.9%w/v

25. The volume of 45 g of glycerin is 36 mL and the volume of 45 g of water is 45 mL under the same conditions. Find out the specific volume of the glycerin.

Ans: 0.8

5

CALCULATION RELATED TO CAPSULE FILLING, SUPPOSITORY MOLDS, DRY POWDERS AND DOSES

Pharmaceutical compounding is the process by which therapeutically active ingredients along with other materials (excipients) are combined together to prepare a dosage form, so that the specific needs of patients are met. In practice pharmaceutical compounding is being rarely practiced by the pharmacists. They are mostly involved in dispensing activity. In place of compounding large-scale production of pharmaceutical products (pharmaceutical manufacturing) are being done to meet the needs of the general population.

This chapter shall discuss the calculations involved in

- Capsule filling,
- Making dry powders for oral and parenteral administration,
- Making suppositories and finally
- Calculating the doses.

Calculation Related to Capsule Filling

Empty capsule shells, made of gelatin, are readily available in a variety of sizes; capsules of the largest size are numbered as '000' and the smallest size as '5'.

Capsules should neither be under-filled nor over-filled, should be filled with the ingredients snugly. Various drug powders have different densities, and thus, powders of different weights can be packed into a capsule of particular size. In other words, same weight of different powders cannot be filled in capsule of same capacity or size. Before filling one should select an appropriate capsule size that can accommodate the required amount of powders (fill) and the convenience of swallowing.

Capsule size	Approx. Fill volume (ml)	Approx. weight of Powder, can be filled in
5	0.13	65 – 130 mg
4	0.21	100 – 260 mg
3	0.30	120 – 390 mg
2	0.37	200 – 520 mg
1	0.50	225 – 650 mg
0	0.68	325 – 900 mg
00	0.95	390 – 1300 mg
000	1.40	430 – 1800 mg

Many drugs given orally have relatively small doses; thus, a suitable inert diluent, such as lactose is commonly mixed with the drug to increase the bulk for filling into the capsules.

The steps used in calculating the proper capsule-fill are:

- Choose an approximate capsule size.
- Pour each drug and diluent into the capsule shell separately and record the weights of each capsule.
- Calculate the *diluent displacement weight* for each drug (illustrated in the following example).
- Calculate finally the amount of diluent required per capsule.
- Calculate the total quantities of drug and the diluent required for the lot.

Illustrative Example

Determine the total quantities of each drug and lactose required to fill 50 numbers of size 2.

Each capsule contains

Pantaprazole	40 mg
Domperidone	30 mg
Lactose	q.s.

Solution

- Say, size 2 capsule is chosen for filling.
- Each component is filled in 10 or 20 capsule of size 2 and average weights are recorded as follows (arbitrary values);

  Capsule can accommodate 450 mg of Pantaprazole

  Capsule can accommodate 337.5 mg of Domperidone

  Capsule can accommodate 236.25 mg of Lactose

- Calculation of diluent displacement weight for each drug

  Say, diluent displacement weight for Pantaprazole = x mg

  $$\text{Then, } \frac{450 \text{ mg of Pantaprazole/capsule}}{236.25 \text{ mg of lactose/capsule}} = \frac{40 \text{ mg Pantaprazole}}{x \text{ mg lactose}}$$

  $$x = \frac{236.25 \times 40}{450} \text{mg} = 21 \text{ mg}$$

  Similarly, assume that the diluent displacement weight for Domperidone = y mg

  $$\text{Then, } \frac{340 \text{ mg of Domperidone/capsule}}{236.25 \text{ mg of lactose/capsule}} = \frac{30 \text{ mg Domperidone}}{y \text{ mg lactose}}$$

  $$y = \frac{236.25 \times 30}{337.5} \text{ mg} = 21 \text{ mgs}$$

- Diluent (lactose) required per capsule

  Lactose required per capsule = 336.25 mg – (21 mg + 21 mg)

  = 336.25 mg – 42 mg

  = 294.25 mg

- Calculation of the total quantities of each drug and the diluent required for 50 capsules.

  Pantaprazole 40 mg × 50 = 2000 mg = 2 g

  Domperidone 30 mg × 50 = 1500 mg = 1.5 g

  Lactose 294.25 mg × 50 = 14712.5 mg

Ans. 14.71 g

According to the composition of the above formulation total drug content is only 70 mg per capsule. For such a small content size 4 capsules would have been sufficient. The size 4 capsule can accommodate 100 – 260 mg of powders depending on the density of the powders. Hence, if size 2 capsules are used more lactose would be required and the cost of the product would increase.

There is another method to select appropriate size of capsule. The steps involved are;

- Select the minimum size of capsule.
- Fill the capsule with the drugs by hand.
- Fill the capsule with diluent just sufficient to fill the capsule.
- The content of the filled capsule is removed and weighed
- Then the amount of diluent required is calculated by subtracting the content of diluent – total drug content.

This is illustrated with the help of following example:

Illustrative Example

Determine the quantity of lactose required per capsule.

Each capsule contains

Pantaprazole	40 mg
Domperidone	30 mg
Lactose	q.s.

Solution

- Total amount of drug to be filled in each capsule is 70 mg. To accommodate 70 mg of drugs size 5 or size 4 capsules would be sufficient.
- Assume that size 5 capsule can contain 105mg of lactose. Size 5 capsule can contain 65–130 mg of powders.
- Thus, 105–70 = 35 mg of lactose is required for snug fill of capsule.

Ans. Thus, 35 mg of lactose would be sufficient per capsule

But, this method cannot provide correct answer. The correct procedure is:

- Determine the tapped densities of the drug or of the mixture of drug and of proposed diluent (lactose) separately.

- Calculate the volume of the required amount of drug or of the mixture of drugs on the basis of tapped density (V) and fill volume of the capsule (V_1).
- Compare the fill volume of the selected capsule and the volume of required amount of drug or drugs; that is whether $V > V_1$ or $V < V_1$.
- Analyze the volume difference; if (1) $V > V_1$, capsule of greater fill-volume to be selected, (2) $V < V_1$, diluent is required.
- Calculate $V - V_1$ or $V_1 - V$, as the case may be.
- Determine the tapped density of the proposed diluent (lactose) and calculate the amount of diluent equivalent to $V - V_1$ or $V_1 - V$.

Illustrative Example

Each capsule should contain 50mg of a drug having tapped density of 0.6551g/ml, capsule size 5 having fill-volume of 0.13 ml is selected. Say whether lactose is to be added or not. If yes, the density of lactose available is 0.8976g/ml; find out the amount of lactose required per capsule.

Solution

Given that the quantity of drug to be filled/capsule = 50mg = 0.050g

The tapped density of drug = 0.6551g/ml

The tapped density of lactose = 0.8976g/ml

The fill-volume of capsule size 5 = 0.13ml (V_1)

The volume of 50mg of drug $= \frac{0.050}{0.6651} = 0.075$ml (V);

1. Minimum size of the capsule is 5 and has the fill volume of 0.13ml which much larger than the volume of drug powder, 0.075ml.

   Ans. Hence, addition of lactose is necessary

2. $V_1 - V = 0.13 - 0.075 = 0.055$ml

   Tapped density of lactose = 0.8976g/ml

   Volume of lactose equivalent to 0.055ml = 0.055ml × 0.8976g/ml

   = 0.04937 g per capsule.

   Ans. Hence, per capsule 49.37mg of lactose would be required

Example

A batch of 1.0 lac of Ampicillin Trihydrate 268 mg equivalent to 250 mg of Ampicillin capsule is to be filled in size 2 capsules. The fill volume of size 2 capsules is 0.37 ml and the tapped density of Ampicillin Trihydrate powder is 0.745g/ml. The tapped density of starch is 0.75 g/ml. Calculate the amount of starch to be mixed with the drug for lot.

Solution

Given that the tapped density of Ampicillin Trihydrate powder = 0.745g/ml

Tapped density of starch = 0.70g/ml

Batch size = 1.0 lac

Fill volume of the capsule = 0.37 ml

According to the tapped density, the volume of 268 mg

$$= \frac{1\ \text{ml} \times 0.268\text{g}}{0.745\text{g}} = 0.359 \text{ ml or } 0.36 \text{ ml}$$

The difference between fill volume and volume of drug

$$= 0.37 - 0.36 \text{ ml} = 0.01 \text{ ml}$$

Volume to be occupied by starch in each capsule = 0.01 ml

Amount of starch equivalent to 0.01 ml

$$= 0.01\text{ml} \times 0.70\text{g/ml} = 0.007 \text{ g per capsule}$$

Amount of starch required for 1.0 lakh capsules

$$= 0.007\text{g} \times 100000 = 700 \text{ g (Answer)}$$

Example

Each capsule contains 500mg of a drug, 5 mg of lactose and 2 mg of talcum. The fill volume of capsule is 0.50 ml. Tapped density of lactose is 0.695g/ml and that of talcum is 0.60g/ml. Find out the tapped density of the drug.

Solution

Given that the tapped density of lactose = 0.695 g/ml

The tapped density of talcum = 0.60 g/ml

Fill volume of capsule = 0.50 ml

Each capsule contains

Drug 500 mg

Lactose 5 mg

Talcum 2mg

The volume of 5mg or 0.005g of lactose = $\frac{1\text{ml} \times 0.005\text{g}}{0.695\text{g}}$ = 0.0072ml

The volume of 2mg or 0.002g of talcum = $\frac{1\text{ml} \times 0.002\text{g}}{0.6\text{g}}$ = 0.0033ml

The volume occupied by 500mg of drug

$$= 0.50\text{ml} - (0.0072 + 0.0033)\text{ ml} = 0.4895\text{ml}$$

Thus, 0.4895ml is the volume of 0.500g of the drug

The density of the drug = weight of unit volume of drug

$$= \frac{0.5\text{g}}{0.4895\text{ml}} = 1.021\text{g/ml (Answer)}$$

Calibration of Suppository Molds

Suppository is a solid dosage form used for insertion into body cavity. After it is inserted it softens, melts, or dissolves and releases the active ingredient (drug) to the surrounding tissues. There are number of suppository bases that can be used as vehicle for preparing suppository. Cocoa butter (also called theobroma oil) is commonly used as vehicle. Cocoa butter is solid at room temperature but melts at body temperatures.

Suppositories can be prepared by molding process. In this process calibration of mold must be done.

Calibration of suppository mold for preparing suppositories:

- Pour the melted base into all the cells of the suppository mold, allow to cool and harden; then remove the suppositories and weigh.
- Determine the total and average weights of the suppositories.
- Divide the total weight and average weight of the suppositories by the density of the base;
- Determine the volume of the suppository mold and the average volume of each cell.

Calculation and Preparation of Suppositories

- Calculate and weigh the active ingredient for the preparation of a single suppository.
- Mix the active ingredient with a portion of melted base for a single suppository, the amount of the base would be insufficient to fill one cell of the mold.
- Pour the mixture of drug and base into a cell, add additional melted base to completely fill the cell.
- When the suppository is hardened, remove it from the mold and weigh.
- Subtract the amount of the drug from the weight of the molded suppository and calculate the weight of the base present.
- By multiplying the amounts of the drug and base required to prepare for a single suppository with the required number of suppositories total amounts required may then be calculated.

The volume of base required may also be calculated, if desired, by the use of its known density.

Example

Calculate the amounts of drug and cocoa butter (density is 0.86g/ml) required to prepare 10 numbers of suppositories for rectal administration. Each suppository contains 375 mg of the drug. Assume that the average weight of suppositories would be about 2 g.

Solution

The amount of cocoa butter to be required

$= 2\text{ g} - 0.375\text{ g (drug)} = 1.625\text{ g (cocoa butter)}$

The volume of 1.65 g of cocoa butter

$= 1.625\text{ g} \div 0.86\text{ g/mL (density of cocoa butter)}$

$= 1.889\text{ mL}$

Place the mixture of 350 mg of drug and 1 mL of melted cocoa butter in a cell, and add sufficient amount of melted cocoa butter to fill the cell completely.

Say the weight of the suppository = 1.98 g.

Then the amount of the cocoa butter in one suppository

= 1.98 g – 0.375 g = 1.605 g

The amount of drug required for 10 suppositories

= 0.375 × 10 = 3.75 g

The amount of cocoa butter required for 10 suppositories

Ans. 1.605 g × 10 = 16.05 g

Calculation Related to Dry Powders for Oral Use

Dry powders are prepared and packaged in self-contained bottles of adequate size. By adding required volume of vehicle, the suspension is constituted at the time of dispensing. The powder contains the drug and other pharmaceutical ingredients such as suspending agents, stabilizers, colorants, sweeteners, flavoring agents, etc.

The instructions for constitution are provided in the label. Usually purified water is used to prepare oral suspension.

Depending on the formulation and certain other factors, the final preparation may be a clear solution; for example, dispersible granules or tablets. The final volume of product is the sum of the volume of solvent added and the volume occupied by the dissolved or suspended powder mixture. These products generally are intended for infants, children, and for those patients who cannot swallow any tablet or capsule.

For children and adults, it is an oral solution or suspension and the usual child dose of the drug is contained in a teaspoonful amount (5ml), while adult dose can be provided in a tablespoonful amount; for infants, pediatric drops are provided which is generally preconstituted preparation.

Example

The label for a dry powder of a drug for oral suspension directs to add 45 mL of purified water to prepare 60 mL of suspension. If the bottle contains 3.0 g of the drug, how many milligrams of the drug would be contained in each teaspoonful dose of the constituted suspension?

Solution

It is considered that the single dose of the drug is present in 5 ml (1 teaspoonful) and final volume of the product is 60 ml.

Then 60 ml contains $\frac{60}{5} = 12$ doses.

Hence, 12 doses is equivalent to 3.0 g = 3000 mg of the drug

or, $$\frac{12\text{ doses}}{1\text{ dose}} = \frac{3000\text{ mg of the drug}}{x\text{ mg of the drug}}$$

$$x = \frac{3000\text{mg} \times 1\text{ dose}}{12\text{doses}}$$

Ans. 250 mg

Example

A bottle of 50 ml suspension contains 1.25 g of Ampicillin and the 125 mg of Ampicillin is the single dose. The patient is advised to take 1teaspoonful thrice a day. Calculate in how many days the bottle would finish.

Solution

1 teaspoonful thrice daily = 5 ml of the suspension × 3 = 125 mg of Ampicillin × 3 = 375 mg

Hence, 375 mg of Ampicillin is administered in a day

If it is consumed in x days

Then, $$\frac{1250\text{ mg}}{375\text{ mg}} = \frac{x\text{ days}}{1\text{ day}}$$

$$x = \frac{1250\text{ mg} \times 1\text{ day}}{375\text{ mg}}$$

Ans. 3.3 days

Example

A 60 ml suspension contains 1.5 g of Ampicillin; if a physician advises to administer Ampicillin 100 mg/5 mL instead of 125 mg/5 mL, what should be final volume of the suspension?

Solution

The final volume of the suspension is 60 ml and each 5ml contain 125 mg of drug.

Let, the final volume of suspension would be x ml if the dose is 100 mg/5ml

Now, $$\frac{125\text{ mg}}{100\text{ mg}} = \frac{x\text{ ml}}{60\text{ ml}}$$

$$x = \frac{125\text{ mg} \times 60\text{ ml}}{100\text{ mg}} = 75\text{ ml}$$

Ans. Thus, the final volume of the suspension would be 75 ml

Calculation Related to Dry Powders for Parenteral Use

The USP/NF (United States Pharmacopeia/National Formulary) provides the steps necessary for safe preparation, storage, stability, and use of compounded sterile preparations. It also defines the levels of risk for the compounding of single-dose and multiple-dose sterile preparations.

Some preparations (mostly antibiotics) intended for parenteral administration are not stable in liquid form; hence, prepared and supplied as dry powder in vials. These are subsequently constituted with sterile water for injection, or other specified solvent immediately before administration. Generally, these preparations are small-volume parenterals intended for injection or administered as additives to large-volume parenterals.

Injectable products may contain specified ingredients other than active constituent to increase the stability and therapeutic effectiveness of the drug. No colorant, flavoring agent, or sweetener is added. Thus, the bulk volume of the dry contents of a vial is mainly or entirely of the drug.

When the amount of the dry drug powder is small the volume of solvent used will be estimated as the final volume of the solution. For example, 1000 units of an antibiotic in dry form are to be dissolved and injected; if the amount of powder does not contribute significantly to the final volume, addition of 5 mL of solvent will produce a solution of 200 units/ml.

On the other hand, bulky dry powder can increase the final volume of the constituted solution and the increase in volume produced by the drug must be considered in calculating the amount of solvent to be used to prepare the solution of a desired concentration. For example, to prepare penicillin G potassium solution of 500 000 units/ml, 20,000,000 units of a sterile powder of penicillin G potassium should be present in 40 ml of solution. Addition of 32 mL of sterile water for injection produces the final volume of 40 mL. Thus, 8 mL of the final volume is accounted for the dry powder.

Example

A vial contains 128.5 mg of potassium penicillin G having potency of 1556.5 units/mg. How many milliliters of sterile water for injection should be added to the dry powder for preparing a solution of 20,000 units/mL?

Solution

1 mg contains 1556.5 units of potassium penicillin G

128.5 mg contains 128.5 × 1556.5 = 200010.25 units of potassium penicillin G

Let us assume that x ml of sterile water for injection should be added to prepare a solution containing 20000 units of potassium penicillin G per ml

Then,

$$\frac{20{,}000 \text{ units}}{200\ 010.25 \text{ units}} = \frac{1 \text{ ml}}{x \text{ ml}}$$

Ans. x = 10.00 ml (approximately)

Example

A vial contains 1.0 g of a sterile powder drug which is to be reconstituted before administration so that 200mg of drug/ml is produced. Calculate the final volume of preparation.

Solution

Given that, total amount of drug powder = 1.0g

Final concentration of the reconstituted preparation = 200 mg/ml = 0.2g/ml, and

Say, final volume = x ml

Then, $$\frac{0.2\text{g}}{1.0\text{g}} = \frac{1 \text{ ml}}{x \text{ ml}}$$

$$x = \frac{1 \times 1}{0.2}$$

Ans. 5 ml

Calculation Related to Dose

The quantitative amount of a drug is either administered to a patient or is taken by a patient for an expected therapeutic effect is called *dose*. The dose taken at one time is called *single dose;* for example, 250 mg of Ciprofloxacin or 4 mg of Salbutamol sulphate. The total amount taken daily is called daily dose; for example, 250 mg of Ciprofloxacin 4 times daily, i.e., 4×250mg =1 g per day and the total amount of a drug taken during the course of therapy is called a *total dose;* 4×250 mg of Ciprofloxacin ×5 days, i.e. 5 g. Depending on the characteristics of the drug and extent of the illness, daily dose may be taken in *divided doses*; that is, two or more times in a day. The schedule of dosing (e.g., *three times per day for 5 days*) is called the *dosage regimen*.

One of the primary responsibilities of the pharmacist is to check doses specified in the prescriptions based on the knowledge of the usual dose ranges and dosage regimens of the drugs prescribed.

$$\text{Number of doses} = \frac{\text{Total amount of drug to be administered}}{\text{Amount of drug per dose(Dose size)}}$$

The dose of a drug may be small or relatively large. The dose of a drug depends on:

- its biochemical and pharmacologic activity,
- its physical and chemical properties,
- the dosage form used,
- the route of administration,
- Patient factors.

Usually the dose of a drug may be calculated on the basis of:

- The age of patient,
- Body weight,
- Body surface area,
- Physiological conditions such as liver and kidney function, drug metabolism and elimination, and
- The severity of the illness being treated.

Dose

The amount of a drug that usually produces the desired therapeutic effect on an adult patient is called *adult dose* of a drug. Similarly the *pediatric dose* is the amount of a drug that usually produces the desired therapeutic effect on the infant or child patient. The term *infant* is defined differently. Usually, young child having age within 1 month to 12 months is called infant. Sometimes, a newborn being few hours old is considered as an infant. The upper age limit for an infant is extended up to 2 years even. Generally a newborn baby up to first 28 days is called neonate who is also an infant. The child refers to human being below 18years old.

The doses are called 'usual' when they are administered to the patients who have normal physiologic conditions such as renal function, drug metabolic activity, etc. except the disease being treated.

The dose of a drug is calculated on the basis of ability of a patient to metabolize and eliminate drugs from the body, liver or renal function. If such physiologic functions are not normal, dose may be reduced. This is called *pharmacokinetic dosing*. Usually in the package label or through inserts the information about the use and dose of the drug is provided. There are various references through which necessary information about a drug is available. The dose response of individuals varies and may require dosage adjustment in a given patient; for example, during treatment of cancer patient drug dosing is highly specialized and individualized. Sometimes combinations of drugs are used and the dose of each drug is fixed according to the patient's response. Many anticancer drugs are administered *cyclically*, usually for 21 to 28 days. A rest period between the dosing cycles is given for recovery from the toxic effects of the drugs. Anticancer drugs are most commonly dosed on the basis of the patient's body surface area.

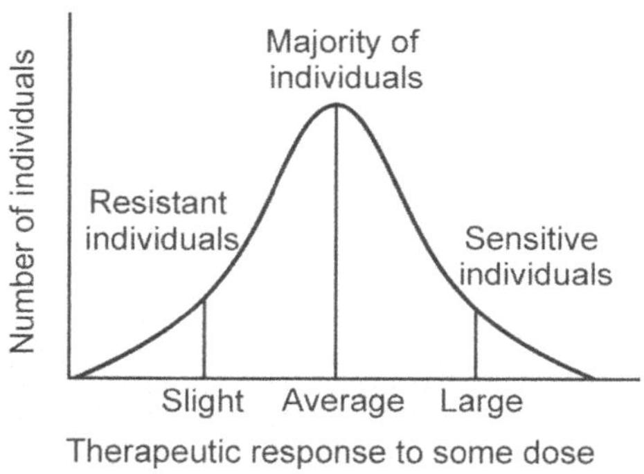

Figure 5.1 Therapeutic effect of drug in a sample population.

There are some terms commonly used and closely related to dose calculation. These are defined below.

- The amount of a drug that produces the desired intensity of effect in 50% of the individuals tested is called ***median effective dose***.
- The amount of a drug that produces toxic effects in 50% of the individuals tested is called ***median toxic dose***.
- The minimum concentration of a drug in the patient's blood that produces the desired therapeutic effects in a patient is called the ***minimum effective concentration*** (MEC).
- The minimum concentration of a drug in the patient's blood that produces dose-related toxic effects is called ***minimum toxic concentration*** (MTC).

The patients may be categorized into three classes – resistant, normal and sensitive to a particular drug. Accordingly the therapeutic effect of that drug can be observed as shown in Figure 5.1

Optimal therapeutic effect of a drug is achieved when its concentration remain within the therapeutic window (in between MTC and MEC). The serum concentration of a hypothetical drug is shown in Figure 5.2. The serum concentration of the drug reaches the MEC 2 hours after its administration, reaches a peak concentration in 4 hours, and falls below the MEC in 10 hours. This dose is referred to as the *priming* or *loading dose*. To maintain the serum concentration above the MEC for a longer period, a second dose or a *maintenance* dose of the same size would be required after 8 hours. When rapid effect is desired, the loading dose may be administered as an injection and the subsequent maintenance doses may be administered in other forms, such as tablets or capsules.

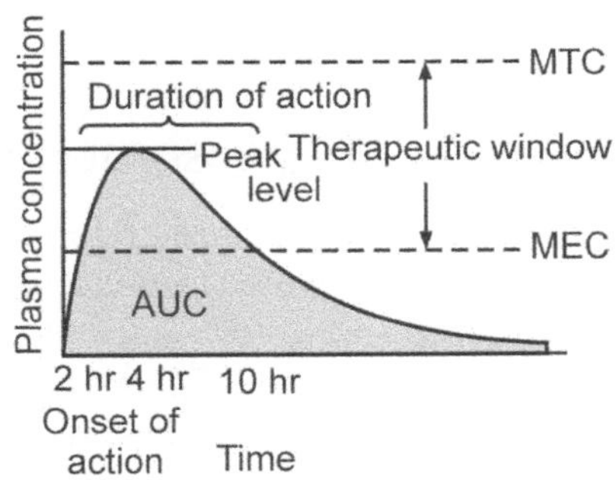

Figure 5.2 Plasma concentration vs. Time curve.

In some cases *low-dose therapy* or *high-dose therapy* is prescribed for a particular patient. For certain drugs different doses are required depending on whether the use is for *monotherapy* (the primary drug treatment), or *adjunctive therapy* (additional to or supportive) of a different primary treatment.

To protect the patient from contacting a specific disease certain biologic or immunologic products, such as vaccines, may be administered in *prophylactic doses*. To fight against a disease after exposure or contraction other products, such as antitoxins, are administered in *therapeutic doses*.

When the products are prepared on a large scale within the pharmaceutical manufacturing industry, these are called *prefabricated* products and there is no provision for compounding in the pharmacy. When the product is prepared by careful weighing, measuring, and mixing of individual ingredients on a smaller scale, in community and hospital pharmacies are called *compounding*. Pharmaceutical products may be prepared to contain one or more therapeutic agents. Products containing more than one therapeutic agent are termed *combination products*.

Whether a pharmaceutical product is prepared on a large or small scale or is compounded individually in the pharmacy, the dose of a drug must be calculated by the pharmacist to ensure proper treatment and welfare of the patient.

Routes of Drug/Dose/Dosage Form Administration

There are variety of dosage forms and routes of administration. A dosage form contains *pharmaceutical ingredients,* in addition to the drug. These ingredients such as solvents, vehicles, preservatives, stabilizers, solubilizers, binders, fillers, disintegrants, flavors, colors, and others to provide the physical features, stability requirements, and aesthetic characteristics desired for optimal therapeutic effects.

Measurement of Dose

Various measuring devices such as calibrated cups for oral liquids and syringes and intravenous sets for parenteral medication are used to measure the dose. Liquid dosage form is usually measured in terms of teaspoonful (5 ml) and tablespoonful (15 ml) at homes. Although oral dispensers are available for administering calibrated quantities of liquid medication to children. For calculating doses, equivalent measures are necessary.

Teaspoon and Tablespoon

In fact, one teaspoonful measures 5 mL and one tablespoonful measures 15 mL. In reality the capacities of household teaspoons may vary from

3 to 7 mL and those of tablespoons may vary from 15 to 22 mL. Depending on the viscosity and surface tension of a given liquid, as well as the technique of measuring the liquid by a person, the actual volume held by a household spoon the volume can again vary.

To avoid such variation and to ensure uniform measurement, an American Standard Teaspoon has been established by the American National Standards Institute which contains 4.93 ± 0.24 mL. The *United States Pharmacopeia* has also recognized the same. Preparations intended for administration by teaspoon are being formulated on the basis of 5 mL unit dose. However any dropper, syringe, medicine cup, special spoon, or other device used to administer liquids should deliver 5 mL. Most of the pharmaceutical manufacturers provide cup marked at 5-mL and 15 mL along with the formulation.

Due to habit and tradition, the f□ -symbol for fluidram is still being written by some physicians in the prescriptions to indicate teaspoonful dose. While dispensing, the pharmacist should interpret this symbol as a teaspoonful. Doses less than a teaspoonful (usually for children) are often indicated on the labeling as fractions of a teaspoonful, such as 1⁄4 or 1⁄2 of a teaspoonful. Special medicinal spoons for these amounts are available.

The Drop as a Unit of Measure

Sometimes, the drop is used as a measure for small volumes of liquid medications. A drop does not represent a definite quantity. Depending on the viscosity and surface tension of the liquid and orifice through which it falls, the size and volume of drops vary greatly. To standardize the drop as a unit of volume, the *United States Pharmacopeia* defines the official medicine dropper. The delivery end should have a round opening with an external diameter of about 3 mm. When held vertically, the dropper should deliver water in drops and the weight of each drop must be 50 ± 5 mg.

Accordingly, the official dropper is calibrated to deliver approximately 20 drops of water per milliliter (1 mL of water = 1gram or 1000 mg ÷ 50 mg = 20 drops).

Since the surface and flow characteristics of few medicinal liquids may differ from that of water, the size of drops varies from one liquid to another. Until the volume of the drop represents 0.05 ml of the liquid the drop should not be used as a measure for a specific liquid medication. Thus, calibration of the dispensing dropper is highly necessary before use. Most manufacturers provide a specially calibrated dropper along with their prepackaged medications for measuring dosage by the patients. A dropper may be calibrated by counting the number of drops of a liquid when they fall into a graduated cylinder until a measurable volume is obtained. The number of drops per mL is then calculated and established.

Example

If 40 drops of a liquid medication measure 2.5mL, how many drops per milliliter did the dropper deliver?

Solution

Given that, 40 drops constitute 2.5 ml

That is, 2.5ml constitute 40 drops

1 ml constitutes $\frac{40}{2.5}$

Ans. 16 drops

Example

Intended dose is 0.05ml. The dropper used delivers 40 drops that make 2.5 ml. Calculate the percentage error, if one drop is administered.

Solution

Given that, 40 drops constitute 2.5 ml

Correct dose is 0.05ml

1 drop constitutes $\frac{2.5\text{ml}}{40} = 0.0625\text{ml}$

The dropper delivers excess dose, which is 0.0625ml – 0.05ml = 0.0125ml

The error in delivery = $\frac{0.0125 \times 100}{0.05}$

Ans. 25%v/v

Low-Dose and High-Dose Therapies

The low-dose or high-dose therapy refers to administration of doses smaller or higher than the normal dose of a drug. The variation in a dose is done on the basis of:

- Patient's age,

- Weight,
- Renal function,
- Other physiologic parameter, or
- Therapeutic requirement.

The usual dose of aspirin is 325 mg. To lower the risk of heart attack and clot-related stroke 81mg of aspirin is administered. This is a common example of low-dose therapy. Similarly, in case of postmenopausal hormone therapy, the dose administered is 50% of the usual dose.

High-dose therapy is usually found in case of chemotherapeutic treatment of cancer, to kill tumor cells. Other example is the use of high-dose progestin during the treatment of endometriosis. During high-dose therapy the patient must be kept under strict supervision for consequent drug overdose. Such circumstance may occur in case of multiple medications also; where common medicines in total may exceed a safe level. The drug acetaminophen, which is a component of a great number of products, is a common example.

General Methods of Dose Calculation

A pharmacist often needs to calculate the size of a dose, the number of doses, or the total quantity of medication to dispense. For these calculations the following equation is useful. In using the equation, the units of weight or volume must be the same for the total quantity and size of the dose.

$$\text{Number of doses} = \frac{\text{Total Quantity}}{\text{Size of Dose}}$$

Example

If the total quantity of the drug to be taken is 9 g and the dose size of the drug for an adult is 300 mg. How many doses are to be administered?

Solution

Total quantity of drug to be taken = 9g = 9000 mg

$$\text{Number of doses} = \frac{\text{Total Quantity}}{\text{Size of Dose}} = \frac{9000}{300} = 30$$

Ans. Hence, 30 doses of the drug are to be administered

Dose Calculation

There are various rules for conversion of adult dose to child dose. The rules are given below:

Young's Rule: Child dose = $\frac{\text{Age in year}}{\text{Age + 12}}$ × Adult dose

Fried's Rule: Child dose = $\frac{\text{Age in month} \times \text{Adult dose}}{150}$

Drilling's Rule: Child dose = $\frac{\text{Age in year} \times \text{Adult dose}}{12}$

Clark's Rule: Child dose = $\frac{\text{Weight in lbs} \times \text{Adult dose}}{150}$

Child dose = $\frac{\text{Body surface area of child} \times \text{Adult dose}}{\text{Body surface area of adult}}$

Child dose = $\frac{\text{Body surface area of child} \times \text{Adult dose}}{173M^2}$

Example

The adult dose of a drug is 500mg thrice a day. What would be the daily dose for a child of 8 years old?

Solution

According to the Drilling's Formula the child dose

$$= \frac{\text{Age in year} \times \text{Adult dose}}{12}$$

Given that the adult dose of the drug = 500 mg

The age of the child = 8 years

Then the dose for a child = $\frac{\text{Age in year} \times \text{Adult dose}}{12}$

$$= \frac{8 \times 500 \text{ mg}}{12}$$

= 333.33mg.

Ans. Hence, the daily dose for the child would be 333.33 mg thrice daily

Example

A bottle contains 10 ml of an eye-drop. Each drop constitutes 0.05 ml and two drops four times a day are to be instilled. In how many days 10 ml would be exhausted?

Solution

Total volume of the eye-drop = 10 ml

1 drop = 0.05 ml

Thus, $10\text{ml} = \frac{1 \times 10}{0.05}$ drops = 200 drops

2×4 = 8 drops are consumed in 1 day

200 drops would be consumed $\frac{1 \times 200}{8}$ = 25 days.

Ans. The bottle would be exhausted in 25 days

Example

If the dose of a drug is 250 mg, how many doses shall be contained in 10 g?

Solution

Total quantity of drug = 10g = 10000mg

Size of the dose = 250mg

Then, the number of doses = $\frac{\text{Total quantity}}{\text{Size of dose}}$

$= \frac{10000\text{mg}}{250\text{mg}}$

Ans. 40

Example

If 1 tablespoon measuring 15ml has been used to administer a liquid preparation; calculate the approximate number of doses present in 1.2 pint of the medicine? (1 pint = 473 ml)

Solution

The measure of 1 tablespoon = 15 ml

1 pint = 473ml

1.2 pint = 1.2 × 473ml = 567.6ml (total quantity)

$$\text{Number of doses} = \frac{\text{Total quantity}}{\text{Size of dose}}$$

$$= \frac{567.6\text{ml}}{15\text{ml}}$$

Ans. 37.84

Example

If the dose of a drug is 500 μg, how much drug would be there in 10 doses?

Solution

Size of the dose = 500 μg

Number of doses = 10

$$\text{Number of doses} = \frac{\text{Total quantity}}{\text{Size of dose}}$$

Then, total quantity of drug = size of the dose × number of doses

= 500μg × 10 = 5000μg/1000

Ans. 5 mg

Example

The adult dose of a drug is 25mg. If the age of an infant is 8months; how many milligrams of drug should be given?

Solution

Given that, the adult dose = 25 mg

The age of the infant = 8 months

According to the Fried rule, the infant's dose

$$= \frac{\text{Age in month} \times \text{Adult dose}}{150}$$

$$= \frac{8 \times 25\text{ mg}}{150}$$

Ans. 1.33 mg

Example

If a child weighs 15 lbs and the child dose is 2.5mg, what would be the adult dose according to the Clark's formula?

Solution

Given that, the weight of a child = 15 lbs

The child dose of the drug = 2.5mg

According to the Clark's formula Child's dose

$$= \frac{\text{Weight in lbs} \times \text{Adult dose}}{150}$$

$$2.5\text{mg} = \frac{15 \times \text{adult dose}}{150}$$

$$\text{Adult dose} = \frac{2.5\text{mg} \times 150}{15}$$

Ans. 25 mg

Example

The child dose of a drug is 2mg and the age of the child 5years. Calculate the adult dose using Young's formula and Drilling's formula.

Solution

Given that, the age of child = 5 years

Child dose of the drug = 2 mg

According to Young's formula, child dose

$$= \frac{\text{Age in year}}{\text{Age} + 12} \times \text{Adult dose}$$

$$2\text{ mg} = \frac{5}{5+12} \times \text{Adult dose}$$

$$= 0.294 \times \text{Adult dose}$$

$$\text{So, adult dose} = \frac{2\text{ mg}}{0.294} = 6.80\text{mg (Answer)}$$

According to Drilling's formula, Child dose

$$= \frac{\text{Age in year} \times \text{Adult dose}}{12}$$

$$2 \text{ mg} = \frac{5 \times \text{Adult dose}}{12}$$

$$\text{The adult dose} = \frac{2 \text{ mg} \times 12}{5} = 4.8 \text{ mg (Answer)}$$

Example

The body surface area of a child is 1.7 sq m and adult dose of a drug is 200mg. Calculate the child's dose.

Solution

Given that, body surface area of a child = 1.7 sq m

Adult dose = 200mg

$$\text{Child dose} = \frac{\text{Body surface area of child} \times \text{Adult dose}}{173\text{M}^2}$$

$$= \frac{1.7 \text{ sqm} \times 200\text{mg}}{173 \text{ sqm}}$$

Ans. 1.965 mg

Example

The surface area of a child is 1.55 sq m and adult dose of a drug is 200 mg. If the child dose is 2 mg; calculate the body surface area of the adult.

Solution

Given that, the body surface area of the child = 1.55 sq m

Adult dose = 200 mg

Child dose = 2 mg

$$\text{Child dose} = \frac{\text{Body surface area of child} \times \text{Adult dose}}{\text{Body surface area of adult}}$$

$$\text{or, } 2\text{mg} = \frac{1.55 \text{ sqm} \times 200 \text{ mg}}{\text{Body surface area of adult}}$$

$$\text{Body surface area of adult} = \frac{1.55 \text{ sqqm} \times 200 \text{ mg}}{2 \text{ mg}}$$

Ans. 155 sq m

Exercise

1. Each tablet contains 150 μg of drug. How many tablets may be prepared from 0.3 g of the drug?

Ans: 2000 tablets

2. A dropper that can deliver 4 drops per ml is used to deliver a solution containing 50 mg of drug per 5ml; if 10 drops are delivered how many milligrams of the drug would be administered?

Ans: 25 mg

3. A solution contains 200 mg of drug per 5 ml. If 250 mg of the drug is to be administered, how many milliliters of the solution are to be administered?

Ans: 6.25 ml

4. How many drops are to be administered in each dose of a liquid medicine if 5 mL contained 15 doses; if the dispensing dropper delivers 3 drops/mL.

Ans: 1 drop

5. How many milliliters of a suspension would be required for a patient who needs to take one teaspoonful dose three times a day for 5 days?

Ans: 75 ml

6. If 0.075mg of a drug substance is required in preparing 15 capsules, what would be the drug content (in micrograms) in each capsule?

Ans: 5 mcg

7. Each tablet contains spironolactone 50 mg and hydrochlorothiazide 50 mg. How many such tablets would be required to prepare 100ml of suspension containing formula spironolactone 5 mg/ml and hydrochlorothiazide 5 mg/ml?

Ans: 10 tablets

8. Each 1g suppository contains Progesterone 20mg and silica gel 20 mg. Calculate the amount of suppository base required to prepare 150 suppositories.

Ans: 144 g

9. If 1 tablespoon measuring 15ml has been used to administer a liquid preparation, calculate approximate number of doses present in 0.7 pint of the medicine? (1 pint = 473ml)

Ans: 22.07 doses

10. A bottle contains 5 ml of an eye-drop. Each drop constitutes 0.05 ml and two drops three times a day are to be instilled. In how many days 5 ml would be exhausted?

Ans: 16.7 days

11. If the dose of a drug is 200 μg, how many milligrams of drug would be there in 15 doses?

Ans: 3 mg

12. A bottle contains 50 ml of syrup; if 3 teaspoonful of the syrup is administered each day for 10 days how many bottles are to be procured?

Ans: 3 bottles

13. The adult dose of a drug is 500 mg thrice a day. What would be the daily dose for a child of 9 years old?

Ans: 375 mg

14. If 1 tablespoon of a suspension has been administered in a day, calculate approximate number of doses present in 60ml of the suspension?

Ans: 4 days

15. Daily adult dose of a drug is 650 mg of paracetamol. Calculate the dose for a child weighing 25 pounds. Use the Clark's formula.

Ans: 108.33 mg

16. If 30 drops of a liquid medication measure 1.5 mL; how many drops per milliliter should be delivered by the dropper?

Ans: 2 drops/ml

17. Daily adult dose of a drug is 1000 mg. How many milligrams of the drug should be administered to an infant of 9 months? (Use the Fried's rule)

Ans: 60 mg

18. If the total quantity of the drug to be taken is 5 g and the dose size of the drug for an adult is 500 mg. How many doses are to be administered?

Ans: 10 doses

19. The label for a dry powder of a drug for oral suspension directs to add 40 mL of purified water to prepare 50 mL of a suspension. If the bottle contains 2.5 g of the drug, how many milligrams of the drug would be contained in each teaspoonful dose of the constituted suspension?

Ans: 250 mg

20. Each capsule should contain 75 mg of a drug having tapped density of 0.7002 g/ml, capsule size 5 having fill-volume of 0.13ml is selected. Say whether lactose is to be added or not. If yes, find out the amount of lactose required per capsule. The tapped density of lactose available is 0.8156g/ml.

Ans: Yes, 18.76 mg of lactose/capsule

21. Each capsule should contain 250 mg of a drug having tapped density of 0.685g/ml, capsule size 2 having fill-volume of 0.37 ml is selected. Find out the amount of lactose required for 1.0 lac capsules. The tapped density of lactose available is 0.8156 g/ml.

Ans: 490 g

22. Each capsule should contain 267.5 mg of a drug having tapped density of 0.7505g/ml; determine the appropriate capsule size and the amount of dry starch required per capsule. The tapped density of starch is 0.568g/ml.

Ans: Size 2 capsule & 7.95 mg/capsule

23. A vial contains 50 mg of a drug having potency of 956.5 units/mg; how many milliliters of sterile water for injection should be added to the dry powder to prepare a solution of 1000 units/mL?

Ans: 47.825 ml

24. Calculate the amounts of drug and cocoa butter (density is 0.85g/ml) required to prepare 20 numbers of suppositories for rectal administration having average weight of about 1.5 g. Each suppository contains 350 mg of the drug.

Ans: 23 g of cocoa butter and 7.0 g of drug

25. To prepare 150mg of a drug in 5 ml a tablet containing 500mg of the drug is dissolved in sufficient water. In how many milliliters of water the tablet should be dissolved?

Ans: 100 ml

6

CALCULATION INVOLVING ISOTONIC BUFFER SOLUTIONS

When two solutions of different concentrations are separated by a semipermeable membrane, the solvent from the dilute solution passes through the membrane into the concentrated one. This process continues till the concentrations of the two solutions become equal and the phenomenon is called *osmosis*. The driving force for this movement of solvent is the *osmotic pressure;* it varies with the nature and concentration of the solute.

If the solute is a nonelectrolyte, its solution contains only molecules. If the solute is an electrolyte, its solution contains ions (more number of species) and molecules depending on the degree of dissociation. Since, the osmotic pressure depends on (1) the concentration of the solute (nonelectrolyte) and (2) its degree of dissociation in case of ionizable solute; solution of electrolyte produces greater numbers of particles in solution and concentration gradient is higher; hence, produces greater osmotic pressure than *un*dissociated or non-ionizable solutes.

Since osmotic pressure of a solution depends on the amount of solutes in a solution, it is one of the *colligative properties* of solutions. Other colligative properties are vapour pressure, boiling point, and freezing point. As the colligative properties depend on the number of particles present in solution, these properties are interrelated. If any one of these properties is changed, a corresponding change in the others will also take place.

Two solutions having the same osmotic pressure are called *isosmotic.* For better patient comfort, efficacy, and safety, the solutions intended to be infused into the body are designed to have the same osmotic pressure with the body fluid. A solution having the same osmotic pressure as a *specific* body fluid is called *isotonic* (of equal tone) with *thats* specific body fluid. Solutions having osmotic pressure *lower* than that of a body fluid are called *hypotonic*, and solutions having osmotic pressure *higher* than that of a body fluid are termed *hypertonic*.

Pharmaceutical dosage forms intended to be infused directly to the blood or mixed with biological fluids of the eye, nose, and bowel are of principal concern to the pharmacist for their preparation and clinical applications. Basic information is given so that calculations related to this area can be done confidently. Hence, this chapter will enable the student to understand:

- The terms - isosmotic, isotonic, hypertonic, and hypotonic; and distinguish one from other.
- How to apply physicochemical principles in the calculation of isotonic solutions.
- Calculation related to isotonic solution.
- The buffer equation and its application in calculations.

Clinical Consideration of Tonicity

It is generally accepted that isotonic solutions are preferred for ophthalmic and parenteral administration than hypotonic and hypertonic solutions. These are better tolerated by the patient and a homeostasis with the intracellular body fluids is maintained. However, there are exceptions. Hypertonic solutions are used to 'draw' fluids out of edematous tissues or hypertonic solution is mixed with the solution being administered intravenously.

Most ophthalmic preparations formulated are isotonic, or approximately isotonic. Duplicate ophthalmic tears are sometimes prepared for the comfort of the patient. Injections that are not isotonic should be administered slowly and in small quantities to reduce irritation of tissue, pain, and cell fluid imbalance. Most of the large-volume parenteral preparations contain sodium chloride or dextrose. Sodium chloride and dextrose are generally used to adjust the tonicity of the preparations. Thus, hypertonic small-volume injections can be mixed with these and administered.

On the other hand, hypotonic or hypertonic intravenous infusions, if administered can exert adverse effects because they generally are administered in large volumes. Large volumes of *hypertonic* infusions containing dextrose, for example, can cause in hyperglycemia, osmotic diuresis, and excessive loss of electrolytes. When *hypotonic infusion* is administered in excess, osmotic hemolysis of red blood cells can occur because the body cannot absorb large amount of such fluids safely. In fact, excessive volumes of an isotonic fluid, if infused intravenously or infused at excessive rates, deleterious effects may take place.

Preparation of Isotonic Solutions

Physical and Chemical Consideration

For preparation of isotonic solutions calculations can be done using the colligative property of solutions. For example, freezing point depression is a colligative property and it is used for determining tonicity of a solution. The freezing point of both blood serum and lachrymal fluid is -0.52°C.

The freezing point of one molal solution of boric acid, a non electrolyte (gram molecular weight dissolved in 1000 g of water) is about 1.86°C below the freezing point of pure water. Hence, by using simple law of proportion, we can calculate the weight of any nonelectrolyte that should be dissolved in each 1000 g of water to make isotonic with body fluids. For example,

$$\frac{1.86\ (^{o}C)}{52\ (^{o}C)} = \frac{61.8\ (g)}{x\ (g)}$$

$$x = 17.3\ g$$

Thus, 17.3 g of boric acid in 1000 g of water, or approximately 1.73% solution shall be isotonic with lachrymal fluid.

In case of electrolytes, it is not so simple; because osmotic pressure depends more on the number than on the kind of particles, substances present in a solution. The tonic effect will increase with the degree of dissociation. With greater degree of dissociation, a smaller amount can produce any required osmotic pressure. Say, a weak solution of sodium chloride dissociates up to 80%; then each 100 molecules produce 180 particles. In other words, in comparison to a nonelectrolyte the number of particles available in the solution would be 1.8 times. This dissociation factor, commonly symbolized by the letter *i,* and it must be included in the proportion used to determine the strength of an isotonic solution of sodium chloride (mol. wt. 58.5).

$$\frac{1.86\ (^{o}C) \times 1.8}{52\ (^{o}C)} = \frac{58.5\ (g)}{x\ (g)}$$

$$x = 9.09\ g$$

Hence, 9.09 g of sodium chloride dissolved in 1000 g of water shall make a isotonic solution. In practice, a 0.90% w/v sodium chloride solution is considered isotonic with body fluids.

Simple isotonic solutions may then be calculated by using this formula:

$$\frac{0.52 \times \text{molecular weight}}{1.86 \times \text{dissociation factor } (i)}$$

= g of solute per 1000 g of water

The experimental value of i for many drug substances are not known. However, dissociation of most of the salts (drugs) and weak solution of sodium chloride are almost similar. In absence of experimental value of i, the following values may be used if the number of ions formed in dissociation is known;

- For nonelectrolytes and substances dissociate slightly - 1.0
- For substances that dissociate into 2 ions- 1.8
- For substances that dissociate into 3 ions - 2.6
- For substances that dissociate into 4 ions - 3.4
- For substances that dissociate into 5 ions - 4.2

To make a 0.5% w/v solution of sodium chloride isotonic, 400 mg of sodium chloride (0.9 g - 0.5 g) should be added per 100 mL. 17.3 g of boric acid in 1000 g of water and 9.09 g of sodium chloride in 1000 g of water are both isotonic with lachrymal fluid. In other words, 17.3 g of boric acid are equivalent in tonicity to 9.09 g of sodium chloride. Then 1 g of boric acid must be the equivalent of 9.09 g ÷17.3 g or 0.52 g of sodium chloride. Similarly, 1 g of sodium chloride must be 'tonicic equivalent' of 17.3 g ÷ 9.09 g or 1.90 g of boric acid.

We have seen that one quantity of any substance should in theory have a constant tonic effect if dissolved in 1000 g of water: 1 g molecular weight of the substance divided by its i or dissociation value. Hence, the relative quantity of sodium chloride that is the tonicic equivalent of a quantity of boric acid may be calculated by these ratios:

$$\frac{58.5 \div 1.8}{61.8 \div 1.0} = \frac{58.5 \times 1.0}{61.8 \times 1.8}$$

It becomes difficult to prepare isotonic solution using ingredients other than the active ingredient; how much sodium chloride should be used in preparing 100 mL of a 1% w/v solution of atropine sulfate, to make it isotonic with lachrymal fluid.

Thus, a convenient rule can be stated as: *Quantities of two substances that have tonicic equivalents are proportional to the molecular weights of each multiplied by the i value of the other.*

To return to the problem involving 1 g of atropine sulfate in 100 mL of solution:

Molecular weight of sodium chloride = 58.5 and i =1.8

Molecular weight of atropine sulfate = 695 and i =2.6

Then, $$\frac{695 \times 1.8}{58.5 \times 2.6} = \frac{1\ (g)}{x\ (g)}$$

x = 0.12 g of sodium chloride equivalent to 1.0 g of atropine sulphate

Because a solution isotonic with lachrymal fluid should contain the equivalent of 0.90 g of sodium chloride in each 100 mL of solution, the difference to be added must be 0.90 g ÷ 0.12 g = 0.78 g of sodium chloride.(Answer)

The sodium chloride equivalents (*E* values) of some of the substances are listed below.

Substance	Mol. Weight	ions	*i*	E value
Antazoline phosphate	363	2	1.8	0.16
Antipyrine	188	1	1.0	0.17
Atropine sulfate H_2O	695	3	2.6	0.12
Benoxinate hydrochloride	345	2	1.8	0.17
Benzalkonium chloride	360	2	1.8	0.16
Benzyl alcohol	108	1	1.0	0.30
Boric acid	61.8	1	1.0	0.52
Chloramphenicol	323	1	1.0	0.10
Chlorobutanol	177	1	1.0	0.24
Chlortetracycline hydrochloride	515	2	1.8	0.11
Cocaine hydrochloride	340	2	1.8	0.16
Cromolyn sodium	512	2	1.8	0.11
Cyclopentolate hydrochloride	328	2	1.8	0.18
Demecarium bromide	717	3	2.6	0.12
Dextrose (anhydrous)	180	1	1.0	0.18
Dextrose H_2O	198	1	1.0	0.16
Dipivefrin hydrochloride	388	2	1.8	0.15
Ephedrine hydrochloride	202	2	1.8	0.29
Ephedrine sulfate	429	3	2.6	0.23
Epinephrine bitartrate	333	2	1.8	0.18

Table *contd...*

Epinephryl borate	209	1	1.0	0.16
Eucatropine hydrochloride	328	2	1.8	0.18
Fluorescein sodium	376	3	2.6	0.31
Glycerin	92	1	1.0	1.34
Homatropine hydrobromide	356	2	1.8	0.17
Hydroxyamphetamine	232	2	1.8	0.25
hydrobromide	354	1	1.0	0.09
Idoxuridine	289	2	1.8	0.22
Lidocaine hydrochloride	182	1	1.0	0.18
Mannitol	759	3	2.6	0.11
Morphine sulfate 5H_2O	247	2	1.8	0.27
Naphazoline hydrochloride	297	2	1.8	0.20
Oxymetazoline hydrochloride	497	2	1.8	0.12
Oxytetracycline hydrochloride	353	2	1.8	0.20
Phenacaine hydrochloride	254	2	1.8	0.24
Phenobarbital sodium	204	2	1.8	0.32
Phenylephrine hydrochloride	413	2	1.8	0.16
Physostigmine salicylate	649	3	2.6	0.13
Physostigmine sulfate	245	2	1.8	0.24
Pilocarpine hydrochloride	271	2	1.8	0.23
Pilocarpine nitrate	136	2	1.8	0.43
Potassium biphosphate	74.5	2	1.8	0.76
Potassium chloride	166	2	1.8	0.34
Potassium iodide	101	2	1.8	0.58
Potassium nitrate	372	2	1.8	0.18
Potassium penicillin G	273	2	1.8	0.21
Procaine hydrochloride	331	2	1.8	0.18
Proparacaine hydrochloride	438	2	1.8	0.12
Scopolamine hydrobromide 3H_2O	170	2	2.8	0.33
Silver nitrate	84	2	1.8	0.65
Sodium bicarbonate	381	5	4.2	0.42
Sodium borate10H_2O	106	3	2.6	0.80
Sodium carbonate	124	3	2.6	0.68
Sodium carbonate H_2O	58.5	2	1.8	1.00
Sodium chloride	294	4	3.4	0.38
Sodium citrate 2H_2O	150	2	1.8	0.39
Sodium iodide	112	2	1.8	0.52
Sodium lactate	142	3	2.6	0.53
Sodium phosphate, dibasic,	268	3	2.6	0.29
anhydrous	120	2	1.8	0.49

Table *contd...*

Sodium phosphate, dibasic $7H_2O$	138	2	1.8	0.42
Sodium phosphate, monobasic,	301	2	1.8	0.18
anhydrous	481	2	1.8	0.12
Sodium phosphate, monobasic	237	2	1.8	0.25
H_2O	432	2	1.8	0.14
Tetracaine hydrochloride	468	1	1.0	0.07
Tetracycline hydrochloride	284	1	1.0	0.11
Tetrahydrozoline hydrochloride	60	1	1.0	0.59
Timolol maleate	136	3	2.6	0.62
Tobramycin	288	2	1.4	0.15
Tropicamide	136	3	2.6	0.62
Urea	288	1.4	1.4	0.15
Zinc chloride				
Zinc sulfate $7H_2O$				

These values have been calculated according to the rule stated earlier. *If the number of grams of a substance is multiplied by its sodium chloride equivalent, the amount of sodium chloride represented by that substance is determined.*

The steps involved in calculation of isotonic solutions with sodium chloride equivalents are:

Step I: Calculate the amount (in grams) of sodium chloride represented by the ingredient; multiply the amount (in grams) of each substance by its sodium chloride equivalent.

Step II: Calculate the amount (in grams) of sodium chloride to be contained in a specific volume of its isotonic solution; for example, *450 mg of sodium chloride in 500 ml of 0.9% solution.*

Step III: Deduct the amount of sodium chloride represented by the ingredient (Step I) from the amount of sodium chloride alone that would be present in the specific volume of an isotonic solution (Step II). The answer would be the amount (in grams) of sodium chloride to be added to make the solution isotonic.

Step IV: If any substance such as boric acid, dextrose, or potassium nitrate, other than sodium chloride, is to be used to make the solution isotonic, divide the amount of sodium chloride (Step III) by the sodium chloride equivalent of that substance.

Calculations of the *i* Factor

Example

Zinc sulfate ($ZnSO_4$) is an electrolyte that produces two ions. It dissociates 40% of its concentration. Calculate its dissociation factor, *i*.

Solution

On the basis of 40 % dissociation the solution of $ZnSO_4$ will contain,

40 zinc ions

40 sulfate ions.

60 undissociated particles

Total 140 particles

Before dissociation there were 100 particles and after dissociation140 particles,

Thus, the dissociation (*i*) factor $= \frac{140}{100}$

Ans. 1.4

Example

Zinc chloride ($ZnCl_2$) produces three ions when dissociates. It dissociates up to 80% of its concentration. Calculate its dissociation factor, *i*.

Solution

Due to 80% dissociation, 100 particles of zinc chloride will produce

80	zinc ions
$2 \times 80 = 160$	chloride ions
20	undissociated particles
Total	260 particles

Before dissociation there were 100 particles and after dissociation 260 particles,

Thus, the dissociation (*i*) factor $= \frac{260}{100}$

Ans. 2.6

Calculation of Tonicic Agent Required [Using Sodium Chloride Equivalent (E value)]

The sodium chloride equivalent of a substance may be calculated as:

$$\text{Sodium Chloride Equivalent (E value)} = \frac{\text{Mol wt of Sodium Chloride}}{i \text{ factor of Sodium Chloride}}$$

$$= \frac{i \text{ factor of the substance}}{\text{Mol wt of the substance}}$$

Example

Papaverine hydrochloride (mol wt. 376) dissociates into two ions in aqueous medium and 80% of a given concentration dissociates. Calculate its sodium chloride equivalent.

Solution

Papaverine hydrochloride is a 2-ion electrolyte and dissociates up to 80%.

100 particles of Papaverine hydrochloride will produce

$2 \times 80 = 160$ ionic particles

<u>20</u> undissociated particles

Total 180 particles produced from 100 particles

Thus, its *i* factor is $\frac{180}{100} = 1.8$

E value of Papaverine hydrochloride $= \frac{58.5}{1.8} \times \frac{1.8}{376}$

Ans. 0.15

Example

The molecular weight of glycerin is 92 and it is a nonelectrolyte, its *i* factor is 1.0. Calculate its sodium chloride equivalent.

Solution

The *i* factor of glycerin is 1.0

Then its E value $= \frac{58.5}{1.8} \times \frac{1.0}{92}$

Ans. 0.35

Example

The molecular weight of timolol maleate is 432, dissociates into two ions and its *i* factor is 1.8. Calculate the sodium chloride equivalent (E value) for timolol maleate.

Solution

The E value of timolol maleate $= \frac{58.5}{1.8} \times \frac{1.8}{432}$

Ans. 0.14

Example

Fluorescein sodium dissociates into three ions, its *i* factor is 2.6 and its molecular weight is 376. Calculate the sodium chloride equivalent (E value) for Fluorescein sodium.

Solution

The molecular weight of Fluorescein sodium = 376

The *i* factor = 2.6

The E value of timolol maleate $= \frac{58.5}{1.8} \times \frac{2.6}{376}$

Ans. 0.23

Example

How many grams of sodium chloride should be used to prepare 30 ml of 1% solution of pilocarpine nitrate isotonic to body fluids? E value of pilocarpine nitrate is 0.23.

Solution

E value of pilocarpine nitrate:

Step I: 0.23×0.3 g = 0.069 g of sodium chloride represented by pilocarpine nitrate

Step II: 30×0.009 g = 0.27 g of sodium chloride required for 30 ml of isotonic solution of sodium chloride

Step III: 0.27 g (Step II)

– 0.069 g (Step I)

0.201 g of sodium chloride would be required for making 30 ml of isotonic solution of pilocarpine nitrate (1%) (Answer)

Example

How many grams of boric acid should be used for preparing 50 ml solution of Phenacaine HCl (1%) and chlorobutanol (0.5%).

Solution

The prescription calls for 0.5 g of Phenacaine hydrochloride and 0.25 g of chlorobutanol in 50ml.

Step I: 0.20×0.5 g = 0.10 g of sodium chloride represented by Phenacaine hydrochloride

0.24 × 0.25 g = 0.06 g of sodium chloride represented by chlorobutanol

Total: 0.16 g of sodium chloride represented by both ingredients

Step II: 50 × 0.009 = 0.450 g of sodium chloride in 50 mL of an isotonic solution of sodium chloride

Step III: 0.450 g (from Step II)

– 0.16 g (from Step I)

0.29 g of sodium chloride required to make the solution isotonic

Since boric acid is used for making isotonic solution

Step IV: 0.29 g ÷ 0.52 (E value of boric acid) = 0.56 g of boric acid would be required. *Answer.*

Example

How many grams of potassium nitrate could be required to prepare 50 ml of isotonic solution of silver nitrate using 0.2% Silver nitrate sol? The E value of silver nitrate is 0.33.

Solution

Amount of sodium chloride represented by silver nitrate = E value of silver nitrate × amount of silver nitrate required.

= 0.33 × 0.10 g = 0.033 g (Step I)

Amount of sodium chloride required for 50 ml of its isotonic solution = 50×0.009 g = 0.45 g (Step II)

Amount of sodium chloride required for 50 ml isotonic solution of silver nitrate (Step III) = Step II – Step I

= 0.45g – 0.033g

Ans. 0.417 g or 0.42 g

Preparation of Isotonic Solutions (Using an Isotonic Sodium Chloride Solution)

Isotonic solution of sodium chloride refers to 0.9% w/v sodium chloride solution. This may be used to prepare isotonic solutions of other drug substances as follows:

- **Step I:** Calculate the quantity of the drug substance required to make the specified volume of the solution.
- **Step II:** Calculate the volume of water required to make the solution of the drug substance isotonic by using following equation:

  Volume of water required to prepare the isotonic solution of the drug (assuming that the volume of the drug is negligible)

  $$= \frac{\text{Amount of drug required} \times \text{E value of the drug}}{0.009} \text{ ml}$$
- **Step III:** The volume of 0.9% w/v sodium chloride solution to be added

  = volume of the preparation – volume of water added

Example

How much quantity of purified water and 0.9% w/v sodium chloride solution to be required to prepare 20 ml of a 1% w/v solution of hydromorphone hydrochloride (E value 0.22).

Solution

Step I: The amount of hydromorphone hydrochloride required for 20 ml of 1% solution

$= 20 \text{ ml} \times 1\% \text{ w/v soln} \quad [20 \text{ ml} \times \frac{1 \text{ g}}{100 \text{ ml}} = 0.2 \text{ g}]$

= 0.2 g.

Step II: Volume of water required to make 20 ml solution

$$= \frac{\text{Amount of drug required} \times \text{E value of the drug}}{0.009}$$

$$= \frac{0.2 \times 0.22}{0.009}$$

$= 4.9$ ml

Step III: Volume of 0.9% sodium chloride solution required

= volume of the preparation – volume of water added

= 20 ml – 4.9 ml

= 15.1 ml (Answer)

Calculation of Tonicic Agent Required (Using Freezing Point Depression Data)

Isotonicity calculations can be done by using freezing point depression data (ΔT_f). The freezing point depression data can be used when the agent has a tonicic effect and does not penetrate the biologic membranes in question (e.g., red blood cells). It has been mentioned earlier that the freezing point of both blood and lachrymal fluid is -0.52°C. Thus, a pharmaceutical solution that has a freezing point of -0.52°C can be considered isotonic.

The freezing point depression data ($T_f^{1\%}$) of some drug and other pharmaceutical substances are presented below. The strengths of the solution of these substances are 1%.

Substance	$T_f^{1\%}$
Atropine sulfate	0.07
Boric acid	0.29
Butacaine sulfate	0.12
Chloramphenicol	0.06
Chlorobutanol	0.14
Dextrose	0.09
Dibucaine hydrochloride	0.08
Ephedrine sulfate	0.13
Epinephrine bitartrate	0.10
Ethylmorphine hydrochloride	0.09
Glycerin	0.20

Table *contd...*

Homatropine hydrobromide	0.11
Lidocaine hydrochloride	0.063
Lincomycin	0.09
Morphine sulfate	0.08
Naphazoline hydrochloride	0.16
Physostigmine salicylate	0.09
Pilocarpine nitrate	0.14
Sodium bisulfite	0.36
Sodium chloride	0.58
Sulfacetamide sodium	0.14
Zinc sulfate	0.09

Calculations using Freezing Point Data

Example

How many milligrams of each of sodium chloride and dibucaine hydrochloride are required to prepare 30 mL of a 1% solution of dibucaine hydrochloride isotonic with tears?

Solution

To make this solution isotonic, the freezing point must be lowered to -0.52. It is determined that a 1% solution of dibucaine hydrochloride shows a freezing point depression of 0.08°. Thus, sufficient sodium chloride must be added to lower the freezing point for additional 0.44° (0.52° - 0.08°).

1% solution of sodium chloride lowers the freezing point of water by 0.58 °C.

$$\frac{1\% \text{ Sodium chloride}}{x\% \text{ Sodium chloride}} = \frac{0.58^{o}}{0.44^{o}}$$

$$x = 0.76\%$$

Thus, 0.76% sodium chloride is required to lower the freezing point by 0.44° and 0.76g of sodium chloride is required to make 100ml of the solution isotonic.

To make 30 mL of solution, 30 mL ×1% = 0.3 g = 300 mg dibucaine hydrochloride, and

30 mL × 0.76% = 0.228 g = 228 mg sodium chloride would be required. (Answer)

Buffers and Buffer Solutions

Addition of a trace amount of hydrochloric acid to pure water brings about a significant increase in *hydrogen-ion* concentration instantly. Similarly if a trace amount of sodium hydroxide is added to pure water, the *hydroxyl-ion* concentration increases immediately. Such changes occur because water alone cannot neutralize even traces of acid or base. Pure water does not the ability to resist changes in hydrogen-ion concentration or pH. Even a solution of a neutral salt, such as calcium chloride or potassium chloride, does not have this ability.

When certain substances or combinations of substances are present in aqueous solution the system can resist change in pH and maintain the pH at a relatively constant level. This happens even after addition of materials that may change the hydrogen–ion concentration or pH. These substances or combinations of substances are called *buffers*. Their ability to resist the changes in pH is called *buffer action* and their efficiency is measured in terms of the function called *buffer capacity*. The solutions of these substances are called *buffer solutions*. Thus, a *buffer solution* is a system, usually an aqueous solution that possesses the ability to resist the changes in pH with the addition of small amounts of a strong acid or base.

Applications of Buffers

Buffers are used to create and maintain an ion activity within almost a definite range. In pharmacy, the most common buffer systems are used for the following purposes;

- For preparation of dosage forms such as injections and ophthalmic solutions, which are placed directly into pH-sensitive body fluids;
- To manufacture formulations in which the pH must be maintained at a relatively constant level to ensure maximum product stability; and
- Pharmaceutical tests and assays those require adjustment or maintenance of a specific pH for analytic purposes.

Usually a buffer is a mixture of a weak acid and a salt of the acid, such as acetic acid and sodium acetate, or a weak base and a salt of the base, such as ammonium hydroxide and ammonium chloride. The buffer systems commonly used in pharmaceutical formulations are - acetic acid and sodium acetate, boric acid and sodium borate, and disodium phosphate and sodium acid phosphate, etc.. The *United States*

Pharmacopeia provides a list of standard buffer solutions used in pharmaceutical analysis.

During selection of a buffer system the dissociation constant of the weak acid or base must be considered to achieve maximum buffer capacity. The strength of the acid is measured by its dissociation constant. If the dissociation constant is high, the acid dissociates more readily. The dissociation constant is expressed as k_a and it is given by the equation;

$$k_a = \frac{[H^+][A^-]}{[HA]}$$

Where HA is an acid which dissociates as: $HA \leftrightarrow H^+ + A^-$; HA is the acid and A^- is salt.

Most dissociation constants have smaller numeric values and may vary over many powers of 10; hence, it would be more convenient to express them as negative logarithms. That is, $p^{k_a} = - \log k_a$

$$k_a = \frac{[H^+][A^-]}{[HA]}$$

or, $$- \log k_a = - \log \frac{[H^+][A^-]}{[HA]}$$

or, $$p^{k_a} = - \log [H^+] - \log \frac{[A^-]}{[HA]}$$

$$= pH - \log \frac{[salt]}{[acid]} \qquad (pH = - \log [H^+])$$

Or, $$pH = p^{k_a} + \log \frac{[salt]}{[acid]}$$

This is known as Henderson-Hasselbalch equation for weak acids.

Buffer Equation

The Henderson-Hasselbalch equation for weak acids is commonly known as the ***buffer equation***. The dissociation of a base BOH can be expressed as;

$$BOH \leftrightarrow [B^+] + [OH^-]$$

The dissociation constant of a weak base, K_b is given by the equation:

$$K_b = \frac{[B^+][OH^-]}{[BOH]}$$

Where BOH is the base and B^+ is the salt.

Hence, the buffer equation for base can be written as;

$$pH = pk_w - pk_b + \log \frac{\text{base}}{\text{salt}}$$

Application of the Buffer Equation

The above buffer equation is valuable for calculating

- The pH of a buffer system if its composition is known and
- The molar ratio of the components of a buffer system required to give a solution of a desired pH.
- The change in pH of a buffered solution with the addition of a given amount of acid or base.

Calculation of pK_a Value of a Weak Acid with known Dissociation Constant

Example

The dissociation constant of lactic acid is 1.38×10^{-4} at 25 °C. Calculate its pK_a value.

Solution

$k_a = 1.38\times10^{-4}$

$\log k_a = \log 1.38 - 4 \log 10$

$= 0.\ 1399 - 4 = -3.86$

$pK_a = -\log K_a = -(-3.86) = 3.86$

The pk_a value of lactic acid is 3.86 (Answer)

Example

The dissociation constant of salicylic acid is 1.06×10^{-3} at 25°C. Calculate its pK_a value.

Solution

$k_a = 1.06\times10^{-3}$

$\log k_a = \log 1.06 - 3 \log 10$

$= 0.\ 0253 - 3 = -2.97$

$pK_a = -\log K_a = -(-2.97) = 2.97$

The pk_a value of salicylic acid is 2.97 (Answer)

Calculation of pH Value of Buffer System

Example

What is the pH of a buffer solution prepared with 0.01 M sodium borate and 0.002 M boric acid?

The pK_a value of boric acid is 9.24 at 25°C.

Solution

Note that the ratio of the components of the buffer solution is given in molar concentrations.

Using the buffer equation for weak acids:

$$pH = pK_a + \log \frac{\text{salt}}{\text{acid}}$$

$$= 9.24 + \log \frac{0.01}{0.002}$$

$$= 9.24 + \log 5$$

$$= 9.24 + 0.6990$$

Ans. 9.939 or 9.94

Example

Boric acid-sodium borate buffer of pH 10.24 was prepared using 0.005M solution of boric acid. Find out the molar concentration of sodium borate to be present in the buffer. The pK_a value of boric acid is 9.24 at 25°C.

Solution

Suppose the concentration of sodium borate solution is *x* M.

Then, by using the buffer equation for weak acids:

$$pH = pK_a + \log \frac{\text{salt}}{\text{acid}}$$

$$10.24 = 9.24 + \log \frac{x}{0.005}$$

$$\log \frac{x}{0.005} = 10.24 - 9.24$$

$$= 1$$

$$\log x - \log 0.005 = 1$$

$$\log x = 1 + \log 0.005$$

$$= 1 + \bar{3}.6990$$

$$= \bar{2}.6990$$

$$x = \text{antilog } \bar{2}.6990 = 0.05$$

Ans. The molar concentration of sodium borate is 0.05

Example

What would be the pH of a buffer solution containing 2 M ammonia and 1 M ammonium chloride? The dissociation constant, K_b of ammonia is 1.80×10^{-5} at 25°C.

Solution

The buffer equation for weak bases is;

$$pH = pK_w - pK_b + \log \frac{\text{base}}{\text{salt}}$$

The K_w for water at 25°C is 10^{-14}; thus, $pK_w = 14$

$$K_b = 1.80 \times 10^{-5}$$

$$\log K_b = \log 1.80 \times 10^{-5}$$

$$= \log 1.80 + \log 10^{-5}$$

$$= 0.2553 - 5$$

$$= -4.74$$

$$-\log K_b = -(-4.74)$$

$$pK_b = 4.74$$

$$\text{So, } pH = pK_w - pK_b + \log \frac{\text{base}}{\text{salt}}$$

$$= 14 - 4.74 + \log \frac{2}{1}$$

$$= 9.26 + \log 2$$

$$= 9.26 + 0.3010$$

Ans. 56

Example

Find out the pH of a buffer solution containing 0.25 moles of formic acid per liter and 0.1 mole of sodium formate per liter. (ka for formic acid is 1.8×10^{-4})

Solution

$$k_a = 1.8\times10^{-4}$$

$$pk_a = -\log 1.8 \times 10^{-4}$$

$$= 4 - \log 1.8 = 3.7447$$

$$\text{Now, } pH = pk_a + \log \frac{[\text{Salt}]}{[\text{Acid}]} = 3.7447 + \log \frac{0.1}{0.25}$$

$$= 3.7447 - 0.3979$$

Ans. $3.3468 \approx 3.35$

Example

Find out the molar ratio of salt/acid required to prepare a sodium acetate-acetic acid buffer solution with a pH of 5.72? The pK_a value of acetic acid is 4.76 at 25°C.

Solution

The buffer equation is $pH = pK_a + \log \frac{\text{salt}}{\text{acid}}$

Given that, pK_a = 4.76 and the desired pH = 5.72

Then, $$5.72 = 4.76 + \log \frac{\text{salt}}{\text{acid}}$$

$$\log \frac{\text{salt}}{\text{acid}} = 5.72 - 4.76 = 0.96 = 0.96:1$$

Ans. Thus, the ratio of salt: acid = 0.96:1

Calculation of Volume to Prepare Buffer Solution

Sometimes the amounts of the components of a buffer system are to be calculated to prepare a desired volume of buffer solution for a given molar ratio and the total buffer concentration.

Example

The molar ratio of sodium acetate to acetic acid in a buffer solution with a pH of 5.74 is 9:1. The total buffer concentration is 2.4×10^{-2} mol/L, Calculate how many grams of sodium acetate (mol wt 82) and how many grams of acetic acid (mol wt 60) would be required to prepare 1000 ml of the solution?

Solution

Given that,

The molar ratio of sodium acetate to acetic acid = 9:1,

Total concentration of buffer = 2.4×10^{-2} mol/L,

The pH of the buffer solution = 5.74,

Final volume = 500 ml

Molecular weight of sodium acetate = 82, and

Molecular weight of acetic acid = 60

Thus, the mole fraction of sodium acetate = $\frac{9}{9+1} = \frac{9}{10}$

The mole fraction of acetic acid = $\frac{1}{9+1} = \frac{1}{10}$

The molar concentration of sodium acetate = $\frac{9}{10} \times 2.4 \times 10^{-2}$ mol/L = 2.16×10^{-2} mol/L

The molar concentration of acetic acid = $\frac{1}{10} \times 2.4 \times 10^{-2}$ mol/L = 0.24×10^{-2} mol/L

So, the amount of sodium acetate required per 1000 ml of solution = $2.16 \times 10^{-2} \times 82$

= 1.77 g (Answer)

Similarly, the amount of acetic acid required per 1000 ml of solution = $0.24 \times 10^{-2} \times 60$

= 0.144g (Answer)

The efficacy of buffer solutions is the specific ability to resist the changes in pH; measured in terms of *buffer capacity*. If the pH changes in small amount on addition of a given amount of acid or base, the buffer capacity of the system is considered *greater*. The buffer capacity of a system depends on the following factors;

- The relative concentration of the buffer components and
- The ratio of the components.

For example, a 0.1 M-acetate buffer at a pH of 4.76 would have a higher buffer capacity than a 0.05 M-buffer.

Change in pH with Addition of an Acid or Base

If a strong base such as sodium hydroxide is added to a buffer system consisting of equimolar concentrations of sodium acetate and acetic acid, the base is neutralized by the acetic acid forming more sodium acetate, and the pH increases slightly. Actually, the addition of the base increases the concentration of sodium acetate and decreases *by an equal amount* of the concentration of acetic acid. In a similar manner, if a strong acid is added to a buffer system consisting of a weak base and its salt, it would decrease the pH slightly.

Example

To a liter of 0.2 M sodium acetate and 0.2M acetic acid buffer solution 2 g of sodium hydroxide is added. Calculate the change in pH. The pK_a value of acetic acid is 4.76 at 25°C.

Solution

The buffer equation for weak acid and its salt: $pH = pK_a + \log \frac{\text{salt}}{\text{acid}}$

Given that, pK_a of acetic acid = 4.76

Molar concentration of buffer = 0.2

$$\text{Thus, } pH = 4.76 + \log \frac{0.2}{0.2}$$

$$= 4.76 + \log 1$$

$$= 4.76 + 0 = 4.76$$

On addition of 2 g of sodium hydroxide (2/40 = 0.05 mol) to this buffer, sodium hydroxide will react with acetic acid forming equivalent amount of sodium acetate. As a result, the concentration of acetic acid will decrease and that of sodium acetate will increase. That is, the concentration of acetic acid will be 0.2 – 0.05 = 0.15 mol and the concentration of sodium acetate will be 0.2 + 0.05 = 0.25 mol.

$$\text{Thus, pH} = 4.76 + \log \frac{0.25}{0.15}$$

$$= 4.76 + \log 1.667$$

$$= 4.76 + 0.2219$$

$$= 4.98$$

Ans. Change in pH would be 0.22

Example

The pH of a buffer solution containing 0.5 mole/Lt of acetic acid and 0.5 mole/Lt of sodium acetate is 4.76. What will happen to the pH of this solution if 0.1 mole of hydrochloric acid is added per liter? Assume that the volume of the solution does not change. The pk_a of acetic acid is 1.75×10^{-5}

Solution

When 0.1 mole of HCl is added to the buffer, it reacts with CH_3COONa and forms 0.1 mole of CH_3COOH; thus, the concentration of CH_3COONa is increased by 0.1 mole/liter.

Thus, the concentration of acetic acid and acetate ions in the solution would be as follows;

$[CH_3COOH] = 0.5 \text{ mole} + 0.1 \text{ mole} = 0.6 \text{ moles/liter}$

$[CH_3COO^-] = 0.5 \text{ mole} - 0.1 \text{ mole} = 0.4 \text{ moles/liter}$

$$\text{Then, } k_a = \frac{[H^+][[CH_3COO^-]}{[CH_3COOH]}$$

$$= \frac{[H^+]\times 0.4}{0.6} = 1.75\times 10^{-5}$$

$$[H^+] = \frac{0.4 \times 1.75 \times 10^{-5}}{0.6}$$

$$pH = -\log [H^+] = -\log \left(\frac{0.4 \times 1.75}{0.6}\right) - \log 10^{-5}$$

$$= -\log 1.167 + 5\log 10 = 5 - \log 1.167 = 4.93$$

Ans. The pH of the buffer will decrease from 4.76 to 4.93

Example

What would be the pH of 1 Lt of a solution containing 0.1N acetic acid and 0.1N sodium acetate, if 10.0 ml of 1N hydrochloric acid is added to it? (pK_a of acetic acid = 4.74)

Solution

Given that the concentration of [Acid] = 0.1moles/lt

The concentration of [Salt] = 0.1moles/lt

The pH of acetic acid-sodium acetate buffer is given by;

$$pH = pKa + \log \frac{[salt]}{[acid]}$$

$$= 4.74 + \log \frac{0.1}{0.1} = 4.74 + \log 1.0 = 4.74 + 0 = 4.74$$

On addition of 10.0ml of HCl to 1.0 Lt of the buffer, the volume becomes 1010ml (0.01moles of HCl). Let us ignore the change in volume. The HCl shall react with acetate ions and the change in concentration of acetic acid and of acetate ions are as follows;

The concentration of [Acid] = 0.1 – 0.01 = 0.09

The concentration of [salt] = 0.1 + 0.01 = 0.11

$$\text{Thus, } pH = pKa + \log \frac{[salt]}{[acid]}$$

$$= 4.74 + \log \frac{0.11}{0.09} = 4.74 + 0.0871$$

= 4.827 (Answer)

Example

What would be the pH of a buffer solution contains 0.25 mole of ammonium chloride and 0.20 moles of ammonium hydroxide. The dissociation constant of ammonium hydroxide is 1.80×10^{-5}.

Solution:

$$pOH = pK_b + \log \frac{[Salt]}{[Base]} = -\log Kb + \log \frac{[Salt]}{[Base]}$$

$$= -\log (1.80 \times 10^{-5}) + \log \frac{0.25}{0.20}$$

$$= 4.7447 + 0.0969$$

Ans. 4.841

Example

The dissociation constant of propionic acid is 1.34×10^{-5}. Calculate the pH of a solution containing 0.5 moles of propionic acid and 0.75 moles of sodium propionate in one liter.

Solution

Given that, [Acid] = 0.5 and [Salt] = 0.75

$$Ka = 1.34 \times 10^{-5}$$

$$pKa = -\log Ka = -\log (1.34 \times 10^{-5})$$

$$= 4.87$$

According to Henderson-Hasselbach equation

$$pH = pK_a + \log \frac{[Salt]}{[Acid]}$$

$$= 4.87 + \log \frac{0.75}{0.50}$$

$$= 4.87 + \log 1.5$$

$$= 4.87 + 0.1761$$

Ans. 5.046

Example

A buffer solution contains 0.25M formic acid and 0.10M sodium formate. The dissociation constant of formic ion of formic acid is 1.8×10^{-4}. Find out the pH of the buffer solution.

Solution

Given that, molar concentration of formic acid = 0.25

Molar concentration of sodium formate = 0.10

The dissociation constant of formic ion of formic acid, $K_a = 1.8 \times 10^{-4}$

$$pKa = -\log Ka = -\log 1.8 \times 10^{-4}$$

$$= 4 - \log 1.8$$

$$= 3.7447$$

According to Henderson-Hasselbach equation

$$pH = pK_a + \log \frac{[Salt]}{[Acid]}$$

$$= 3.7447 + \log \frac{0.10}{0.25}$$

$$= 3.7447 - 0.3979$$

Ans. $3.3468 \approx 3.35$

Example

To one liter of a buffer solution of 0.1ic acid and 0.1M of sodium acetate, 0.8g of sodium hydroxide was added. Calculate the pH of the solution. The dissociation constant of acetic ion of formic acid is 1.8×10^{-5}.

Solution

Given that the molar concentration of acetic acid = 0.1

The molar concentration of sodium acetate = 0.1

Ka of acetic acid = 1.8×10^{-5}

Sodium hydroxide added = 0.8g = $\frac{0.8}{40}$ = 0.02 moles

On addition of 0.02 moles of NaOH, 0.02 moles of OH^- ions will be produced and these ions will shift the equilibrium of dissociation reaction of CH_3COOH.

The molar concentration of acetic acid shall become 0.1 – 0.02 = 0.08

The molar concentration of sodium acetate shall become 0.1 + 0.02 = 0.12

Thus, the changed equilibrium can be expressed as

$$Ka = \frac{[H^+][CH_3COO^-]}{[CH_3COOH]} = 1.8 \times 10^{-5}$$

or, $$\frac{[H^+] \times 0.12}{0.08} = 1.8 \times 10^{-5}$$

$$[H^+] = 1.2 \times 10^{-5}$$

$$pH = -\log [H^+] = -\log 1.2 \times 10^{-5}$$

Ans. = 4.92

Exercise

1. What would be pH of a solution containing 0.5 moles of acetic acid and 0.5 moles of sodium acetate per liter? The ka of acetic acid is 1.34×10^{-5}.

Ans: 4.87

2. A liter of solution contains 0.1 mole of acetic acid and 0.1 mole of sodium acetate; the pH of this buffer is 4.74. What would be pH if 80 mg of sodium hydroxide is added to the buffer? The dissociation constant of NaOH is 1.8×10^{-5}.

Ans: 4.75

3. What would be hydrogen ion concentration of solution having pH
   (i) 5.0, and
   (ii) 7.8.

Ans:

(i) 1.0×10^{-5}M

(ii) 1.584×10^{-8} M

4. How many grams of ammonium chloride have to be added to one liter of 0.2M ammonium hydroxide solution to make a buffer of pH 9.0? The pk_b of ammonia is 4.75

Ans: 19.26 g of NH_4Cl would be required

5. The pH of a liter of buffer solution containing 1.0 mole of acetic acid and 1.0 mole of sodium acetate is 4.76. What will happen to the pH of this solution if 0.2 mole of hydrochloric acid is added to the solution? Assume that the volume of the solution does not change. The pk_a of acetic acid is 1.75×10^{-5}.

Ans: 3.58

6. Calculate the pH of a solution produced by adding 10.0ml of 1N hydrochloric acid to a liter of solution containing 0.1N acetic acid and 0.1N sodium acetate ($K_a = 1.82 \times 10^{-5}$).

Ans: 4.65

7. Sodium Iodide (NaI) is an electrolyte that produces two ions. It dissociates 80% of its concentration. Calculate its dissociation factor, *I*.

Ans: 1.80

8. Sodium phosphate, monobasic (anhydrous) produces two ions in water. It dissociates 80% of its concentration. Calculate its dissociation factor, *I*.

Ans: 1.80

9. Physostigmine sulfate (mol wt. 649) dissociates into three ions in aqueous medium and 80% of a given concentration dissociates. Calculate its sodium chloride equivalent (E value).

Ans: 0.13

10. The molecular weight of Tropicamide is 136, dissociates into three ions and its *i* factor is 2.6. Calculate the sodium chloride equivalent (E value) for Tropicamide.

Ans: 0.62

11. The molecular weight of Mannitol is 182 and it is a nonelectrolyte, its *i* factor is 1.0. Calculate its sodium chloride equivalent.

Ans: 0.18

12. How many grams of sodium chloride should be used to prepare 40 ml of 1% solution of pilocarpine nitrate isotonic to body fluids? E value of pilocarpine nitrate is 0.23.

Ans: 0.268

13. The molecular weight of urea is 288, dissociates into two ions and its *i* factor is 1.4. Calculate the sodium chloride equivalent (E value) for urea.

Ans: 0.15

14. How many milligrams of sodium chloride ($T_f^{1\%} = 0.58$) would be required to prepare 50 mL of a 1% solution of Pilocarpine nitrate ($T_f^{1\%} = 0.14$) isotonic with tears?

Ans: 0.3275g of sodium chloride

15. Calculate the pH of a 0.01M solution of acetic acid if its degree of dissociation is 12.5%.

Ans: 2.903

16. Molecular weights of sodium chloride and benzalkonium chloride are 58.5 and 360 respectively; the dissociation factors, *i* of 1% solution of sodium chloride and of 1% solution of benzalkonium chloride are 1.8 and 1.8 respectively. Find out the sodium chloride equivalence of 1% benzalkonium chloride solution.

Ans: 0.16

17. The *i*-values of sodium chloride and atropine sulphate are 1.8 and 2.6 respectively, and 0.12 g of sodium chloride equivalent to 1.0 g of atropine sulphate. If the molecular weight of sodium chloride is 58.5; find out the molecular weight of atropine sulphate and how much sodium chloride is to be added to 100ml of 1% solution of atropine sulphate isotonic to body fluids.

Ans: Mol wt of atropine sulphate is 695 and 0.78g of sodium chloride is to be added

18. The freezing point depression of 1% solution of ephedrine sulphate is 0.13° and that of sodium chloride is 0.58 °. How many milligrams of sodium chloride are to be added to prepare 25ml of 1% solution of ephedrine sulphate isotonic to body fluids?

Ans: 167.5mg

19. The molecular weight of nonelectrolyte substance shows sodium chloride equivalent of 0.35, its *i* factor is 1.0. Calculate its molecular weight.

Ans: 92

20. How many milliliters of 0.9% solution of sodium chloride would be required to prepare 20 ml of 1% solution of phenylephrine hydrochloride isotonic to tear fluid? E-value of phenylephrine hydrochloride is 0.32.

Ans: 12.89ml

21. The pH of a buffer solution is 9.94. It is prepared with 0.01 molar solution of the salt of a weak acid; if the pK_a value of the weak acid is 9.24 at 25°C, find out the molar concentration of the acid used.

Ans: 0.002 M

22. Calculate the moles a weak acid required to prepare a buffer solution having pH of 5.72; if 0.96 moles of its salt is used and pK_a value of the acid is 4.76 at 25°C.

Ans: 1 mole

23. Boric acid-sodium borate buffer of pH 10.2 was prepared using 0.15M solution of boric acid. The pK_a value of boric acid is 9.24 at 25°C.Find out the molar concentration of sodium borate required to prepare the buffer.

Ans: 1.368

24. Find out the molar ratio of salt/acid required to prepare a acetic acid- sodium acetate buffer solution with a pH of 5.74? The pK_a value of acetic acid is 4.76 at 25°C.

Ans: 4.9:5

25. The molar ratio of acetic acid to sodium acetate in a buffer solution with a pH of 5.76 is 1:9. If the total buffer concentration is 2.39×10^{-2} mol/L, calculate how many grams of acetic acid (mol wt 60) and how many grams of sodium acetate (mol wt 82) would be required to prepare 250 ml of this solution?

Ans: 0.4409 g of sodium acetate and 0.0358 g of acetic acid

7

CALCULATION INVOLVING ELECTROLYTE SOLUTIONS

It is known that in solution the molecules may dissociate into *ions*, or they may remain undissociated. The ions carry an electric charge. The substances that do not dissociate in solution are called *nonelectrolytes*, and those dissociate with varying degrees are called *electrolytes*. For example, urea, dextrose, sucrose are nonelectrolytes; while sodium chloride, potassium chloride, carbonic acid are electrolytes.

Sodium chloride produces Na^+ and Cl^- ions in solution, these carry electric charges. If electrodes carrying a weak current are placed in the solution, the ions move in a direction opposite to the charges. For example, Na^+ ions migrate towards the negative electrode (*cathode*) and are called *cations*. On the other hand, Cl^- ions migrate towards the positive electrode (*anode*) and are called *anions*. Electrolyte ions in the blood plasma include the cations Na^+, K^+, Ca^{2+}, and Mg^{2+} and the anions Cl^-, HCO_3^-, HPO_4^{2-}, SO_4^{2-}, organic acids$^-$, and proteinate$^-$. In body fluids electrolytes play an important role;

- Maintain the acid-base balance in the body,
- Control body water volumes, and
- Help to regulate body metabolism.
- This chapter provides the basic information about:
- The milliequivalent weight and its calculation from an atomic or formula weight.
- Conversion from milligrams to milliequivalents and vice versa.
- Calculations involving milliequivalents, millimoles and milliosmoles.

The electrolyte preparations are used in the treatment of disturbances of the electrolyte and fluid balance in the body.

These may be administered in the form of oral solutions and syrups, or by dissolving the dry granules in water or in juice to make an oral solution, as oral tablets and capsules and, if necessary, as intravenous infusions.

Milliequivalents

The *milliequivalent (mEq)* is a *chemical unit,* used to express the concentration of electrolytes in solution. It is related to the total number of ionic charges in solution, and valence of the ions. It is a unit of measurement of the amount of *chemical activity* of an electrolyte. In the International System (SI), molar concentrations such as milli-moles per liter (mmol/L) and micromoles per liter (μmol/L) are used by the most clinical laboratories to express the values, including those of electrolytes.

Blood plasma contains 154 mEq of cations and an equal number of anions under normal conditions. The electrolytes present in blood plasma are given below.

Electrolyte concentration in plasma			
Cations	mEq/L	Anions	mEq/L
Na^+	142	Cl^-	105
K^+	5	HCO_3^-	24
Ca^{2+}	5	Proteinate⁻	16
Mg^{2+}	2	Organic Ac⁻	6
		HPO_4^{2-}	2
	154	SO_4^{2-}	1
			154

Due to difference in unit used the figure (electrolyte values) may vary from laboratory to laboratory. However, for any compound, the milliequivalents of cation shall be equal to that of the anion, and their sum shall be equal to the milliequivalents of the chemical compound. For example, if 0.5 mol of sodium chloride is dissolved in 1 L of water, the solution will contain 0.5 mol of Na^+ ions/L and 0.5 mol of Cl^- ions/L.

Calculations of Milliequivalents

A milliequivalent is $\frac{1}{1000}$*th part of a gram equivalent weight, expressed as mEq wt. The milliequivalent represents the chemical activity or combining power of a substance relative to the activity of 1 mg of hydrogen.*

Hence, depending on the atomic weight and valence of the species, 1 mEq may be represented by 1 mg of hydrogen, 20 mg of calcium,

23 mg of sodium, 35.5 mg of chlorine, 39 mg of potassium, etc. The concentration of electrolytes in intravenous infusion fluids is most often stated in mEq/L.

The concentration of electrolytes in solution expressed as milliequivalents per unit volume can be converted to weight per unit volume and vice versa by using the following: formula.

From milligrams (mg) to milliequivalents (mEq):

$$\text{mEq} = \frac{\text{mg} \times \text{valence}}{\text{Atomic wt or Mol wt or Formula wt}}$$

From milliequivalents (mEq) to milligrams (mg):

$$\text{mg} = \frac{\text{mEq} \times \text{Atomic wt or Mol wt or Formula wt}}{\text{Valence}}$$

From mEq/mL to mg/mL:

$$\text{mg/ml} = \frac{\text{mEq/ml} \times \text{Atomic wt or Mol wt or Formula wt}}{\text{Valence}}$$

Example

A solution contains 5 mEq of sodium chloride (NaCl) per milliliter. What is the concentration, in milligrams per milliliter?

Solution

Molecular weight of sodium chloride = 58.5

Equivalent weight of sodium chloride = 58.5

$$1 \text{ mEq of sodium chloride} = \frac{1}{1000} \times 58.5 \text{ g} = 0.0585 \text{ g}$$

$$= 58.5 \text{ mg}$$

$$\text{mg/ml} = \frac{5 \text{ mEq/ml} \times 58.5 \text{ mg}}{1 \text{ mEq}} = 292.5$$

So, 5 mEq/ml

Ans. 292.5 mg/ml

Example

Express the concentration of a solution containing 10 mEq of calcium chloride ($CaCl_2, 2H_2O$) per ml in grams per milliliter.

Solution

$$\text{Equivalent weight of } CaCl_2, 2H_2O = \frac{\text{Mol wt of Formula weight}}{\text{Valence}}$$

Formula weight = 147

$$\text{Equivalent weight of } CaCl_2, 2H_2O = \frac{147}{2} = 73.5$$

$$1 \text{ mEq of } CaCl_2, 2H_2O = \frac{1}{1000} \times 73.5 = 0.0735 \text{ g}$$

$$10 \text{ mEq/ml of } CaCl_2, 2H_2O = 0.0735 \text{ g} \times 10$$

Ans. 0.735 g/ml

Example

In 540ml of water 75g of potassium hydroxide is dissolved. How many moles of KOH are present per liter of the solution?

Solution

Given that, Amount of KOH dissolved = 75g

Volume of water = 540ml

Molecular weight of KOH = 39.1 + 16.0 + 1.0 = 56.1

Thus, 56.1g of KOH = 1 mole of KOH

$$75\text{g of KOH} = \frac{1 \times 75}{56.1} = 1.337 \text{ moles}$$

Ignoring the change in volume, we can say that 540 ml of solution contains 75 g of KOH

In other words, 540ml solution contains 75g or 1.337 moles of KOH

$$1000 \text{ ml solution contains } \frac{1.337 \text{ moles} \times 1000 \text{ ml}}{540\text{ml}}$$

Ans. 2.476moles of KOH

Example

A solution contains 0.2mole of potassium carbonate per 240ml. Calculate the concentration in terms of %w/v.

Solution

Given that, volume of the solution = 240ml

Amount of K_2CO_3 present in the solution = 0.2 mole of K2CO3

$= 138.2 \times 0.2$

$= 27.64g$

Molecular weight of $K_2CO_3 = 2\times39.1 + 1\times12 + 3\times16$

$= 78.2 + 12 + 48$

$= 138.2$

Hence, 1 mole of K_2CO_3 = 138.2g of K_2CO_3

0.2 mole of $K_2CO_3 = 138.2 \times 0.2 = 27.64g$ of K_2CO_3

240 ml of solution contains 27.64g of K_2CO_3

100 ml of the solution contains $\frac{27.64 \times 100}{240}$ g = 11.516g

Thus, the concentration of the solution is

Ans. 11.52%w/v

Example

25ml of 5% solution of sodium carbonate is mixed with 15ml of water. Calculate the concentration (1) in terms of molarity and (2) how many mEq of Na_2CO_3 are there in 100ml.

Solution

Given that, initial volume of solution = 25ml

Final volume of solution = 25 + 15ml = 40ml

Concentration of the solution = 5%

(1) That is, 100ml of the solution contains 5g of Na_2CO_3

25 ml of the solution contains $\frac{5 \times 25}{100} = 0.5g$

On addition of 15 mml water to 25ml 0f 5% solution, the volume becomes 40 ml

Thus, 40 ml solution contains 0.5g of Na_2CO_3

1000 ml solution contains $\frac{0.5g \times 1000ml}{40ml} = 12.5$ g

Molecular weight of $Na_2CO_3 = 2\times23 + 1\times12 + 3\times16$

$= 46 + 12 + 48$

$= 106$

When 106g of Na_2CO_3 in 1000ml solution = 1 M

12.5g in 1000ml = $\frac{1 \times 12.5}{106}$ M = **0.118M** (Answer)

(2) Equivalent weight of $Na_2CO_3 = \frac{\text{Mol wt}}{\text{Valence}} = \frac{106}{2} = 53$

1 mEq of $Na_2CO_3 = \frac{53}{1000} = 0.053$g

or, 0.053g of Na_2CO_3 = 1 mEq

12.5g of $Na_2CO_3 = \frac{1 \times 12.5}{0.053} = 235.85$ mEq

The solution contains **235.85 mEq of Na_2CO_3** (Answer)

Example

A solution of magnesium chloride contains 0.5 g of $MgCl_2$ in 100 ml. Calculate the number of mEq of $MgCl_2$ present in the solution.

Solution

Given that, the concentration of $MgCl_2$ solution = 0.5%w/v

Molecular weight of $MgCl_2$ = 95.2

Valency of $MgCl_2$ = 2

Equivalent weight of $MgCl_2 = \frac{\text{Mol wt}}{\text{Valence}} = \frac{95.2}{2} = 47.6$

1 mEq of $MgCl_2 = \frac{47.6}{1000} = 0.0476$g

Concentration of solution of $MgCl_2$ = 0.5g in 100ml

0.0476g of $MgCl_2$ = 1 mEq of $MgCl_2$

0.5g of $MgCl_2 = \frac{1 \times 0.5}{0.0476}$ mEq

Ans. $10.638 \approx 10.504$ mEq of $MgCl_2$

Example

Express the concentration of a solution containing 50 mEq of calcium chloride ($CaCl_2$) per liter in the percent (w/v).

Solution

Molecular weight of calcium chloride = 111

Equivalent weight of calcium chloride $= \frac{\text{Mol wt}}{\text{Valence}} = \frac{111}{2} = 55.5$

1 mEq of calcium chloride $= \frac{1}{1000} \times 55.5 \text{ g} = 0.0555 \text{ g}$

50 mEq of calcium chloride = 50 × 0.0555 g = 2.775 g/L

That is, 1000 ml contain 2.78 g

In 100 ml $\frac{2.78 \times 100}{1000} \text{ g} = 0.278 \text{ g}$

Ans. Hence, the concentration is **0.278 %w/v**

Example

A solution contains 10 mg of Na^+ ions per 100 mL. What would be this concentration in terms of mEq per liter?

Solution

Atomic weight of Na^+ ion = 23

Valence of Na^+ ion = 1

Equivalent weight of Na^+ ion = 23

1 mEq of Na^+ ion $= 23 \times \frac{1}{1000} = 0.023 \text{ g} = 23 \text{ mg}$

10 mg of Na^+ ion per 100 ml = 100 mg of Na^+ ion per liter

So, 100 ÷ 23

Ans. 4.35 mEq/L

Example

A solution contains 200 mEq of magnesium chloride per liter. What is the percent (w/v) concentration?

Solution

Molecular weight of $MgCl_2$ = 95.2

Valence of $MgCl_2$ = 2

Equivalent weight of $MgCl_2 = \frac{\text{Atomic wt}}{\text{Valence}} = \frac{95.2}{2} = 47.6$

1 mEq of $MgCl_2 = \frac{1}{1000} \times 47 = 0.0476$ g

200 mEq of $MgCl_2$ = 200 × 0.0476 = 9.52 g per liter

Thus, 1000 ml of the contain 9.52 g of $MgCl_2$

100 ml contain $\frac{9.52 \times 100}{1000} = 0.952$ g of $MgCl_2$

The concentration of $MgCl_2$ solution is

Ans. 0.952%

Example

How many milliequivalents of sodium hydroxide are present in a 10% solution of it?

Solution

Given that the concentration of sodium hydroxide solution = 10%

Molecular weight of NaOH = 23 + 16 + 1 = 40

Valence of NaOH = 1

Equivalent weight of NaOH $= \frac{40}{1} = 40$

1 mEq of NaOH $= \frac{40}{1000} = 0.040$g

That is, 0.04g of NaOH = 1mEq

10 g of NaOH $= \frac{1 \times 10}{0.04}$

Ans. 250 mEq

Example

A solution contains 10 mg% of Ca^{2+} ions. Express the concentration in terms of mEq per liter.

Solution

Atomic weight of Ca^{2+} ion = 40

Valence of Ca^{2+} ion = 2

10 mg% of Ca^{2+} ions = 10 mg of Ca^{2+} ions per 100 ml

= 100 mg of Ca^{2+} ion per L

$$\text{mEq/L of } Ca^{2+} \text{ ions} = \frac{\text{mg/L} \times \text{Valence}}{\text{Atomic wt}} = \frac{100 \times 2}{40} = 5$$

Thus, the concentration of Ca^{2+} ion in the solution is

Ans. 5 mEq/L

Example

A solution contains 25mg% of Mg^{2+} ions. How many mEq of Mg^{2+} ions are present per liter?

Solution

Given that, the concentration of the solution of Mg^{2+} ions = 25 mg in 100 ml

Atomic weight of magnesium ion = 24.3

Valence of Mg = 2

25 mg% of Mg^{2+} ions = 25 mg of Mg^{2+} ions per 100 ml

= 250 mg of Mg^{2+} ion per L

$$\text{mEq/L of } Mg^{2+} \text{ ions} = \frac{\text{mg/L} \times \text{Valence}}{\text{Atomic wt}} = \frac{250 \times 2}{24.3} = 20.576 \approx 20.58$$

Thus, the concentration of Mg^{2+} ion in the solution is

Ans. 20.58 mEq/L

Example

In blood plasma the concentration of phosphate ion (HPO_4^{2-}) was found to be 2.5 mEq/L. Express the concentration in terms of mg%.

Solution

The formula weight of HPO_4^{2-} = 97

$$\text{Equivalent weight of } HPO_4^{2-} = \frac{97}{2} = 48.5$$

Concentration of HPO_4^{2-} in plasma = 2.5 mEq/L

$$mg/L = \frac{mEq/L \times Formula\ wt}{Valence} = \frac{2.5 \times 97}{2} = 121.25$$

That is, 121.25 mg of HPO_4^{2-} ion is present in 1000 ml of plasma

In 100 ml of plasma 12.125 mg of HPO_4^{2-} ion is present.

So, the concentration of HPO_4^{2-} ion in plasma

Ans. 12.12 mg%

Example

How many milliequivalents of sodium chloride are represented in 1.5 g of anhydrous sodium Chloride (NaCl)?

Solution

Molecular weight of NaCl = 58.5

Valence of NaCl = 1

1.5 g = 1.5 × 1000 mg = 1500 mg

Equivalent weight of NaCl = 58.5

1 mEq of NaCl = $\frac{1}{1000}$ × 58.5 g = 0.0585 g = 58.5 mg

mEq present in 1500 mg of NaCl = $\frac{mg \times Valence}{Mol\ w} = \frac{1500 \times 1}{58.5} = 25.64$

So, 1.5 g of NaCl contain 25.64 mEq (Answer)

Example

An ORS formulation contains 2.9 g of anhydrous sodium citrate ($Na_3C_6H_5O_7$) per 27.9 g. Calculate the concentration of Na^+ ion and $C_6H_5O_7^{3-}$ ions in terms of mEq.

Solution

Molecular weight of $Na_3C_6H_5O_7$ = 258

Valence = 3

Equivalent weight = $\frac{258}{3}$ = 86

2.9 g = 2900 mg

1 mEq of $Na_3C_6H_5O_7 = \frac{1}{1000} \times 86 = 0.086$ g = 86 mg

1 mEq of $C_6H_5O_7^{3-}$ ion or 3Na^+ ions in 2900 mg of $Na_3C_6H_5O_7$

$= \frac{2900}{86} = 33.72$

Thus 2.9 g of sodium citrate contains 33.72 mEqs of $C_6H_5O_7^{3-}$ ion and 33.72 mEqs of Na^+ ions are present. (Answer)

Example

Calculate how many mEq of dextrose is there in 5% Dextrose Injection.

Solution

Given that the concentration of dextrose solution = 5%

It is a nonelectrolyte.

Molecular weight of $C_6H_{12}O_6 = 180$

Valence = 1

Equivalent weight of dextrose ($C_6H_{12}O_6$) $= \frac{180}{1} = 180$

1 mEq of dextrose $= \frac{1}{1000} \times 180 = 0.18$ g = 180 mg

5% dextrose solution means 5 g of dextrose is present in 100ml solution

Or, 5000 mg of dextrose is present in 100ml solution

180 mg of dextrose = 1 mEq

5000 mg of dextrose $= \frac{1 \times 5000}{180}$ mEq $= 27.777 \approx 27.8$ mEq

Hence, 5% dextrose injection contains

Ans. 27.8 mEq of dextrose in 100ml

Example

Each 100ml of Mannitol Injection IP contains 20.0g of mannitol. Calculate (1) the molar concentrations and (2) how many mEq of mannitol are present.

Solution

Given that, the concentration of mannitol injection = 20.0g in 100ml

1. Molecular weight of mannitol, $C_6H_{14}C_6$ = 182.2

   Valence = 1

   $$\text{Equivalent weight of } C_6H_{14}C_6 = \frac{\text{Molecular weight}}{\text{Valence}}$$

   $$= \frac{182.2}{1} = 182.2$$

   $$1 \text{ mEq of } C_6H_{14}C_6 = \frac{1}{1000} \times 182.2 = 0.1822\text{g} = 182.2\text{mg}$$

   Thus, 182.2mg of $C_6H_{14}C_6$ = 1 mEq

   20g = 20000mg of $C_6H_{14}C_6$

   $$= \frac{1}{182.2} \times 20000 = 109.769 \approx 109.77\text{mEq}$$

2, 1 molar solution means 1 gm mol wt of solute in 1000 ml of solution

   So, 182.2 g of $C_6H_{14}C_6$ in 1000 ml = 1 M solution

   20 g of $C_6H_{14}C_6$ in 100 ml = 200 g in 1000 ml

   200g of $C_6H_{14}C_6$ in 1000 ml

   $$= \frac{1}{182.2} \times 200 = 1.0976 \approx 1.098 \text{ M solution}$$

   Molar concentration of the solution is 1.098 M and it contains 109.77mEq of $C_6H_{14}C_6$ (Answer)

Example

In an ORS formulation 27g of anhydrous dextrose is there. Calculate the amount of dextrose present in terms of mEqs.

Solution

Molecular weight of dextrose, $C_6H_{12}O_6$ = 180

It is a nonelectrolyte.

Valence = 1

Weight of $C_6H_{12}O_6$ present in ORS = 27 g = 27000 mg

Equivalent weight of $C_6H_{12}O_6 = \frac{180}{1} = 180$

1 mEq of $C_6H_{12}O_6 = \frac{1}{1000} \times 180 = 0.18$ g = 180 mg

180 mg of $C_6H_{12}O_6$ = 1 mEq

27000 mg of $C_6H_{12}O_6 = \frac{27000}{180}$

Ans. 150 mEqs

Example

The composition of a liquid formulation is as follows;

Each 15 ml contains

Disodium hydrogen phosphate (Na_2HPO_4, $7H_2O$) 2.7 g

Sodium biphosphate (NaH_2PO_4, H_2O) 7.2 g

Calculate milliequivalents of Na^+ ions present in 15 ml.

Solution

1. Molecular weight of Na_2HPO_4, $7H_2O$ = 268

   Valence = 2

   Equivalent weight $= \frac{268}{2} = 134$

   1 mEq of Na_2HPO_4, $7H_2O = \frac{1}{1000} \times 134 = 0.134$ g = 134 mg

   That is, 134 mg of Na_2HPO_4, $7H_2O$ = 1 mEq

   2.7 g = 2700 mg of Na_2HPO_4, $7H_2O = \frac{2700}{134} = 20.15$ mEq

   Thus, on dissociation 2.7 g of Na_2HPO_4, $7H_2O$ produces 20.15 mEqs of HPO_4^{2-} ion and 20.15 mEqs of Na^+ ions.

2. Molecular weight of NaH_2PO_4, H_2O = 138

   Valence = 1

   Equivalent weight $= \frac{138}{1} = 138$

   1 mEq of NaH_2PO_4, $H_2O = \frac{1}{1000} \times 138 = 0.138$ g = 138 mg

That is, 138 mg of NaH_2PO_4, H_2O = 1 mEq

7.2 g of NaH_2PO_4, H_2O = 7200 mg of NaH_2PO_4, H_2O = $\frac{7200}{138}$ = 52.2 mEqs of NaH_2PO_4,

Thus, in solution 52.2 mEqs of $H_2PO_4^-$ ions and 52.2 mEqs of Na^+ ions are present.

The total Na^+ ions in 15 ml of the solution = 20.15 mEq + 52.2 mEq = **72 35 mEqs** shall be present. (Answer)

Millimoles and Micromoles

A **mole** is defined as the molecular weight of a substance expressed in grams.

One **millimole** (mmol) is $\frac{1}{1000}$ th of a mole, and

One **micromole** (μmol) is $\frac{1}{1000}$ th of a millimole or one millionth of a mole.

That is, 1 m mol = 10^{-3} mol and 1 μmol = 10^{-3} mmol = 10^{-6} mol.

Example

The molecular weight of monobasic sodium phosphate is 138. How many millimoles of monobasic sodium phosphate are present in 100 g of it?

Solution

Mol wt of monobasic sodium phosphate =138

1 mole of it = 138 g

1 mmol of it = $\frac{1}{1000} \times 138$ g = 0.138 g = 138 mg

Or, 0.138 g of monobasic sodium phosphate = 1 mmol

100 g of monobasic sodium phosphate = $\frac{1 \times 100}{0.138}$ mmol

Ans. 724.64 mmol

Example

The concentration of acetic acid in a solution is 2.4g in 300ml; calculate how many moles, millimoles, micromoles and mEq of acetic acid are present per ml.

Solution

Given that the concentration of acetic acid in a solution is 2.4 g in 300 ml

1ml of the solution contains $\frac{2.4g}{300} = 0.008$ g = 8 mg of acetic acid

Molecular weight of acetic acid, CH_3COOH

$= 1 \times 12 + 3 \times 1 + 1 \times 12 + 2 \times 16 + 1 \times 1$

$= 12 + 3 + 12 + 32 + 1 = 60$

Valence of acetic acid = 1

$$\text{Equivalent weight} = \frac{\text{Molecular weight}}{\text{Valence}} = \frac{60}{1} = 60g$$

$$1 \text{ mEq of acetic acid} = \frac{1}{1000} \times 60 = 0.060g = 60 \text{ mg}$$

In other words, 60mg of acetic acid = 1 mEq

$$8 \text{ mg of acetic acid} = \frac{1 \times 8}{60} = 0.133 \text{ mEq}$$

60 g of acetic acid = 1 mole

$$0.008g \text{ of acetic acid} = \frac{1 \times 0.008}{60} = 1.33{\times}10^{-4} \text{ moles}$$

1 mole = 10^3 millimoles

$1.33{\times}10^{-4}$ moles = $1.33{\times}10^{-4}{\times}10^3$ millimoles = 0.133 mmole

1 mole = 10^6μmoles

$1.33{\times}10^{-4}$ moles = $1.33{\times}10^{-4}{\times}10^6$ μmoles = $1.33{\times}10^2$μmole

Thus, each ml of acetic acid solution contains $1.33{\times}10^{-4}$ moles, 0.133 mmole, $1.33{\times}10^2$μmole and 0.133 mEq of acetic acid. (Answer)

Example

The molecular weight of magnesium sulphate is 120. How many micrograms of it would be present in 1μmol?

Solution

The molecular weight of magnesium sulphate is 120

One mole of $MgSO_4$ = 120 g

One m mol of it $= \frac{1}{1000} \times 120 = 0.120$ g of $MgSO_4$ = 120 mg

One µmol of it $= \frac{1}{1000} \times 120$ mg = 0.120 mg = 0.120 mg × 1000

Ans. 120 µg of $MgSO_4$

Example

In two solutions (A and B) the concentrations of lead ion have been found 5µg/ml and 0.5µg/ml respectively. Express the concentrations in terms of µmol/L. (Atomic weight of lead is 207.2).

Solution

Atomic weight of lead is 207.2

One mole of lead = 207.2 g

One mmol of lead $= \frac{1}{1000} \times 207.2 = 0.2072$ g = 207.2 mg

One µmol of lead $= \frac{1}{1000} \times 207.2$ mg = 0.2072 mg = 207.2 µg

That is, 207.2 µg = 1 µmol of lead

Or, 5 µg $= \frac{1}{207.2} \times 5 = 0.0241$ µmol of lead

The concentration of lead in solution A is 5 µg/ml = 0.02413 µmol/ml

So, per liter the concentration of lead would be 0.02413 µmol/ml × 1000 ml = 241.3 µmol

Similarly, in solution B the concentration of lead = 0.5 µg/ml

$= 0.02413 \times \frac{1}{10} = 0.002413$ µmol/ml

Per liter the concentration of lead = 0.002413 µmol/ml × 1000 ml = 2.413 µmol

Hence, the concentrations of lead in solution A and B are 241.3µmol/L and 2.413µmol/L respectively. (Answer)

Osmolarity

Osmotic pressure in important to biological processes. The diffusion of solutes or the transfer of fluids through semipermeable membranes takes place through this process. According to the *United States Pharmacopeia* the parenteral preparations such as intravenous replenishment of fluid, nutrients, or electrolytes, and the osmotic diuretic mannitol must mention the composition of each formulation in their labels in terms of osmolar concentration. This information helps the practitioner to understand whether a solution is hypo-osmotic, iso-osmotic, or hyper-osmotic to the biologic fluids. For example, dextrose is a nonelectrolyte; 180 mg of it = 1 mmol or 1 mOsmol. However, this is not true with electrolytes; because the total number of particles in a solution depends on the degree of dissociation of the solute. For example, 1 mmol of NaCl dissociates completely into two ions – Na^+ and Cl^- ion. Hence, its osmolar concentration becomes 2 mOsmol. Again 1 mmol of $MgCl_2$ represents one Mg^{2+} ion and $2Cl^-$ ions, total 3ions or 3particles; hence, 1 mmol represents 3 mOsmol.

The osmotic concentration is expressed in terms of *milliosmoles* (mOsmol). Osmotic pressure being a colligative property of dilute solutions is proportional to the *total number* of particles present in the solution. In case a nonelectrolyte 1 mmol is equal to 1 mOsmol. In case of electrolyte the milliosmolar value of separate ions of an electrolyte may be calculated as;

$$\frac{\text{Concentration (mg/L)}}{\text{Atomic weight}}$$

The milliosmolar value of the whole electrolyte in solution is equal to the sum of the milliosmolar values of the separate ions.

According to the *United States Pharmacopeia,* the osmolar concentration may be calculated according to the following equation:

$$\text{mOsmol/L} = \frac{\text{Weight of substance (g/L)}}{\text{Mol wt (g)}} \times \text{No of species} \times 1000$$

Actually physicochemical interaction among solute particles increases with increase in concentration of the solute in a solution; and the practical osmolar values decrease in comparison to ideal values. When the concentration of solutes is either within the physiologic range or less, deviation from ideal conditions becomes slight or negligible. For highly concentrated solutions, the actual osmolarity may be appreciably lower than ideal values. For example, the ideal osmolarity of 0.9% sodium chloride injection is calculated as:

$$\text{mOsmol/L} = \frac{9\ \text{g/L}}{58.5\ \text{g}} \times 2 \times 1000$$

$$= 307.69$$

The measured value is 286 mOsmol/L; around 7% less than the theoretical value. This may be due to lower value of the bonding forces, n. When the concentration of sodium chloride is 0.9% the value of n is about 2. In many cases the label of the electrolyte solution mentions the theoretical or ideal or stoichiometric osmolarity, not the actual values.

There are two terms – osmolarity and osmolality; and there is difference between these terms.

Osmolarity is the milliosmoles of solute per liter of solution; whereas osmolality is the milliosmoles of solute per kilogram of solvent. For dilute aqueous solutions, osmolarity and osmolality are almost identical.

When the concentration of solutions is higher, the values of osmolarity and osmolality may be quite different.

However, care should be taken on the statement of a label regarding molarity and molality. Commercially Osmometers are available to measure osmolality. The osmolality of normal serum lies within 275 to 300 mOsmol/kg. Deviation from the values may be observed in case of shock, trauma, burns, water intoxication (overload), electrolyte imbalance, hyperglycemia, or renal failure. Different constituents of normal human serum have different concentration as well as osmotic pressure; the major concentration and contributions are of sodium and chloride ions.

Calculations of Milliosmoles

Example

Dextrose Injection contains 5% of anhydrous dextrose in water for injection. Express the concentration in terms of milliosmoles per liter.

Solution

Molecular weight of dextrose = 180

1 mmol of dextrose = 180 mg = 1mOsmol

5% solution contains 5 g in 100 ml,

Or, 50 g in 1000 ml (1 L)

Or, 50 g/L × 1000 = 50000 mg/L = $\frac{50000}{180}$ mmol/L = 277.8 mmol/L

277.8 mmol of dextrose/L = 277.8 mOsmol/L.

Hence, 5% solution of dextrose contains

Ans. 277.8 mOsmol/L.

Example

Each ml of Mannitol Injection contains 100 mg of mannitol. Calculate how many mOsmol of it are there in one liter?

Solution

Given that the concentration of solution = 100mg of mannitol/ml

The amount of mannitol in 1000ml = 100mg×1000 =100g

The molecular weight of mannitol = 182.2

1 mole of $C_6H_{14}O_6$ = 182.2g

1 millimole (mmol) of $C_6H_{14}O_6$ = 182.2mg = 1 mOsmol

That is, 182.2mg of $C_6H_{14}O_6$ = 1 mOsmol

100g of $C_6H_{14}O_6$ = $\frac{1 \times 100 \times 1000}{182.2}$ mOsmol

= 548.847 ≈ 548.85mOsmol

Hence, one liter of solution of $C_6H_{14}O_6$ contains 548.85 mOsmol of mannitol. (Answer)

Example

A solution contains 106 mg of Na^+ ions in 100 mL. How many milliosmoles would be there in a liter of this solution?

Solution

Atomic weight of Na^+ = 23

1 mole of Na^+ ion = 23 g

1 mmol of Na^+ ion = 23 mg = 1 mOsmol

In other words, 23 mg of Na^+ ion =1mOsmol

So, 106 mg of Na^+ ion/100 ml = $\frac{106}{23}$ = 4.61mOsmol/100 ml

That is, 100 ml of the solution contains 4.61 mOsmol of Na^+ ion

1000 ml of the solution contains $4.61 \times \frac{1000}{100}$

Ans. 46.1mOsmol of Na^+ ion

Example

A solution of potassium chloride contains 15 mg% of K^+ ion. How many milliosmoles of K^+ would be in a liter of Solution?

Solution

Atomic weight of K^+ = 39

1 mmol of K^+= 39 mg = 1 mOsmol

The concentration of the solution is 15 mg%.

That is, 100 ml of the solution contains 15 mg of K^+ ion.

Or, 1000 ml contains 150 mg of K^+ ion

39 mg of K^+ ion = 1mOsmol of K^+ ion

150 mg of K^+ ion = $\frac{150}{74.5}$ = 2.01 mmol of K^+ ion = 2.01 mOsmol of K^+ ion

Hence, the solution would contain

Ans. 2.01 mOsmol of K^+ ion per liter

Example

The concentration of solution of calcium chloride ($CaCl_2$) is1.5%. How many milliosmoles of ions would be in a liter of solution? Assume complete dissociation of the electrolyte.

Solution

Osmotic concentration (in terms of milliosmoles) is a function of the total number of particles or ions present. Assuming complete dissociation, 1 mmol of calcium chloride ($CaCl_2$) represents 3 mOsmol of total particles (Ca^{2+} + $2Cl^-$).

Molecular weight of $CaCl_2$ = 111

1 mmol of $CaCl_2$ = 111 mg of $CaCl_2$ = 3 mOsmol

1.5% of $CaCl_2$ = 1.5g of $CaCl_2$ in 100 ml

In other words, in 100 ml solution, 1.5 g = 1500 mg of $CaCl_2$ is present

In 1000 ml of solution, 1500 mg $\times \frac{1000}{100}$ = 15000 mg of $CaCl_2$ is present

111 mg of $CaCl_2$ is = 3 mOsmol

15000 mg of $CaCl_2$ = $\frac{3 \times 15000}{111}$ = 405.4 mOmol

Thus, osmotic concentration of one liter of solution 405.4 mOmol/L (Answer)

Example

A solution is prepared by dissolving 2.0g of sodium chloride in 50ml of water. How many mOsmol of ions would be produced in the solution?

Solution

Given that the solution contains 2 g in 50 ml

Dissociation of NaCl is NaCl = Na^+ + Cl^-

Thus, 2 particles (Na^+ and Cl^-) are formed from each molecule of NaCl

Molecular weight of NaCl = 58.45

1 mole of NaCl = 58.45 g

1 mmol NaCl = 58.45 mg NaCl = 2 mOsmol

Or, 58.45mg of NaCl = 2 mOsmol

2 g or 2000 mg of NaCl = $\frac{2 \times 2000}{58.45}$ = 68.43 mOsmol

Thus, **68.43 mOsmol of Na+** ions and **68.43 mOsmol of Cl- ions** would be there in the solution.

Water and Electrolyte Balance in the Body

For good health maintenance of water and electrolyte balance in the body is essential. Water is the primary medium for survival of cells, for the intake of nutrients and the excretion of metabolic waste products. Usually, the osmolality of body fluid is maintained within narrow limits. Water is supplied through intake of food, the regulatory endocrine processes. Balance of water is maintained by excretion through the kidneys, lungs, skin, and the gastrointestinal system. In clinical practice, fluid and electrolyte therapy is carried out either to supply maintenance requirements or to restore serious losses. There are various reasons for loss of water and/or electrolytes from the body such as vomiting, diarrhea, profuse sweating, fever, chronic renal failure, diuretic therapy, surgery, etc. Depending on the patient's specific requirements the type of therapy is undertaken such as oral or parenteral and the content of the fluid administered. For example;

- A daily oral potassium supplement along with adequate intake of water would be sufficient for a patient taking diuretics.
- Rehydration with or without added electrolytes would be adequate for an athlete.
- Parenteral administration of fluids and electrolytes to a hospitalized patient is ordinarily sufficient to restore metabolic function.
- Patients with severe loss of fluid require immediate and substantial replacement of fluids and electrolytes through intravenous administration of electrolytes and fluids. Such loss of fluids may result from surgery, trauma, burns, or shock.

Under normal conditions the total body water ranges between 55% and 65% of body weight in adult males. In case of adult women, total body water ranges within 45% and 55%. Body water of newborn infants is about 75%. However, the amount of body water depends on the amount of fat present in body. If the amount of fat is more, the proportion of water would be less. With growth and increase in body fat the proportion of water decreases. Two thirds of the body water of an adult is intracellular and one third is extracellular. The extracellular body water decreases in infants in the first year from approximately 45% to 30% while the intracellular portion increases with gradual growth of the infant.

Average daily requirements of water intake for healthy individuals can be calculated

- On a weight basis- about 32 mL/kg for adults and 100 to 150 mL/kg for infants.
- On average body surface area basis - about 1500 mL of water per square meter of body surface area for adults.

These estimated requirements differ greatly in persons with clinical disorders affecting water and electrolyte homeostasis and in conditions of acute deficit. Approximately 2500 mL of daily water intake (from ingested liquids and foods and from oxidative metabolism) would be sufficient for an adult to balance the daily water output.

The composition of body fluids generally depends on the body compartments:

- Intracellular (within cells),
- Intravascular (blood plasma), or
- Interstitial (between cells in the tissue).
- Extracellular *(*intravascular and interstitial fluids commonly grouped together*)*

Although all electrolytes and nonelectrolytes in body fluids contribute to osmotic activity, major contributions are by sodium and chloride ions in *extra*cellular fluid, and potassium and phosphate predominate in *intra*cellular fluid.

In general, water can freely permeate through all cell membranes. The osmolality of the extracellular fluid (about 290 mOsm/kg water) is almost equal to that of the intracellular fluid. Therefore, the plasma osmolality is a convenient and accurate reference to intracellular osmolality and may be estimated by using the formula;

$$\text{Plasma osmolality (mOsm/kg)} = 2\ ([\text{Na}] + [\text{K}])\ \text{plasma} + \frac{[\text{BUN}]}{2.8} + \frac{[\text{Glucose}]}{18}$$

Where, sodium [Na] and potassium [K] are in mEq/L, and blood urea nitrogen [BUN] and [Glucose] concentrations are in mg/100 mL.

Example

What would be the daily requirement of water for a healthy adult with a body surface area of 2.0 m^2?

Solution

As per body surface area water requirement for a healthy adult is 1500 ml/sq.m

In other words, for 1 sq m body surface water requirement is 1500 ml

For 2 sq.m body surface water requirement $\frac{1500 \times 2}{1}$ ml

Ans. 3000 ml

Example

The body weight of a male person is 65 kg. Calculate the average daily requirement of water.

Solution

As per body weight the daily water requirement = 32 ml per kg

The weight of the person = 65 kg.

Then, the daily water requirement = $\frac{32 \text{ ml} \times 65 \text{ kg}}{1 \text{ kg}}$

Ans. 2080 ml

Example

The body weight of an infant is 4.5 kg. What would be the approximate daily requirement of water?

Solution

For a healthy infant the approximate daily requirement of water

= 125 ml per kg.

For a healthy infant the approximate daily requirement of water

$= \frac{125 \text{ ml} \times 4.5 \text{ kg}}{1\text{kg}}$

Ans. 562.5 ml

Example

The plasma contains 135 mEq of sodium/L, 4.5 mEq of potassium/L, 14 mg of blood urea nitrogen/dL, and 90 mg of glucoses/dL. Calculate the plasma osmolality.

Solution

As the standard formula

Plasma osmolality (mOsm/kg)

$$= 2\ ([Na] + [K])\ \text{plasma} + \frac{[BUN]}{2.8} + \frac{[Glucose]}{18}$$

$$= 2(135\ mEq/L + 4.5\ mEq/L) + \frac{14}{2.8}\ mg/dL + \frac{90}{18}\ mg/dL$$

(1 dL = 100 ml)

$$= 2 \times 139.5 + 5 + 5$$

Ans. 289

Example

A solution is prepared by dissolving 0.25g of copper sulphate and 0.5g of sodium hydroxide in 100ml. Calculate how many (1) milliequivalents, and (2) mOsmol of each ion are present in the solution. Assume complete dissociation.

Solution

Given that, in 100ml solution $CuSO_4$ present = 0.25g and NaOH present = 0.5g

1. Molecular weight of $CuSO_4$ = 63.54+ 32.07+4×16 = 159.61

   Valence = 2

   Equivalent weight of $CuSO_4 = \frac{159.61}{2} = 79.80$

   So, 79.80mg of $CuSO_4$ = 1mEq

   0.25g = 250mg of $CuSO_4 = \frac{1 \times 250}{79.80}$

   = 3.132 mEq of $CuSO_4$ (Answer)

   Molecular weight of NaOH = 40

   Valence = 1

   Equivalent weight of NaOH = 40

   So, 40 mg of NaOH = 1 mEq

   0.5g = 500mg of NaOH $= \frac{1 \times 500}{40}$

Ans. 12.5 mEq of NaOH

2. On dissociation 1 molecule of NaOH produces 2 ions (Na^+ and OH^-)

   Molecular weight = 40

   1 mole of NaOH = 40g

   1 mmol of NaOH = 40mg of NaOH = 2mOsmol

   Or, 40mg of NaOH = 2mOsmol

   So, 500mg of NaOH = $\frac{2 \times 500}{40}$

   Ans. 25 mOsmol of Na^+ and 25 mOsmol of OH^- ions

   Dissociation reaction of $CuSO_4$ is $CuSO_4 = Cu^{2+} + SO_4^{2-}$

   Nos. of ions formed = 2

   Molecular weight of $CuSO_4$ = 179.80

   1 mole of $CuSO_4$ = 179.80g of $CuSO_4$

   1 mmole of $CuSO_4$ = 179.80mg of $CuSO_4$ = 2 mOsmol

   So, 250mg of $CuSO_4$ = $\frac{2 \times 250}{179.80}$

   Ans. 2.78mOsmol of Cu^{2+} and 2.78mOsmol of SO_4^{2-} ions.

Example

The composition of a parenteral solution is given below;

Dextrose, Anhydrous	25.0 g
Sodium chloride	2.25 g
Potassium chloride	0.745 g
Sterile Water for Injection	q.s. 500 ml

Calculate how many milliequivalents of dextrose, sodium chloride, potassium and chloride, dextrose present and the total osmolarity of the preparation.

Solution

Milliequivalents of sodium chloride:

Molecular weight of NaCl = 58.5

Equivalent weight = 58.5

$1 \text{ mEq of NaCl} = 58.5 \times \frac{1}{1000} = 0.0585\text{g} = 58.5 \text{ mg}$

That is, 58.5 mg of NaCl = 1 mEq

$2.25 \text{ g of NaCl} = \frac{2.25 \times 1000}{58.5} \text{ mEq} = 38.46 \text{ mEq of NaCl;}$

Thus, 38.5 mEq of Na^+ ions and 38.5 mEq of Cl^- ions are present.

Milliequivalents of Potassium chloride:

Molecular weight of KCl = 74.5

Equivalent weight = 74.5

$1 \text{ mEq of KCl} = 74.5\text{g} \times \frac{1}{1000} = 0.0745 \text{ g} = 74.5 \text{ mg}$

That is, 74.5 mg of KCl = 1 mEq

$0.745 \text{ g of KCl} = \frac{0.745 \times 1000}{74.5} \text{ mEq} = 10 \text{ mEq of KCl}$

Thus, 10mEq of K^+ ions and 10mEq of Cl^- ions are there

Na^+ ion 38.5 mEq

K^+ ion 10 mEq

Cl^- ion (10 mEq + 38.5 mEq) = 48.5 mEq

Millimoles of dextrose anhydrous: Molecular weight of $C_6H_{12}O_6$ = 180

1 mole of $C_6H_{12}O_6$ = 180 g

1 mmol of $C_6H_{12}O_6$ = 180 mg

In other words, 180 mg of $C_6H_{12}O_6$ = 1mmol of $C_6H_{12}O_6$

25 g of $C_6H_{12}O_6$ = 25000 mg of $C_6H_{12}O_6 = \frac{25 \times 1000}{180}$ = 138. 9 mmol

In terms of Osmolarity:

Dextrose, anhydrous: 139 mmol ×1 particle per mmol = 139 mOsmol

NaCl: 38.5 mEq × 2 particles per mEq (or mmol) = 77 mOsmol

KCl: 10 mEq × 2 particles per mEq (or mmol) = 20 mOsmol

Ans. Total 236 mOsmol

Exercise

1. A solution contains 40 mEq of sodium chloride (NaCl) per liter. What is the concentration, in milligrams per milliliter?

   Ans: 2.34 mg/ml

2. A solution contains 50 mEq of sodium hydroxide (NaOH) per milliliter. What is the concentration, in milligrams per milliliter and in %age?

   Ans: 2 mg/ml and 0.2%w/v

3. Express the concentration of a solution containing 0.735g of calcium chloride ($CaCl_2, 2H_2O$) per ml in mEq per milliliter.

   Ans: 10mEq/ml

4. Express the concentration of a solution containing 20 mEq of calcium chloride ($CaCl_2, 2H_2O$) per ml in grams per milliliter.

   Ans: 1.47g/ml

5. Express the concentration of a solution containing 125 mEq of calcium chloride ($CaCl_2$) per liter in %w/v.

   Ans: 0.695%w/v

6. A solution contains 50 mEq of magnesium chloride ($MgCl_2$) per liter. What is the percent (w/v) concentration?

   Ans: 0.235%w/v

7. The concentration of a solution is 2.5 mg % of Na^+. What would be this concentration in terms of mEq per liter?

   Ans: 1.09 mEq/L

8. In a blood sample the concentration of phosphate ion (HPO_4^{2-}) in plasma was found to be 1.5 mEq/L. Express the concentration in terms of mg%.

   Ans: 7.27 mg%

9. How many mEqs of sodium chloride are present in 0.4 g of anhydrous sodium Chloride (NaCl)?

   Ans: 6.84 mEq

10. A liter of solution contains 2.5 g of anhydrous sodium citrate ($Na_3C_6H_5O_7$). Calculate the concentration of Na^+ ion and $C_6H_5O_7^{3-}$ ions in terms of mEq.

    Ans: 29.07mEq of Na^+ ion and 29.07mEq of $C_6H_5O_7^{3-}$ ions

11. A solution contains 1.0 g of Disodium hydrogen phosphate (Na_2HPO_4, $7H_2O$) and 1.2g of dihydrogen sodium phosphate (NaH_2PO_4, H_2O) per ml. Calculate milliequivalents of Na^+ ions present in 5 ml.

Ans: 80.8 mEq of Na^+ ions/5ml

12. The molecular weight of potassium dichromate is 294.18. How many millimoles of potassium dichromate are present in 50 g of it?

Ans: 169.96 mmol

13. On analysis 1.5lts of a solution was found to contain 3.62μmol of lead. How many micrograms of lead were present in 1ml? Atomic weight of lead is 207.2.

Ans: 0.5μg/ml

14. Dextrose Injection IP contains 10g of anhydrous dextrose per 100ml of water for injection. Express the concentration in terms of milliosmoles per liter.

Ans: 555.6 mOsmol/L

15. A solution contains 53 mg of K^+ ions and 53 mg of Na^+ ions per 100 mL. How many milliosmoles of the two ions would be there in a liter of this solution?

Ans: 23.04 mOsmol of Na^+ ions /L &
13.59 mOsmol of K^+ ions /L

16. A solution of potassium chloride contains milliosmoles of K^+ ion/L. How many milligrams of K^+ ion would be present in 100 ml of the solution?

Ans: 3.35 mg%

17. The concentration of solution of magnesium chloride is 2.0%. How many milliosmoles of ions would be in a liter of solution? Assume complete dissociation of the electrolyte.

Ans: 630.18 mOmol/L

18. On analysis a sample of potable water was found to contain 10μmol of iron per ml. Calculate the concentration in terms of micrograms per liter? Atomic weight of lead is 55.845

Ans: 558.4 μgL

19. A sample of potable water was found to contain 0.4mg of copper sulphate per liter. Calculate the concentration of copper in terms of ppm? Atomic weight of copper is 63.55, mol wt of $CuSO_4$ is 159.61 and the density of sample water was 0.9982g/ml at room temperature.

Ans: 0.159ppm

20. A solution contains 10 mg of NaCl ions per mL. What would be this concentration in terms of mEq per liter?

Ans: 170.94 mEq per liter

21. A powder mixture when dissolved in water produces 2% solution of KCl. How many mEqs of K^+ and Cl^- ions would be in a liter of this solution?

Ans: 268.46mEqs of K^+ and Cl^- 268.46mEqs of ions

22. A powder mixture when dissolved in water produces 0.3% solution of $CaCl_2$. How many mEqs of Ca^{2+} and Cl^- ions would be in a liter of this solution?

Ans: 54.05mEqs of Ca^{2+} and 54.05mEqs of Cl^- ions

23. In a solution the concentration of calcium chloride ($CaCl_2$) is1.5mg/ml. How many milliosmoles of the ions would be present in a liter of solution? Assume complete dissociation of the electrolyte.

Ans: 40.54 mOsmol/L

24. A solution of anhydrous dextrose contains is138.9mmol of dextrose. How many grams of dextrose are present in the solution?

Ans: 27 g

25. The composition of a parenteral solution is given below;

Dextrose, Anhydrous	13.50 g s
Sodium chloride	1.90 g
Potassium chloride	1.15 g
Sterile Water for Injection q.s.	500 ml

Calculate the milliequivalents of sodium, potassium and chloride, millimoles of dextrose and total osmolarity per liter of the preparation.

Ans: 32.48mmol of NaCl,
15. 44 mmol of KCl,
75 mmol of dextrose;
Total osmolarity per liter 341.7 mOsmol

8

IV Infusions, Enternal and Parenteral Nutrition, BMI, Food Nutrition Level

Parenteral Preparation

The term ***parenteral*** is defined as any medication route other than the alimentary canal; and thus, includes all routes of injection.

The basic information are provided in this chapter to facilitate the reader to:

- Solve the numerical problems related to pediatric intravenous infusions.
- Perform calculations for intravenous additives.
- Perform rate-of-flow calculations for intravenous fluids.
- Utilize correctly the rate-of-flow tables and nomograms.

Injections

These are sterile solutions or suspensions of a drug substance in an aqueous or nonaqueous vehicle intended to be administered parenterally. These are administered (injected) through a needle into different parts of the body; such as *intra-articular* (into the joints), intrasynovial (joint fluid), *intraspinal* (into spinal column), *intrathecal* (into spinal fluid), *intra-arterial* (into arteries), and in an emergency, even *intracardiac* (the heart).

Most injections are administered

- into a muscle (*intramuscular, I.M., IM*),

- into vein (*intravenous, I.V., IV*),
- into the skin (*intradermal, I.D., ID, intracutaneous*), or
- Under the skin (*subcutaneous, sub-Q, SQ, hypodermic*).

Injections are usually packaged in small volume ampoules or in prefilled disposable syringes for single-dose use; in vials and pen-injectors for single- or multiple-dose use; or in large volume plastic bags or glass containers for administration by slow intravenous infusion depending on the use.

Most injections are available as *ready to use* either in form of solutions or suspensions. The drug content is labeled as, for example, '10 mg/mL.'

Others are dry powder, to be reconstituted to make either a solution or suspension by adding a specified volume of diluent before use. These are labeled as, for example, '10 mg/vial.' To determine the correct volume of diluent to be added to prepare an injection of a certain concentration some calculations are to done. Small-volume injections may be administered as such or they may be used as *additives* to large-volume parenteral fluids for intravenous infusion.

Intravenous (IV) Infusions

are sterile, aqueous preparations. Relatively large volumes of these are administered intravenously. These are used to restore the blood volume and/or to supply electrolytes, nutrients, or medications. Most of these preparations are commonly administered in following circumstances;

- When the patient is under critical care,
- The patient is infirm, dehydrated, or malnourished,
- During and after surgery.

Health care professionals are involved in the infusion therapy. The *United States Pharmacopeia* has established requirements for the compounding of sterile preparations.

Most of the intravenous infusions are solutions; some contain nutrients or therapeutic agents, or blood and blood products in form of very fine dispersions. Some intravenous solutions are isotonic or nearly isotonic with blood. Isotonicity is not absolutely necessary; because the fluid usually administered is almost immediately diluted by the circulating blood. For this reason, these are normally administered slowly.

Commercial infusions are available in glass or plastic bottles or collapsible plastic 'bags'. The volume ranges from 50 mL (a minibag) from 1000 mL. The smaller volume preparations are usually administered in treatment of pediatric patients and adults who need relatively small volumes. When a smaller intravenous bag is attached to the tubing of a larger intravenous preparation being administered, it is called an IV piggyback (IVPB). Commonly a large volume parenteral is abbreviated as LVP and a small-volume parenteral as SVP. Such classification is made on the basis of volume. Additional drugs or additives are sometimes added to these infusions for rapid distribution in the circulation.

Administration Set

Administration set is attached to the bottle or plastic bag to deliver intravenous fluid into a patient's vein. There are two types of sets - standard (macro-drip) and pediatric (micro-drip) used to administer an infusion into a patient's vein. Depending on the particular set used, the drip rate can vary from 10 to 60 drops/mL. The standard set deliver 10 to 15 drops/mL; while a micro-drip set can deliver 60 drops/ml. The drip rate for blood transfusion sets usually varies from 10 to 15 drops/mL and 250 to 500 mL of infusions is administered over a 2- to 4-hour period.

For administration of an infusion, the bag or bottle is hung on a stand well above the patient's portal vein. Flow of the solution is facilitated by gravity and its rate is controlled either by a pinch cock or by an electronic volumetric infusion pump. Some specially designed infusion pumps are able to deliver micro-infusion, such as 0.1 mL per hour, or to deliver as much as 2000 mL per hour. Depending on the drug being administered and the requirements of the patient, the flow rate is controlled. Electronic controllers can also be used to maintain the desired flow rate.

Special needles or catheters such as large, intermediate, and small-gauge are used for administration of infusions. Based on the patient's age and clinical requirement, the size of the needle is selected. The flow rate is slow when narrow gauge needle is used. Intravenous infusions may be administered continuously or intermittently.

Example

For intravenous infusion how many grams of dextrose and sodium chloride are to be used to prepare a 500 mL of D5 1/2NS?

Solution

The full meaning of D51/2NS is 5% Dextrose and ½ of the concentration of Normal saline (0.45% sodium chloride).

500 ml of 5% Dextrose = $500 \times \frac{5}{100}$ g = **25 g** of Dextrose

500 ml of 0.45% Sodium chloride = $500 \times \frac{0.45}{100}$ g

Ans. 2.25 g of Sodium chloride

Example

Calculate (i) the number of drops and (ii) the duration of time (in minutes), required to administer 60 mL of intravenous solutions using a micro-drip set, at 60 drops/mL, and a standard administration set, at 15 drops/mL, in each case the flow rate is one drop per second.

Solution

The micro-drip set delivers 1 ml in 60 drops

(i) Nos. of drops delivered in 60 ml = 60 drops/mL × 60 mL = 3600 drops

The flow rate is 1 drop/sec = 60 drops/minute

(ii) Time required to deliver 3600 drops = $\frac{3600 \text{ drops}}{60 \text{ drops}}$ minute

= 60 minutes (Anss).

The standard set delivers 15 drops/ml

(i) Nos. of drops in 60 ml is delivered = 15 drops/mL × 60 mL = 900 drops

The flow rate is 1 drop/sec = 60 drops/minute

(ii) Time required to deliver 900 drops = $\frac{900 \text{ drops}}{60 \text{ drops}}$ minute

= 15 minutes (Answer)

Example

An intravenous infusion of 540 ml dextrose injection is being administered at a rate of 10 drops per minute using a standard administration set at 15 drops/ml. Find out the time at which the bottle would be finished.

Solution

Flow rate is 10 drops/min

Standard administration set forms 15 drops/ml

Thus, Nos. of drops formed out of 540 ml

$$= 540 \text{ ml} \times 15 \text{ drops/ml} = 8100$$

The flow rate is 10 drops per minute

That is, 10 drops are delivered in min

8100 drops are delivered in $\frac{1}{10} \times 8100 \text{ min} = 810 \text{ min} = \frac{810}{60}$

Ans. 13 hrs 30 min

Enteral and Parenteral Nutrition

In enteral and parenteral nutrition services, in institutional and home care it is necessary to calculate and participate in the selection, preparation, and administration of nutritional formulas. Now a days, the pharmacists are involved in this activity.

In community practice, the pharmacists are supposed to counsel the patients on matters of nutrition. It is well known that obesity and many chronic conditions, including hypertension, coronary heart disease, sleep apnea, and type 2 diabetes mellitus may be due to poor dietary intake. For the maintenance of good health, controlled weight good diet is required. Enteral nutrition may be used for total or supplemental nutrition, or for patients coming off parenteral nutrition as a transitional phase.

Tubes are inserted into the stomach or small intestine to provide nutritional support. This method is called enteral nutrition. It is applied to patients who do not have the ability or who have decreased ability to take food by mouth. However, nasogastric tubes (tube inserted through nose) may be used, or through surgical openings tubes may be inserted into the stomach, duodenum, or jejunum. Surgical insertions are generally applied to cases where relatively long-term feeding of patients, more than 4 weeks, is required. Tube feeding may be intermittent or continuous. In addition to nutritional requirements, they can be used to replace daily water loss through urination, bowel function, respiration, and perspiration.

Patient's caloric requirements can be met by enteral nutrition. The need for protein, carbohydrate and fat, vitamins and minerals, dietary fiber, electrolytes, and fluids can be ingested by this method. Commercial formulations of enteral feed are available with various compositions.

Some are specifically made for pediatric or adult patients. Some provide a balanced or general requirement. Some are of high in calories, containing protein, amino acids, fat, and/or fiber. Others contain low carbohydrate, sodium, or cholesterol. There are some formulations designed to meet the disease-specific requirements such as for renal or hepatic disease or diabetes, lactose intolerance, or allergy to specific foods. However, additional components may be mixed with commercial formulations to meet specific purpose.

The osmolality of an enteral formulation is important. Sometimes hyper-osmolar formulations exhibit intolerance to a patient. This may cause vomiting, osmotic diarrhea, abdominal distention, and other symptoms. Many formulations made for infants have osmolalities within 150 and 380 mOsmol/kg. Adult formulations have osmolalities between 270 and 700mOsmol/kg. The osmolality of extracellular fluid ranges from 285 to 295 mOsmol/kg. If necessary, therapeutic formulations can be administered through the enteral feeding tubes after diluting with liquid dosage forms. Well-diluted slurries can be prepared and administered from the solid contents of tablets or capsules. Liquid medications with high osmolalities, even greater than 1000 mOsmol/kg, can be diluted with 10 to 30 mL of sterile water before administration. However, the feeding schedule should not be disturbed and care should be taken to avoid drug incompatibilities with other medications and nutritional components.

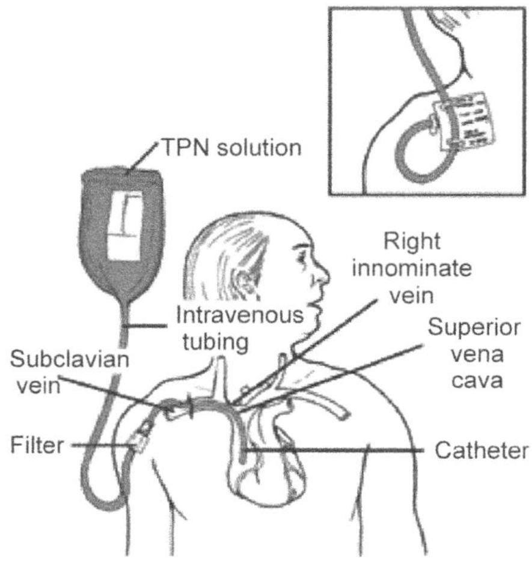

Figure 8.1 Different routes of nutrition – oral, enteral and parenteral.

Parenteral Nutrition

Feeding of a patient by the intravenous infusion of fluids and basic nutrients is called Parenteral Nutrition (PN) or intravenous hyperalimentation (IVH or HAL). When parenteral nutrition is given to supplement the nutrition, it is called partial parenteral nutrition (PPN). It supplements oral intake and provides daily nutritional requirements partially. When complete daily nutritional requirements are provided through intravenous infusion it is called total parenteral nutrition (TPN).

Parenteral nutritions are given to the patients who cannot receive adequate nutrition through oral route. In general, severely malnourished patients who are critically ill and cannot be fed orally are given parenteral nutrition. Central administration lines are inserted into the superior vena cava, while peripheral lines are inserted into veins of the arm or hand. Concentrated dextrose solutions are hypertonic and may damage the veins; hence, central lines are preferred over peripheral lines for higher concentrations of dextrose, 25% or more. Generally, nutritional formulations for peripheral parenteral nutrition are isotonic or almost isotonic.

The composition of parenteral nutrition formulations are given below:

Macronutrients:

Carbohydrate, such as dextrose

Protein, such as amino acids

Fat, such as lipid emulsions

Micronutrients:

Electrolytes

Vitamins

Trace elements

Sterile water for injection

Formulations for parenteral nutrition are available commercially (ready to use) or they may be prepared in a pharmacy as per requirement. The nutritional requirements and formulations differ on basis of the following parameters;

- Age groups, such as neonates, general pediatrics, adults.
- Gender, such as male or female.
- Type of disease, such as renal, liver, pulmonary.
- Current nutritional status, such as acute or mild malnourished.

Electrolytes, vitamins, and minerals, amino acids, dextrose, etc. are available in small and large pack; usually in the form of large-volume parenterals (LVPs) or small-volume parenterals (ampoules and vials).

Typically, infusion rates are kept between about 25 to 50 mL per hour; may be adjusted every 8 to 12 hourly as per the patient's condition and fluid and nutritional status. Infusions may also be administered by gravity flow.

Nutritional Requirements

Nutritional requirements mean the quantities of macronutrients and micronutrients required for a patient to achieve or maintain the desired nutritional condition. The quantitative amounts of fluid and specific nutrients required vary with an individual's age, sex, nutritional status, disease, and physical condition.

Fluid Requirements

The daily fluid or water requirement of a patient is decided by selecting any of the three ways - 30 mL/kg of body weight, 1500 mL per square meter of body surface area, or 1 mL/kcal of nutrition requirement. However, the values may increase, in case of patients who are dehydrated or decrease in case of patients with renal failure or congestive heart failure. In general for adults infusion of 2 to 3 litres per day is sufficient. Otherwise the approximate daily water requirement may be calculated as flows:

Table 8.1 Daily requirement of water with different parameter

Parameter	Daily Requirement of Water
Age	
Neonates	120 – 180 ml/kg
1 – 12 months	150 ml/kg (max. 200 ml)
Weight	
Less than 10 kg	100 ml/kg
10 – 20 kg	1000 ml + 50 ml/kg (above 10 kg)
More than 20 kg	1500 ml + 20 ml/kg (above 20 kg)
Body surface area	
'A' Sq.m	1500 ml/day/Sq.m × 'A' Sq.m
Calorie requirement	
'B kcal'/day	1.2 ml/kcal × 'B kcal'/day

Caloric Requirements

Calorie (Cal) is defined as the amount of heat required to raise the temperature of 1 g of water 1°C. While kilocalorie (kcal) is the amount of heat required to raise the temperature of 1 kg of water 1°C. The unit is used in metabolism studies. The caloric requirements for persons or patients vary, depending on their physical state and medical condition. In general, the Harris-Benedict equations are used to calculate the basal general, the Harris-Benedict equations are used to calculate the basal energy expenditure (BEE) or basal metabolic rate (BMR), the requirements for nonprotein calories. The BEE is also called the resting metabolic energy (RME) or the resting energy expenditure (REE). This is the energy required to carry out primary metabolic functions, such as breathing, ion transport, normal turnover of enzymes and other components of body, etc. This may be calculated by using Harris-Benedict equations. However, any diet having high-calorie value and high-fat content are likely to result in overweight and obesity and consequently illnesses.

The total daily expenditure (TDE) of energy may be calculated for activity and stress factors by using the given formula:

Harris-Benedict equations:

For male

BEE = 66.5 + [13.75 × Weight (kg)] + [5.003 × Height (cm)]
– [6.67 × Age (Yrs)] for female

BEE = 655.1 + [9.56 × Weight (kg)] + [1.86 × Height (cm)]
– [4.68 × Age (Yrs)]

where, **Activity factor** is considered as

1.3 (Ambulatory) and

1.2 (Bed ridden)

1.2 (surgery)

1.4 - 1.6 (Infection)

1.3 – 1.5 (Trauma)

1.5 – 2.1(Burns)

However, without using Harris-Benedict equations the BEE may be roughly estimated as;

- 25 kcal/kg/day for mildly stressed hospitalized patients
- 35 kcal/kg/day for moderately stressed patients,
- 45 kcal/kg/day for postoperative patients,
- 60 kcal/ kg/day for hypercatabolic patients,
- 100 kcal/kg/day for infants,
- 80 - 100 kcal/kg/day for children, and
- 35 - 60 kcal/kg/day for teenagers.

Example

A male person is 60 years old, and is 5ft 6 inch tall. If he weighs 110 lbs, calculate his basal energy expenditure (BEE) according to the Harris-Benedict concept.

Solution

Given that, the weight of male person = 110 lbs = $110 \times \frac{1}{2.2} = 50$ kg

Height = 5ft 6 inches = $5 \times 12 \times 2.54$ cm + 6×2.54cm = 167.64cm

Age = 60 years

According to Harris-Benedict equation the basal energy expenditure (BEE) for a male

$$= 66.5 + [13.75 \times \text{Weight (kg)}] + [5.003 \times \text{Height (cm)}] - [6.67 \times \text{Age (Yrs)}]$$

$$= 66.5 + [13.75 \times 50 \text{ kg}] + [5.003 \times 167.64 \text{ cm}] - [6.67 \times 60 \text{ years}]$$

$$= 66.5 + 687.5 + 838.70 - 400.2$$

Ans. 1192.5 kcal

Example

A female person is 55 years old, and is 5ft tall. If she weighs 100 lbs, calculate his basal energy expenditure (BEE) according to the Harris-Benedict concept.

Solution

Given that, the weight of male person = 101 lbs

$$= 101 \times \frac{1}{2.2} = 45.91 \text{ kg}$$

Height = 5 ft = $5 \times 12 \times 2.54$ cm = 152.4 cm

Age = 55 years

According to Harris-Benedict equation the basal energy expenditure (BEE) for a female

$$= 655.1 + [9.56 \times \text{Weight (kg)}] + [1.86 \times \text{Height (cm)}] - [4.68 \times \text{Age (Yrs)}]$$

$$= 655.1 + [9.56 \times 45.91\text{kg}] + [1.86 \times 152.4\text{cm}] - [4.68 \times 55\text{years}]$$

$= 655.1 + 438.9 + 283.46 - 257.4$

Ans. 1120.06 kcal

The Dietary Guidelines for Americans, 2005 have stated the daily requirements of the caloric in the Table below. In fact, as per the United States Department of Agriculture, the caloric requirements stated are suitable for most of the persons.

Table 8.2 Daily dietary requirements

Age group	Sedentary*		Moderate**		Active***	
	Male	Female	Male	Female	Male	Female
2 – 3	1000	1000	1000-1400	1000-1400	1000-1400	1000-1400
4 – 8	1400	1200	1400-1600	1400-1600	1600-2000	1400-1800
9 – 13	1800	1600	1800-2200	1600-2000	2000-2600	1800-2200
14 – 18	2200	1800	2400-2800	2000	2800-3200	2400
19 – 30	2400	2000	2600-2800	2000-2200	3000	2400
31 – 50	2200	1800	2400-2600	2000	2800-3000	2200
50+	2000	1600	2200-2400	1800	2400-2800	2000-2200

Note:

* Sedentary includes only light physical activity associated with daily life.

** Moderately active includes walking 1.5 to 3 miles per day at 3 to 4 miles per hour or equivalent other activity.

*** Active includes walking more than 3 miles per day at 3 to 4 miles per hour or equivalent other activity.

Unless otherwise mentioned the calorie obtained from different category of food materials may be calculated as the following guidelines;

Carbohydrates provide 4 kcal/g;
Proteins provide 4 kcal/g; and
Fats provide 9 kcal/g.

Carbohydrate Requirements

For physical activity and proper functioning of organs the energy is required. Carbohydrates supply the body with the required energy. The carbohydrates are broken down in the digestive system into sugar molecules which are subsequently used by the body's cells as a source of energy. Diabetics control the intake of carbohydrate. There is a system, called the glycemic index that classifies carbohydrates based on how quickly and how high they boost blood sugar compared to pure glucose.

Carbohydrate is the primary source of cellular energy. Usually, dextrose provides 3.4 kcal of energy per gram. For example, each 100 mL of a 25% dextrose injection provides 85 kcal of energy. For enteral nutrition, the factor used is 4kcal/g.

$$\text{TDE} = \text{BEE} \times \text{Activity factors} \times \text{Stress}$$

Example

A girl is 20 years old and her weight is 120 lbs.; calculate her basal energy expenditure (BEE) without using the Harris-Benedict concept.

Solution

Given that, the girl is 20years old,

The weight = 120 lbs $\times \frac{1}{2.2}$ = 54.54kg

Hence she is a teenager and requires 35 - 60 kcal/kg/day.

Thus, the minimum BEE of the girl = 35× 54.54 kcal = 1908.9 kcal

The maximum BEE of the girl = 60 × 54.54 kcal = 3272.4 kcal

Hence, the basal energy expenditure of the girl is within

Ans. 1908.9 – 3272.4 kcal

Example

A male patient is 48 years old and his height is 5ft 9in.; he weighs 65kg. If the activity factor is 1.5; calculate the total daily expenditure (TDE) ignoring the stress factor.

Solution

Given that, the weight of male person = 65kg

Height = 5ft 9 inches = 5 ×12 × 2.54 cm + 9 × 2.54cm = 175.26cm

Age = 48 years

Activity factor = 1.5

According to Harris-Benedict equation the basal energy expenditure (BEE) for a male

$$= 66.5 + [13.75 \times \text{Weight (kg)}] + [5.003 \times \text{Height (cm)}] - [6.67 \times \text{Age (Yrs)}]$$

$$= 66.5 + [13.75 \times 65 \text{ kg}] + [5.003 \times 175.26 \text{ cm}] - [6.67 \times 48 \text{ years}]$$

$$= 66.5 + 893.75 + 876.82 - 320.16$$

$$= 1516.91 \text{ kcal}$$

Total daily expenditure of energy (TDE) = BEE × Activity factor × Stress factor

$$= 1516.91 \times 1.5 \text{ (ignoring Stress factor)}$$

Ans. 2275.36 kcal

Protein Requirements

In TPN (Total Parenteral Nutrition), protein is provided in form of protein hydrolyzate or amino acids. It is used in these formulations to build tissues and body strength, not to produce energy; although energy is produced by proteins by a factor of 4 kcal/ g. The calorie requirement of a patient should be met by non protein constituents. The amounts of protein required per day by humans of different age group and under different stress conditions are mentioned below:

- 0.8 g/kg of body weight by an unstressed patient,
- 0.8 – 1g/kg for a mildly stressed patient,
- 1.1 – 1.5 g/kg for a moderately stressed patient,
- 1.5 – 2 g/kg for a severely stressed patient and for those with a critical illness or trauma,
- 1.2 g/kg for a patient undergoing renal dialysis, and
- 3 g/kg for a severely burned patient.

Infants may require 2 to 3 g of protein /kg/day, children 1.5 to 2 g of protein /kg/day, and teenagers 1 to 1.5 g of protein/kg/day.

Lipid (Fat) Requirements

When the body cannot get the required energy from carbohydrates, lipids are used to produce energy. The amount of calories supplied by lipids usually range from 30% to 40% of the total daily (requirement) calories. Lipids provide 9 kcal of energy per gram. Lipids are generally present in the form of an emulsion containing carbohydrate-based emulsifying agents, which also provides some calories. It has been found that a 10% lipid emulsion supplies 11 kcal/g of total energy.

Consuming too much fat, saturated fat, *trans* fat, and cholesterol may increase the risk of certain chronic diseases, such as heart disease. Good health guidelines suggest that total daily fat consumed should be less than 65g, saturated fat less than 20 g, and cholesterol less than 300 mg.

Fiber Requirements

In general, 14 g of fibre should be taken daily for each 1000 calories consumed. For women approximately 21 to 25 grams of fiber should be taken daily by women and between 30 to 38 g by men. Insoluble fibre can reach the large intestine and helps in good bowel function. On the other hand, soluble fibre partly dissolves in the upper gastrointestinal tract and reduces absorption of dietary fat and cholesterol.

Calculations of Enteral Nutrition

Example

A patient undergoing renal dialysis weighs 120 lb; calculate the amount of protein to be administered daily and approximate daily fluid requirement.

Solution

Patient undergoing renal dialysis requires 1.2 g/kg of protein in a day.

Body weight of the patient is 120 lb = 120 × 0.454 kg = 54.48 kg

Daily requirement of protein = 54.48 kg ×1.2 g/kg = 65.38 g

So, the protein requirement of the patient undergoing renal dialysis is **65.4g/day**. (Answer)

Fluid requirement calculated on the basis of body weight is: 1500 ml + (54.48 – 20) ×20ml

= 1500ml + 689.6 ml

= 2189.6ml (2190 ml) approximately

So, fluid requirement of the patient is approximately

Ans. 2190 ml/day

Example

The nutritional requirements for an old male of 78 years old whose height is 6 ft and weight is 198 lb. have been determined to be as follows:

Protein: 72.98 g/day

Lipids: 80.93 g/day

Carbohydrates: 267.01 g/day

Water: 2090.00 to 2690.00 mL/day

Total calories: 2075.63 kcal/day

A commercial liquid preparation is selected for enteral nutrition for this patient. A quart of this preparation provides 36.8 g protein, 140 g carbohydrates, 36.7 g lipids, and 1.12 kcal/mL (1 quart = 946 ml).

(a) How many milliliters of the liquid preparation should be given to the patient per day to meet his caloric requirements?

(b) How many grams each of protein, carbohydrates, and lipids would this volume provide?

(c) If the product contains 80% free water, does it meet the patient's daily water requirement?

(d) If the formulation is to be administered continuously over 24-hour, what would be the flow rate in mL/h?

(e) If the patient is administered this formulation at home by intermittent feedings for 4 hours at every 40 min; what volume would be administered in each feeding, and what would be the flow rate in mL/hr?

Solution

(a) Given that the liquid chosen provides 1.12kcal/ml

Daily requirement = 2075.63 kcal/day

The volume (ml) of the liquid to be taken per day

$$= \frac{2075.63 \text{ kcal/day}}{1.12 \text{ kcal/ml}} = 1853.24\text{ml}$$

Hence, the liquid preparation to be given to the patient daily

= 1853.24ml (Answer)

(b) *Protein content*

1 quart or 946 ml of the preparation contains 36.8 g of protein

$$1853.24 \text{ ml would contain} = \frac{36.8 \text{ g} \times 1853.24 \text{ ml}}{946 \text{ ml}} = 72.1\text{g of protein}$$

Hence, 1853.24 ml of the liquid preparation shall contain 72.1 g of protein. (Answer)

Lipid content

946 ml of the preparation contains 36.8 g of lipid

$$1853.24 \text{ ml would contain} = \frac{36.7 \text{ g} \times 1853.24 \text{ ml}}{946 \text{ ml}} = 71.9\text{g of lipid}$$

Hence, 1853.24 ml of the liquid preparation shall contain 71.9 g of lipid. (Answer)

Carbohydrate content

$$1853.24 \text{ ml would contain} = \frac{140 \text{ g} \times 1853.24 \text{ ml}}{946 \text{ ml}}$$

$$= 274.3\text{g of carbohydrate}$$

Hence, 1853.24 ml of the liquid preparation shall contain 274.3 g of carbohydrate. (Answer)

(c) Daily requirement of water for a male person is about 2 to 3 lts.

Water content of 1853.24ml of liquid is 80%,

That is, the water content = 80% of 1853.24ml

$$= 1853.24\text{ml} \times \frac{80}{100} = 1482.6 \text{ ml}$$

Water provided by 1853.24ml of liquid would not be sufficient. (Answer)

(d) When 1853.24 ml of the liquid formulation is administered continuously during 24 hrs, the flow rate per hour would be $\frac{1853.24 \text{ ml}}{24 \text{ hr}} = 77.22$ ml/hr.

(e) When 1853.24 ml of the liquid formulation is administered continuously during 24 hrs, the volume ingested in 4hr = $\frac{1853.24 \text{ ml} \times 4 \text{ hr}}{24 \text{ hr}} = 308.87$ ml (Answer)

That is, 308.87ml is administered during 40 min.

Then the flow rate per hour = $\frac{308.87 \text{ ml}}{40 \text{ min}} \times \frac{60 \text{ min}}{1 \text{ hr}}$ = 463.31 ml/hr.

Hence, the liquid is to be administered at the rate of

Ans. 463.31 ml/hr

Example

A female patient without any stress conditions is being ingested a liquid for enternal nutrition. The liquid contains 0.056 g of protein per ml, 0.08 g of lipids per ml and 0.26 g of carbohydrates per ml. Total volume is 2000 ml and it provides 1.5 kcal/ml. The weight of the patient is 126 lbs, she is 58 yrs old and her height is 5 ft 5 in. Assume that 30ml of water is required per kg of body weight.

Calculate

(a) the volume of the preparation to be ingested to meet the calorie requirement,

(b) the amount of protein, lipid and carbohydrate would be ingested every day,

(c) If the patient requires 0.8g of protein per kg of her body weight, will the amount ingested be sufficient?

Solution

(a) the calorie required per day by the patient is based on BEE, and

BEE for female = 655.1 + [9.56 × 126 ×0.454] + [1.86 × 65× 2.54] – [4.68 × 58]

= 655.1 + 546.87 + 307.09 – 271.44

= 1237.62 kcal/day

The daily requirement of the patient is 1237.62 kcal and

The preparation provides 1.5kcal/ml,

That is, 1.5 kcal is received out of 1 ml of the preparation

1237.62 kcal would be received from $\frac{1 \times 1237.62}{1.5}$

= 825.08 ml of the preparation.

Hence, the volume of the preparation to be administered daily = 825.08 ml (Answer)

(b) Protein, lipid, and carbohydrate to be ingested per day:

Each ml of the preparation contains 0.056 g of protein

Protein content of 825.08 ml of the preparation = 825.08 ml × 0.056g/ml = 46.2 g

Lipids ingested per day:

Each ml of the preparation contains 0.08 g of lipids

Lipids content of 825.08 ml of the preparation

= 825.08 ml × 0.08g/ml = 66.00g

Carbohydrate ingested per day:

Each ml of the preparation contains 0.26 g of carbohydrate

Carbohydrate content of 825.08 ml of the preparation

= 825.08 ml × 0.26g/ml = 214.5g

Hence, the amount of protein, lipid and carbohydrate would be ingested every day are 46.2 g, 66.00 g and 214.5 g respectively. (Answer)

(c) Total volume of the preparation ingested per day = 825.08 ml

It contains 46.2 g of protein

Requirement of protein per day is 0.8g/kg of body weight

The body weight of the patient is 126 lb

= 126 × 0.454 kg = 57.2 kg

Requirement of protein per day = 0.8g/kg × 57.2kg = 45.76 g

Ans. Daily requirement of protein is being met

Calculations Related to Parenteral Nutrition

The steps to be followed for calculating TPN are:

Step I: Calculate the total daily calories required using the Harris-Benedict equations, and apply the appropriate stress or activity factors, if required.

Step II: Calculate the daily quantity (g) of protein required on the basis of 0.8 g/kg of body weight, and adjust as required for stress factors and disease states.

Step III: Calculate the number of calories supplied by the protein (amino acids, from Step 2) at 4 kcal/g.

Step IV: Calculate the kcal of lipids required at 35% of the total daily calories.

Step V: Calculate the grams of lipids required (from Step 4) on basis of 9 kcal/g or on the basis of the lipid emulsion used.

Step VI: Calculate the quantity of carbohydrate required on the basis of 3.4 kcal/g after accounting for the contribution of the lipids.

Step VII: Calculate the daily fluid requirement using 30 mL/kg/day or one of the other methods described earlier in the text.

Notes: In some clinical practices (a) a patient's actual body weight, the ideal body weight, or some arbitrary value is used in the calculations (in Step 1), and (b) in Step 6, the energy provided by the protein, in addition to that from lipids, may or may not be taken into account.

In addition to Steps 1 through 7, TPN calculations also can include:

- Determination of the quantities of the pharmaceutical sources of the macronutrients (e.g., vials) and micronutrients (e.g., LVPs) to use to obtain the required components;
- Determination of the total TPN volume, the number of TPN bags to be prepared, and the rate of flow.

Example

Calculate the parenteral nutrition and fluid requirements for a 45years old woman patient whose height is 5 ft. and weight is 100 lb; she is in hospital and under mild stress.

Solution

The Harris-Benedict equation for female is

$$\text{BEE} = 655.1 + [9.56 \times \text{Weight (kg)}] + [1.86 \times \text{Height (cm)}] - [4.68 \times \text{Age (Yrs)}]$$

Given that, the age of the woman = 45 years

Height of the woman = 5 ft = 5× 12 × 2.54 cm = 152.4 cm

Weight of the woman = 100 lb = 100 × 0.456 g = 45.6 kg

Step I: Total calorie required/day = 655.1 + [9.56 × 45.6kg]

+ [1.86 × 152.4cm] – [4.68 × 45Yrs]

= 655.1 + 435.94 + 283.46 – 210.6

= 1163.9 kcal

Step II: Since the patient is under mild stress,

Protein requirement per day = 0.9g × body weight

= 0.9 × (100 × 0.454) g [1lb = 454g]

= 0.9 × 45.4g

= 40.86g

Step III: Calorie to be provided by protein

Calorie obtained from protein

= protein intake (g)/day × 4kcal

= 40.86g/day × 4 kcal

=163.4kcal/day

Step IV: Lipids required

Requirement of lipids/day can be calculated on the on the basis of 35% calorie intake,

= 35% of 1163.9 kcal/day

$= \frac{35}{100} \times 1163.9$ kcal/day

= 407.4 kcal/day

Step V: Lipid required (g) in form of emulsion

11 kcal of energy is supplied per day by 10% lipid emulsion.

407.4 kcal would be supplied per day $\frac{407.4}{11}$ g = 37.04 g of lipid/day

Step VI: Carbohydrates (dextrose) required (g), for calorie supply:

Total calorie intake = 1163.9 kcal/day

Calorie obtained from protein = 163.4kcal/day

Calorie obtained from lipids = 407.4 kcal/day

1 g of carbohydrate provides 3.4 kcal

Calorie supplied by carbohydrate = total calorie intake –[calorie obtained from protein + calorie obtained from lipids]

= 1163.9 kcal/day – [163.4kcal/day + 407.4 kcal/day]

= 1163.9 kcal/day – 570.8 kcal/day

= 593.1 kcal/day

593.1 kcal would be obtained from carbohydrate

$$= \frac{593.1}{3.4} \text{ g} = 174.4\text{g}$$

Step VII: Fluid requirement per day

The daily fluid requirement on the basis of body weight = 30 ml/kg/day

Weight of the patient = 45.6 kg

Fluid required by the patient = 45.6 kg × 30 ml/kg/day

= 1368 ml

Example

A preparation for TPN requires addition of 3.2 mEq of Mg^{2+} and 18 mEq of K^{+} per liter for adjustment.

How many milliliters of an injection containing 50 mg of magnesium chloride per milliliter and how many milliliters of 17.5% (w/v) of potassium chloride injection should be added for the purpose?

Solution

Molecular weight of $MgCl_2$ = 95.2

1 mEq of Mg^{2+} = 12.15 mg

3.2 mEq of Mg^{2+} = 12.15 mg × 3.2 = 38.88 mg

24.3 mg of Mg^{2+} is contained by 95.2 mg of $MgCl_2$

38.88 mg of Mg^{2+} is contained by $\frac{38.88 \times 12.15}{95.2}$

= 4.96 mg of $MgCl_2$

Given solution contains 50 mg of $MgCl_2$ per ml

4.96 mg of $MgCl_2$ is contained by = $\frac{1 \times 4.96}{50}$ ml

= 0.099 ml, ≈ 0.1 ml (Answer)

Molecular weight of KCl = 74.5

1 mEq of K^+ = 39 mg

18 mEq of K^+ = 39 mg × 18 = 702 mg

39 mg of K^+ ≈ 74.5 mg of KCl

702 mg of K+ ≈ $\frac{74.5 \times 702}{39}$ mg of KCl = 1341 mg of KCl

Given solution contains 17.5 g per 100ml

That is, 175 mg of KCl per ml

Then, 1341 mg of KCl is contained in $\frac{1 \times 1341}{175}$

Ans. 7.66 ml ≈ 7.7 ml

Body Mass Index (BMI)

There is increased of various health problems due to overweight. Particularly gross overweight or obesity brings about greater risk of disease, disease complications, and even mortality. There are different factors in addition to diet that can cause obesity, such as behavioral, cultural, metabolic, and genetic disposition. To begin with the management of overweight or obesity the degree of excessive weight is to be assessed. To measure excessive weight or obesity, body mass index (BMI) has been accepted as the clinical standard. BMI is defined *as the body weight in kilograms divided by the square of height measured in meters*. The National Institutes of Health (NIH) has developed a correlation between BMI and weight of human being:

- If BMI is less than 18.5, it is considered underweight,
- If BMI is within 18.5 to 24.9 it is considered normal weight,
- If BMI is within 25 and 29.9 it is considered overweight,
- If BMI is 30 or more, it is considered obese, and
- If BMI is more than 40, it is considered extremely obese.

An elderly person can be considered suffering from malnutrition if his or her BMI is less than 21. In most of the people BMI is an indicator of high body fat. This may not be true in case of the persons with developed muscles. The NIH also considers waist circumference an important factor in obesity related disease. A waist circumference of more than 40 inches in men and more than 35 inches, in women with BMI between 25 and 35 indicates an increased risk of obesity related diseases. Treatment for overweight and obese patients include dietary therapy, physical activity, behavioral therapy, pharmacotherapy, and, in extreme cases of obesity, weight loss surgery.

Determination of BMI

By using a standardized table as shown in Table 8.3 BMI can be determined. The intercept of a person's height and weight indicates the body mass index. Standard tables are available in units of the common systems of measurement such as feet/inches and pounds or in metric or dual systems for use by the general public. Below a standard table is given which can be used to find out BMI. The table uses feet/inches for height and pounds for weight. The intercepts in the table have been put in three color zones and in a zone without color.

Table 8.3

The dark zone showing BMI within 25 to 29.9 indicates overweight

Light color zone showing BMI less than 18.5 indicates underweight

Another light color zone showing BMI more than 30 indicates obesity

No color zone showing BMI within 18.5 to 24.5 indicates normal weight

	Weight (lbs)															
Height	**100**	**110**	**120**	**130**	**140**	**150**	**160**	**170**	**180**	**190**	**200**	**210**	**220**	**230**	**240**	**250**
5′	20	21	23	25	27	29	31	33	35	37	39	41	43	45	47	49
5′1″	19	21	23	25	26	28	30	32	34	36	38	40	42	43	45	47
5′2″	18	20	22	24	26	27	29	31	33	35	37	38	40	42	44	46
5′3″	18	19	21	23	25	27	28	30	32	34	35	37	39	41	43	44
5′4″	17	19	21	22	24	26	27	29	31	33	34	36	38	39	41	43
5′5″	17	18	20	22	23	25	27	28	30	32	33	35	37	38	40	42
5′6″	16	18	19	21	23	24	26	27	29	31	32	34	36	37	39	40
5′7″	16	17	19	20	22	23	25	27	28	30	31	33	34	36	38	39
5′8″	15	17	18	20	21	23	24	26	27	29	30	32	33	35	36	38
5′9″	15	16	18	19	21	22	24	25	27	28	30	31	32	34	35	37
5′10″	14	16	17	19	20	22	23	24	26	27	29	30	32	33	34	36

Table *contd...*

5′11″	14	15	17	18	20	21	22	24	25	26	27	28	30	32	33	35
6′	14	15	16	18	19	20	22	23	24	26	27	28	30	31	33	34
6′1″	13	15	16	17	18	20	21	22	24	25	26	28	29	30	32	33
6′2″	13	14	15	17	18	19	21	22	23	244	26	27	28	30	31	32
6′3″	12	14	15	16	17	19	20	21	22	24	25	26	27	29	30	31
6′4″	12	13	15	16	17	18	19	21	22	23	24	26	27	28	29	30

A. *Determination of BMI using BMI table*

Example

Using the BMI table, determine the BMI of a person 180 cm in height and weighing 78 kg.

Solution

1 in = 2.54cm

Height is 180cm = $180 \times \frac{1}{2.54}$in = 70.87in = 5ft 10.87in ≈ 5ft 11in

1kg = 2.2lb

Weight is 78kg = 78 × 2.2lb = 171.6lb ≈ 172lb

There is no intercept for 5ft 11in and 172lb in the table, the nearest intercept for 5ft 11in and 170lb is **24**.

Thus, the person is of **normal weight**. (Answer)

B. *Determination of BMI using a formula*

When the table for BMI is not available or the exact values of weight and height are not available in the table, BMI can be calculated using the following equation;

$$\text{BMI} = \frac{\text{Weight (kg)}}{[\text{Height (m)}]^2}$$

Example

The height of a person is 5ft 2.5in and weight is 146 lb, determine the BMI and find whether the person is under weight/normal weight/overweight.

Solution

The BMI table does not provide the intercept for 5ft 2.5 in and 146 lb. Hence, the above formula is to be used.

Weight = 146 lb = $\frac{146}{2.2}$ kg = 66.36 kg [1kg = 2.2 lb]

Height = 5ft 2.5 in = (5 × 12 + 2.5) in = 62.5in

= 62.5 in = 62.5 × 2.54 cm [1 in = 2.54 cm]

= 158.75cm

= 1.5875m ≈ 1.59m

$$\text{BMI} = \frac{\text{Weight (kg)}}{[\text{Height (m)}]^2} = \frac{66.36\text{kg}}{1.59\text{m} \times 1.59\text{m}}$$

$$= \frac{66.36}{2.53} = 26.23$$

Ans. Thus, the person is of overweight

Example

The weight of a person is 179lb and height is 6ft 2in; calculate the BMI and find whether the person is under weight/normal weight/overweight.

Solution

Weight is 179lb = 179 × $\frac{1}{2.2}$ kg [2.21 b =1kg]

= 81.36 kg

Height = 6ft 2 in = (6 × 12 + 2) in

= 74 in

= 74 × 2.54cm

= 187.96 cm

= 1.8796 m ≈ 1.88 m

As per the formula

$$\text{BMI} = \frac{\text{Weight (kg)}}{[\text{Height (m)}]^2}$$

$$= \frac{81.36}{1.88 \times 1.88}$$

$$= 23.02$$

Ans. Thus, the person is of normal weight

C. *Determination of BMI using an alternative formula*

There is an alternative formula for calculating BMI. The units used this formula are pound (lb) and inches (in) of FPS system. A multiplication factor of 704.5, derived by dividing the square of 39.37(1m = 39.37in) by 2.2 (2.2lb = 1kg) is used. This factor is derived by the National Institute of Health. The formula is;

$$\text{BMI} = \frac{\text{Weight (lb)}}{[\text{Height(in)}]^2} \times 704.5$$

Example

A person weighs 182lb and his height is 6ft; calculate the BMI using the alternative formula and examine in which group the person comes under.

Solution

Height = 6ft = 72in

Weight = 182lb

$$\text{According to the formula BMI} = \frac{\text{Weight (lb)}}{[\text{Height(in)}]^2} \times 704.5$$

$$= \frac{182\text{lb}}{72\text{in} \times 72\text{in}} \times 704.5$$

$$= \mathbf{24.73}$$

Ans. The person possesses the normal weight

Example

The weight of a person is 85kg and height is 180cm; what would be the BMI? Use the alternative formula and examine in which group the person comes under.

Solution

Weight is 85kg = 85 × 2.2lb [1kg = 2.2lb]

= 187lb

$$\text{Height} = 180\text{ cm} = 180 \times \frac{1}{2.54}\text{ in}$$

$$= 70.87\text{ in} \approx 70.9\text{ in}$$

According to the formula

$$BMI = \frac{\text{Weight (lb)}}{[\text{Height(in)}]^2} \times 704.5$$

$$= \frac{187 \text{ lb}}{70.9 \text{ in} \times 70.9 \text{ in}} \times 704.5$$

$$= \frac{187}{5026.81} \times 704.5$$

$$= \mathbf{26.21}$$

Ans. The person is of overweight

Example

A person weighs 80kg with a height of 185cm. Calculate the BMI using the alternative formula and examine in which group the person comes under.

Solution

Weight = 80kg = 80 × 2.2 lb

= 176 lb

Height = 185cm = $185 \times \frac{1}{2.54}$ inch = 72.8 inch

According to the formula $BMI = \frac{\text{Weight (lb)}}{[\text{Height(in)}]^2} \times 704.5$

$$= \frac{176\text{lb}}{72.8\text{in} \times 72.8\text{in}} \times 704.5$$

$$= \mathbf{23.4}$$

Ans. The person possesses the normal weight

Example

How many calories are obtained from fat and how many grams of fat should be taken per day for a person on a 2150-calorie diet?

Solution

Out of 2150 calories, calorie obtained from fat

= 35% of 2150 = $2150 \times \frac{35}{100}$ = 752.5, and fat provides 9 calorie/g.

That is, 9 calorie is provided by 1g of fat

700 calorie would be provided by $\frac{1}{9} \times 752.5$ g

Ans. 83.61 g ≈ 83.6 g

Example

A diet consists of 61 grams of fat, 458 grams of carbohydrate, and 175 grams of protein. Calculate the calories provided by the food.

Solution

Calories provided by different types of food are

4 calories per g of carbohydrates

9 calories per g of fat

4 calories per g of protein

Then, calories obtained from 458g of carbohydrates

$= 4 \text{ calories} \times 458 = 1832 \text{ calories}$

Calories obtained from 61g of fat = 9 calories × 61 = 549 calories

Calories obtained from 175g of protein = 4 calories × 175

= 700 calories

Total Calories obtained from the food = 1832 + 549 + 700

Ans. 2581 calories

Example

A person is taking 400 g of carbohydrate, 100g of protein and 90g of fat every day. Find out his calorie-diet per day.

Solution

Given that, daily intake of carbohydrate = 400 g

Daily intake of protein = 100 g

Daily intake of fat = 90 g

Calorie obtained from carbohydrate
= 400g × 4calories = 1600 calories

Calorie obtained from protein = 100 g × 4 calories = 400 calories

Calorie obtained from fat = 90g × 9 calories = 810 calories

Total calories requirement per day = 1600 + 400 + 810

Ans. 2810 calories

Exercise

1. A 50 ml intravenous injection is administered in 50 minutes using a microdrip set. Calculate the total number of drops produced and flow rate. Microdrip set delivers 60 drops/ml.

   Ans: 2500 drops, 1 ml/min

2. What would be duration of infusion to administer 540 ml of an electrolytes solution if it is infused at a rate of 12 drops/min?

   Ans: 4 hr 30 min

3. Dextrose injection is being administered intravenously at a rate of 12 drops per minute using a standard administration set which delivers 14 drops/ml. Find out the time at which 500ml would be administered.

   Ans: 9 hrs 43 min

4. Calculate the daily protein requirement (in g/day) for a moderately stressed patient having weight of 145lb.

   Ans: 85.67g/day

5. How many milliliters of Dextrose Injection (10%) IP should be infused to a neonate weighing 4 lb. 8 oz. on the basis of 60ml/kg/day ?

   Ans: 122.7ml

6. If an administration set that can deliver 50 drops/mL at 20 drops per minute, calculate the total time required for delivery of 122.7 ml of the infusion.

   Ans: 5 hr 6.75min

7. Tetracycline HCl, 50.0 mg/kg, is prescribed for a 1.75-kg neonate. Find out (a) the dose of the drug, and (b) the flow rate, in mL/minute, if the infusion is put in a 60-mL IV bag and administered in 25 minutes.

   Ans: (1) 87.5mg/kg, (2) 2.4ml/min

8. If intravenous solutions are continuously administered during 24 hrs and 4bottles of 540ml are ingested, calculate the flow rate per hour.

   Ans: 90ml/hr

9. If 2liters of an intravenous preparation is continuously administered for 24 hrs, calculate the volume of the preparation ingested in 3 hrs.

Ans: 250ml/3hrs

10. A patient is being given 65g of protein per day. The body weight of the patient is 100 lbs.; calculate the dose of protein being administered.

Ans: 1.43g/kg

11. A solution containing 68g of lipid in 900ml is administered to a patient at a rate of 1.2g/kg. If the weight of the patient is 110 lbs, calculate the volume of the solution is to be administered.

Ans: 794.12ml

12. A patient weighing 56kg has been administered a protein solution at a dose of 8.5g/kg. If the protein solution provides 4kcal/g, calculate how much calories are being received every day by the patient.

Ans: 1904.0 kcal

13. The daily requirement of water is 2.5 lts. A person takes 1800g of diet containing 80% of fluid. Calculate how much water to be taken other than the diet.

Ans: 1060ml

14. A boy is 16 years old, and is 5ft 6 inch tall. If he weighs 110 lbs, calculate his basal energy expenditure (BEE) according to the Harris-Benedict formula, BEE = 66.5 + [13.75 × Weight (kg)] + [5.003 × Height (cm)] – [6.67 × Age (Yrs)].

Ans: 1485.98kcal

15. A girl is 20 years old, she is 5ft 2inchess tall and her weight is 118 lbs. calculate her basal energy expenditure (BEE) using the Harris-Benedict formula, BEE = 655.1 + [9.56 × Weight (kg)] + [1.86 × Height (cm)] – [4.68 × Age (Yrs)].

Ans: 1364.9 kcal

16. A patient undergoing renal dialysis weighs 102 lb; calculate the amount of protein to be administered daily and approximate daily fluid requirement.

Ans: Protein requirement = 55.57g/day, Fluid requirement = 2022 ml

17. The carbohydrate requirement for a person of 47 years old is 250.0g/day and total calories requirement is 2125.0 cal/day. A commercial liquid preparation of 900 ml provides 145 g of carbohydrates, and 1.10 kcal/mL.

    (a) How many milliliters of the liquid preparation should be given to the patient per day to meet his caloric requirements?

    (b) How many milliliters of the preparation can provide the carbohydrate requirement?

Ans: (a) 1931.8ml; (b) 1551.72ml

18. A diet consists of 58 grams of fat, 450 grams of carbohydrate, and 150 grams of protein. Calculate the calories provided by the food.

Ans: 2922 calories

19. How many calories are obtained from protein and how many grams of protein should be taken per day for a person on a 2250-calorie diet?

Ans: 4calories/g of protein and 562.5g of protein to be taken

20. A person is taking 350g of carbohydrate, 180g of protein and 85g of fat every day. Find out his calorie-diet per day.

Ans: 2885 calories per day

21. A person takes 2500 calorie-diet every day. The amount protein present in diet contributes 40% of total calories. How many grams of protein are taken every day?

Ans: 250g of protein

22. A preparation for TPN requires addition of 2.8 mEq of Mg^{2+} and 2.0 mEq of Na^{+} per liter for adjustment.

    How many milliliters of an injection containing 100 mg of magnesium chloride per milliliter and how many milliliters of 10% (w/v) of sodium chloride injection should be added for the purpose?

Ans: (a) 0.0434ml of magnesium chloride

(b) 1.17 ml of 10% sodium chloride

23. A person weighs 68kg with a height of 175cm. Calculate the BMI using the alternative formula and examine in which group the person comes under.

Ans: BMI = 22.19, Normal

24. A person weighs 159lbs with a height of 5ft 9in. Calculate the BMI and examine whether the person comes under normal weight.

Ans: BMI = 23.52, Almost normal

25. The weight of a person is 180lb and height is 6ft; calculate the BMI and find whether the person is under weight /normal weight/overweight.

Ans: BMI=24.4, slightly overweight

9

BIOAVAILABILITY AND PHARMACOKINETICS

The availability of a drug from its formulation into the biologic system is the primary goal of dosage form design and principal requirement for the effectiveness of the medication. Before a drug substance is absorbed by the biologic system, it must be released from its dosage form (*e.g.*, tablet or capsule) or drug delivery system (*e.g.*, transdermal patch) and dissolved in the biological fluids.

Various factors influence the bioavailability of a drug; such as the physical and chemical characteristics of the drug, (*e.g.*, particle size, solubility, etc.), characteristics of the dosage form or delivery system (*e.g.*, the nature of the ingredients used in formulation and the method of manufacture), physiological conditions (e.g., renal function, disease state, etc.).

Biopharmaceutics may be defined as the study of the properties of drug substances and dosage forms that influence the release of the drug for bioavailability. The relative amount of drug that enters the systemic circulation from an administered dosage form is called bioavailability. On the other hand, the study and characterization of the time course of the absorption, distribution, metabolism, and elimination (ADME) of drugs is called pharmacokinetics. The process of passage of the drug from the site of administration into the systemic circulation is called absorption of drug. Drug distribution means the transfer of the drug from the blood to extra vascular fluids and tissues.

The enzymatic or biochemical transformation of the drug substance to (usually less toxic) metabolic products is called *metabolism* of drug; the metabolized drug is then eliminated more readily from the body.

The removal of the drug substance or its metabolites from the body through the kidney (urine), intestines (feces), skin (sweat), saliva, and/or milk is drug elimination.

The relationship among these processes of absorption, distribution, metabolism, and elimination influences the therapeutic and toxic effects of drugs. The application of pharmacokinetic principles in the treatment of individual patients in optimizing drug therapy is referred to as clinical pharmacokinetics.

Availability of Drug from Dosage Form and Delivery System

The availability of a drug from a dosage form or delivery system is determined by two ways – *in vitro* and in vivo. Measurement of the dissolution characteristics outside the biologic system is *in vitro* method; while measurement of drug absorption *in vivo* within the biologic system is *in vivo* method. The results of these experiments provide information on both rate and extent of drug dissolution and absorption. The results collected are plotted on graph paper to represent concentration versus time curves for dissolution and absorption of the drug.

Plotting and Interpreting Dissolution Data

The USP Dissolution Test specifies the apparatus and methods to be used. In general tablets or capsules are tested by this method. Results obtained in *in-vitro* drug dissolution study are presented in tabular form and shown graphically.

Example

Samples of 250-mg capsule of Amoxycillin were subjected to dissolution study. The data obtained are given below. Plot the data on a graph paper and determine the approximate percentage of the drug dissolved in 15, 30, 45, and 60 minutes of the study.

Period (min)	Amount of Amoxycillin (mg), dissolved
0	0
5	22
10	50.7
15	87.7
30	155.9
45	208.2
60	248.3
75	250

Solution

The concentration obtained from the dissolution study refers to the cumulative release of the drug from the dosage form. Hence, the plot would indicate the cumulative release profile of the drug.

Time (min)	Amount of Amoxycilling dissolved (mg)	Drug dissolved (%w/v)
0	0	0
5	22	8.8
10	50.7	20.3
15	87.7	35.1
30	155.9	62.4
45	208.2	83.3
60	248.3	99.3
75	250	100

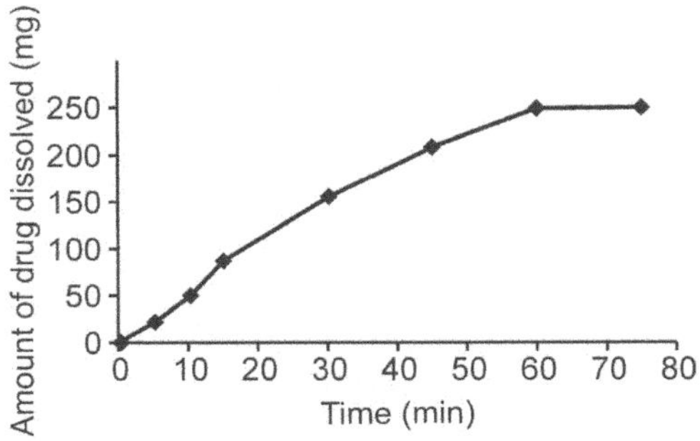

Ans. Drug dissolved in 15, 30, 45, and 60 min are 35.1, 62.4, 83.3 and 99.3% respectively

Example

The dissolution study of a paracetamol tablet 500 mg IP provides the following release data. Plot the data on a graph paper indicating amount released, cumulative release, and percent release of the drug vs. time and find out the percentage of drug released in 15min, 30 min, and 45 minutes.

Period (min)	Amount of Paracetamol (mg), dissolved
0	0
5	102.2
10	175.7
15	287.5
30	425.8
45	488.9
60	499.9
75	499.9

Solution

Period (min)	Cumulative amount of Paracetamol (mg) dissolved	Percentage of drug dissolved (%)
0	0	0
5	102.2	20.44

Table *contd...*

10	175.7	35.14
15	287.5	57.50
30	425.8	98.30
45	488.9	97.78
60	499.9	99.98
75	499.9	99.98

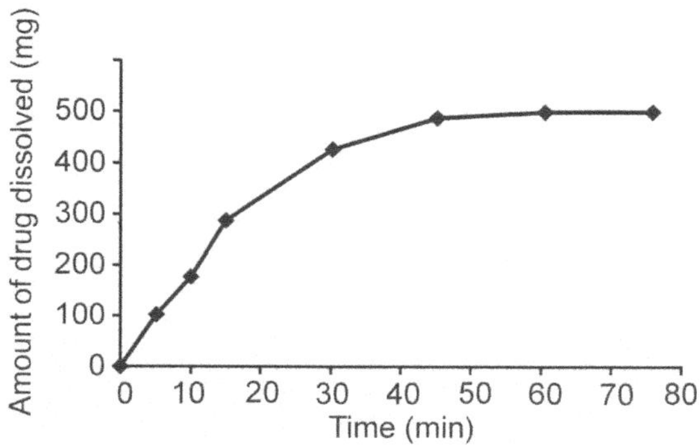

Plot of amount of drug released in milligram

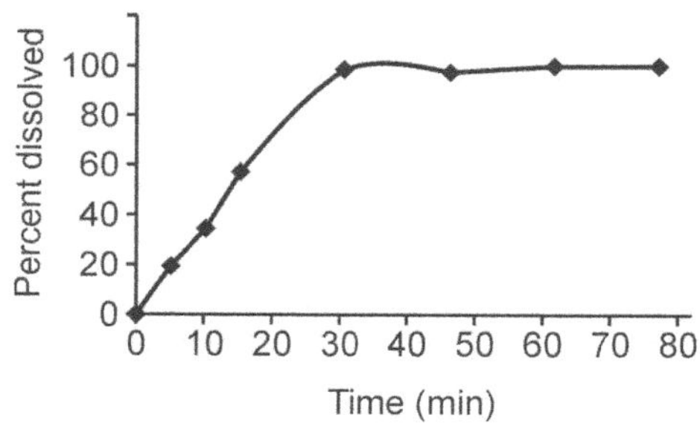

Plot of percent of drug released

In 15 minutes 57.5%, in 30 minutes 98.3% and in 45 minutes 97.78% of drug has been released. (Answer)

Calculations of Bioavailability and Bioequivalence

When the dissolution or absorption studies consistently show that only a portion of a drug substance in a dosage form is available, the bioavailability factor (F) of the drug may be used to calculate bioavailability. The bioavailability factor may represent the decimal percentage of a drug substance available. The value of F may be zero, indicating no absorption, to a maximum of 1, indicating complete absorption.

Example

If the bioavailability factor (F) for a drug substance in a dosage form is 0.60, how many milligrams of drug would be available for absorption from a 100 mg tablet of the drug?

Solution

The bioavailability factor (F) indicates that only 60% of the drug present in the dosage form is available for absorption. Thus:

$$100 \text{ mg} \times \frac{60}{100}$$

Ans. 60 mg

Example

The bioavailability factor (F) for a drug from solid dosage form has been repeatedly investigated and has been found 0.65. Find out how many milligrams of drug would be available for absorption from a 200 mg tablet of the drug?

Solution

The bioavailability factor (F) indicates that only 60% of the drug present in the dosage form is available for absorption. Thus:

$$200 \text{ mg} \times \frac{65}{100}$$

Ans. 130 mg

'Bioequivalent Dose' of 'Bioinequivalent' Dosage Forms

The bioavailability of a drug may vary when it is formulated in different dosage forms or when the same dosage form is prepared by different manufacturers. Thus, it is necessary to measure the equivalent doses for two bioinequivalent products. Let us explain with an example.

Example

If the bioavailability (F) of salbutamol in a 4 mg tablet is 0.70 compared to the bioavailability (F) of 0.80 in salbutamol syrup (4mg/5ml), calculate the dose of the syrup equivalent to the tablet.

Solution

1. Bioavailable amount of salbutamol in the tablet = strength of the tablet × bioavailability

   $= 4 \text{ mg} \times 0.70$

   $= 2.8 \text{ mg}.$

2. The amount of 'bioavailable' salbutamol per millilitre of the syrup

   $= \text{amount of drug/ml} \times \text{bioavailability}$

   $= 0.8 \text{ mg} \times 0.8$

   $= 0.64$ mg/ml. (bioavailable amount of salbutamol per ml of the syrup).

3. The volume of syrup that will provide 2.8 mg of 'bioavailable' salbutamol

   $$= \frac{2.8 \text{ mg}}{0.64 \text{ mg/ml}}$$

Ans. 4.375ml ≈ 4.4ml

Example

If the bioavailability (F) of a drug in a 500 mg tablet is 0.66 and that of the same drug dispersed in water is 0.92 (25 mg/ml), calculate the dose of the syrup equivalent to the tablet.

Solution

1. Bioavailable amount of the drug in the tablet = strength of the tablet × bioavailability

   $= 500 \text{ mg} \times 0.66$

   $= 330 \text{ mg}.$

2. The amount of 'bioavailable' drug per millilitre of the dispersion

   $= \text{amount of drug/ml} \times \text{bioavailability}$

   $= 25 \text{ mg} \times 0.92$

   $= 23 \text{ mg/ml}.$

   (bioavailable amount of drug per ml of the dispersion)

3. The volume of dispersion that will provide 330 mg of 'bioavailable' drug

   $$= \frac{330 \text{ mg}}{23 \text{ mg/ml}}$$

Ans. 14.35 ml ≈ 14.35 ml

Example

The bioavailability (F) of a solution of drug (50 mg/ml) is 0.90 and bioavailability of the same drug when dispersed in water and given orally shows 0.8 (50mg/ml), calculate the dose of the dispersion equivalent to the solution.

Solution

1. Bioavailable amount of the drug per ml of the solution

   = strength of the solution × bioavailability

   = 50 mg × 0.9

   = 45 mg.

2. The amount of 'bioavailable' drug per millilitre of the dispersion

   = amount of drug/ml × bioavailability

   = 50 mg × 0.8

   = 40 mg/ml.

   (bioavailable amount of drug per ml of the dispersion)

3. The volume of dispersion that will provide 330 mg of 'bioavailable' drug

   $$= \frac{45 \text{ mg}}{40 \text{ mg/ml}}$$

Ans. 1.125ml ≈ 1.125ml

Example

If the bioavailability factor (F) for a 100mg tablet of a drug is 0.75 was compared with the bioavailability factor of 1.0 for an intravenous injection of the same drug. How many millilitres of the injection containing 50 mg/mL would be considered bioequivalent to the tablet?

Solution

Bioavailable amount of the drug in the tablet = strength of the tablet × bioavailability

= 100 mg × 0.75

= 75 mg

Bioavailable amount of the drug in the injection = strength of the tablet × bioavailability

= 50 mg/ml × 1.0

= 50 mg/ml

The volume of injection having 50 mg of drug/ml bioequivalent to 75 mg of bioequivalent tablet

Ans. $\frac{75mg}{50mg/ml} = 1.5$ ml

Example

The bioavailability factor (F) for an intravenous injection (40 mg/mL) of a drug is 0.99 and the bioavailability factor was found 0.70 when a 250mg capsule of the same drug was given. How many millilitres of the injection would be bioequivalent to the capsule?

Solution

Bioavailable amount of the drug in the capsule = strength of the capsule × bioavailability

= 250 mg × 0.70

= 175 mg.

Bioavailable amount of the drug in the injection = strength of the capsule × bioavailability

= 40mg/ml × 0.99

= 39.6mg/ml

The volume of injection having 50 mg of drug/ml bioequivalent to 75 mg of bioequivalent tablet

$$= \frac{175mg}{39.6mg/ml}$$

Ans. 4.42ml

Plotting and Interpreting a Plasma-Drug Concentration vs. Time Curve

For in vivo determination, a dosage form is administered and then the blood samples are drawn from the patient at predetermined time intervals. The samples drawn are analyzed for drug content. The results are plotted on ordinary graph paper to prepare a plasma concentration of the drug–time curve. The plasma concentrations of the drug are put on y-axis of the plot and time at which the blood samples were collected are put on the x-axis. In case of oral administration of the drug, it is assumed that at zero-time (just after oral administration), the blood concentration of the drug would be zero. Before absorption of drug after oral administration;

- The dosage form first is to reach the site of absorption (stomach and/or intestine) in GI tract,
- The drug is to be released from the dosage form,
- Complete or partial dissolution of the drug to take place.

Hence, to complete all these processes at least some time is required.

As the time passes the concentration of drug in blood increases, until the maximum (peak) concentration (C_{max}) is attained (on-set of action). For certain time the plasma concentration of the drug remains at around its C_{max}; thereafter, decreases gradually. Subsequently if no dose is administered, the plasma concentration of the drug falls back to zero. After absorption of drug (entering into the circulation) its distribution, metabolism and elimination start. In case of conventional dosage forms, such as tablets and capsules, the C_{max} occurs usually at only a single time point, which is called T_{max}. The concentration of drug in blood, plasma serum may be expressed as g/100 mL, or mg/dL or µg/mL, or mg% (mg/100 mL). The quantity of a dose administered and its dissolution, bioavailability, (absorption) distribution, metabolism, and elimination characteristics influence the concentration of the drug in blood. The rate of absorption of a drug determines the T_{max}, the time required to attain the highest concentration of a drug in the blood after administration. If the rate of absorption is high, T_{max} will be attained shortly.

The total amount of drug present in a systemic circulation is represented by the area under the curve (AUC) in a plasma drug concentration vs. time curve. The area under the curve may be measured mathematically, using various techniques. The procedures may be found in text books and reference books.

Example

The results of an in vivo study, the serum concentrations and time at which samples drawn, are given in the table below; determine (a) the peak height concentration (C_{max}) and (b) the time of the peak height concentration (T_{max}).

Solution

Time (hr)	0.5	1.0	2.0	3.0	4.0	6.0	8.0	10.0	12.0
Plasma Conc. (μg/mL)	1.0	1.9	4.05	3.95	3.0	1.65	0.9	0.3	0.15

Plotting the data and interpretation of the curve:

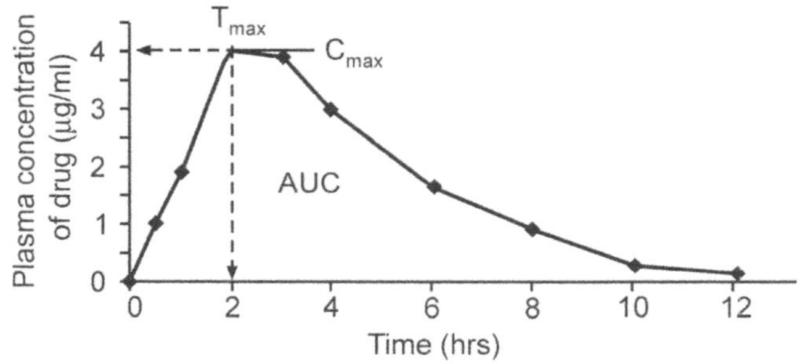

Determining the intercept for C_{max} and T_{max}

C_{max} = 4.05 μg/mL

T_{max} = 2 hours Answer

Calculation of the bioavailability (F) of a drug may be determined by comparison of the AUC data for the particular dosage form against the intravenous form:

$$F = \frac{AUC_{dosage\ form}}{AUC_{iv}} \times 100$$

Example

If the AUC for an oral dose of a drug administered by tablet is 5.2 μg/mL and the intravenous dose is 10.9 μg/mL, calculate the bioavailability of the oral dose of the drug.

Solution

$$F = \frac{AUC_{oral\ tablet}}{AUC_{iv}} \times 100$$

$$= \frac{5.2\ \mu g/ml}{10.9\ \mu g/ml} \times 100$$

$$= 0.477 \times 100$$

Ans. 47.7% or 48%

Example

An oral dose showed the AUC for a drug administered as tablet 7.2 µg /mL; the same dose of the drug when administered intravenously showed the AUC 11.5 µg/mL. Calculate the bioavailability of the oral dose of the drug.

Solution

$$F = \frac{AUC_{oral\ tablet}}{AUC_{iv}} \times 100$$

$$= \frac{7.2\ \mu g/ml}{11.5\ \mu g/ml} \times 100$$

$$= 0.626 \times 100$$

Ans. 62.6% or 63%

Calculations involved in Pharmacokinetics

Plasma Concentration of Unbound Drugs vs. Bound Drugs

After absorption into systemic circulation, a drug remains in plasma in two forms – bound, C_b (bound to plasma proteins, generally albumin), and unbound, C_{ub} or free. The unbound drug is available for further transport to its site of action in the body. The ratio of unbound drug to the bound drug depends mainly on the affinity of the drug molecules to the plasma proteins and the amount of the albumin available for binding. Some people have less and some have more albumin in serum. Thus, in some cases more than 90% of the drug molecules may be bound to plasma proteins, and in some cases the drug molecules may be bound only slightly. Accordingly the distribution, elimination and clinical effects of a drug may change due to the degree of binding of the drug to the plasma protein.

The ratio of unbound drug in the plasma to the total plasma drug concentration, C_t (bound and unbound) is termed *alpha* (or α).

Thus, $$\alpha = \frac{C_{ub}}{C_{ub} + C_b} = \frac{C_{ub}}{C_t}$$

For any drug, if the value of α and total plasma concentration (C_t) are known, the concentration of free or unbound drug can be easily calculated as follows:

$$C_{ub} = \alpha \times C_t$$

Example

If the value of α for a drug is 0.68 and the total plasma concentration of the drug is 0.8 μg/ml, then find out the concentration of free drug in plasma.

Solution

Given that $\alpha = 0.68$ and $C_t = 0.8$ μg/ml

Thus, the concentration of free drug in plasma, $C_{ub} = \alpha \times C_t$

$$= 0.68 \times 0.8 \ \mu g/ml$$

Ans. 0.544 μg/ml

Example

The total plasma concentration and the concentration of free drug were found to be 0.70 μg/ml and 0.49 μg/ml. Calculate the value of α.

Solution

Given that $C_t = 0.7$ μg/ml

$C_{ub} = 0.49$ μg/ml

Thus, $$\alpha = \frac{C_{ub}}{C_t} = \frac{0.49 \ \mu g/ml}{0.7 \ \mu g/ml}$$

Ans. 0.7

Total Amount of Drug Administered, Apparent Volume of Distribution and Plasma Concentration of Drug

The apparent volume of distribution for a drug is not a 'real' volume; it is a hypothetical volume of body fluid required to dissolve the total amount of drug at the concentration same as that found in the blood. The volume of distribution indicates to what extent a drug would be distributed throughout in the body fluids and tissues. When a dose of a drug is infused intravenously the concentration of the drug in the blood changes; this results corresponding change in its concentration in another body fluid or tissue. This helps to understand the pattern of distribution of a drug.

Let us assume a 125 mg amount of a drug substance is dissolved in water, the volume is not known. On analysis the concentration of this solution is found to be 25 mg of drug per litre. The total volume of water required to dissolve the drug can be calculated as follows:

$$\frac{25\ \text{mg}}{125\ \text{mg}} = \frac{1\ \text{litre}}{x\ \text{litre}}$$

$$x = \frac{125}{25} = 5\ \text{litre}$$

Thus, the volume of distribution of this drug is 5 litres and various drugs will indicate various volumes of distribution due to different distribution characteristics. For example, a drug having high affinity towards plasma protein or blood cells is administered intravenously; the concentration of the drug will be high in blood and low in tissues and other fluids. This will result low volumes of distribution. On the other hand, drugs having greater tendency to excrete from the blood will rapidly diffuse into other body fluids and tissues. Hence, there shall be low blood concentrations and high volumes of distribution.

If the volume of distribution of a drug in an adult is 5 litres, it is considered that the drug is present mainly in the circulatory system (blood). This happens immediately after a rapid intravenous injection (IV bolus). The distribution of drugs can be categorized based on the volume of distribution.

- A drug remains distributed mainly in the extracellular fluids, if the volume of distribution is between 10 and 20 litres, or between 15% and 27% of the body weight.
- A drug would be distributed primarily in the intracellular fluid, if the volume of distribution is within 25 and 30 litres, or between 35% and 42% of body weight.
- A drug would be distributed primarily in the whole body fluid, if the volume of distribution is about 40 litres, or 60% of the body weight.
- A drug is thought of being stored in body fat, bound to body tissues, if the apparent volume of distribution exceeds the body weight, or is distributed in peripheral compartments.

The volume of distribution (V_d) can be expressed as a simple volume or as a percentage of body weight and is calculated as:

$$V_d = \frac{\text{total amount of drug in the body (mg)}}{\text{plasma concentration of the drug (mg/litre)}}$$

$$= \frac{D}{C_p}$$

Where D is the total amount of drug in the body and C_p is plasma concentration of the drug (mg/litre or μg/litre).

Example

A dose of 400 mg of a drug substance was administered intravenously. It produced an immediate blood concentration of 10μg of drug per millilitre. Calculate the apparent volume of distribution.

Solution

Given that the plasma concentration,

$$C_p = 10\ \mu g/ml = 10000\ \mu g/1000\ ml \text{ or } 10\ mg/L$$

The total amount of drug in the body, D = 400 mg

Then, the apparent volume of distribution, $V_d = \frac{D}{C_p} = \frac{400\ mg}{10 mg/L}$

Ans. 40 L

Example

A single intravenous dose of 250 mg of a drug was administered and its blood concentration was found 10.52 μg/ml on immediate measurement. What would be the apparent volume of distribution?

Solution

Given that the plasma concentration,

$$C_p = 10.52 \mu g/ml = 10.52\ \mu g \times \frac{1000}{1000} = 10.52\ mg/L$$

The total amount of drug in the body, D = 250 mg

Then, the apparent volume of distribution,

$$V_d = \frac{D}{C_p} = \frac{250 mg}{10.52 mg/L}$$

Ans. 23.76 L

Example

The apparent volume of distribution of a drug is 36 litre and 250 mg of the drug has been administered intravenously. Find out the expected plasma concentration of the drug.

Solution

Given that, the apparent volume of distribution, $V_d = 36$ L

The total amount of drug in the body, D = 250 mg

The plasma concentration of the drug, $C_p = \frac{D}{V_d} = \frac{250\ mg}{36L} = 6.94$ mg/L

Ans. 6.94 μg/ml

Example

A drug was administered intravenously to a patient weighing 72 kg and after administration the plasma concentration was measured and found 9 μg/mL. If the apparent volume of distribution is 12% of body weight, find out the total amount of drug present in body fluids after 4 hours of administration of the drug.

Solution

Given that, the body weight = 72 kg

The apparent volume of distribution, V_d = 12% of body weight

$$= 72 \times \frac{12}{100}$$

$$= 8.64 \text{ L}$$

The plasma concentration of the drug, $C_p = 9$ μg/ml

$$V_d = \frac{D}{C_p}$$

Then the total amount of drug administered, $D = V_d \times C_p$

$$= 8.64\text{L} \times 9\mu\text{g/ml}$$

$$= 8.64 \times 1000 \text{ ml} \times 9 \ \mu\text{g/ml}$$

$$= 77760 \ \mu\text{g}$$

$$= \frac{77760}{1000} \text{ mg}$$

Ans. 77.76 mg

Example

After intravenous administration of a drug to a patient weighing 65 kg the plasma concentration was measured and found 10.5 µg/mL. The apparent volume of distribution is 12.8% of body weight. Calculate the total amount of drug present in the body fluids after 2 hours of administration of the drug.

Solution

Given that, the body weight = 65kg

The apparent volume of distribution, V_d = 12.8% of body weight

$$= 65 \times \frac{12.8}{100}$$

$$= 8.32 \text{ L}$$

The plasma concentration of the drug, C_p = 10.5 µg/ml

$$V_d = \frac{D}{C_p}$$

Then the total amount of drug present in body fluids, $D = V_d \times C_p$

$$= 8.32 \text{ L} \times 10.5 \mu\text{g/ml}$$

$$= 8.32 \times 1000 \text{ ml} \times 10.5 \mu\text{g/ml}$$

$$= 87360 \mu\text{g}$$

$$= \frac{87360}{1000} \text{ mg}$$

Ans. 87.36 mg

Example

A patient weighing 60kg was administered 250 mg of a drug through intravenous route. If the apparent volume of distribution is 15% of the body weight, calculate the plasma concentration of the drug.

Solution

Given that, the body weight = 60kg

The apparent volume of distribution, V_d = 15% of body weight

$$= 60 \times \frac{15}{100} = 9.0 \text{ L}$$

The total amount of drug administered, D = 250mg

(Amount of drug administered = Amount of drug present in the body before elimination)

The apparent volume of distribution,

$$V_d = \frac{\text{total amount of drug in the body (mg)}}{\text{plasma concentration of the drug}\left(\frac{\text{mg}}{\text{litre}}\right)} = \frac{D}{C_p}$$

Then, the plasma concentration of the drug, $C_p = \frac{D}{V_d}$

$$= \frac{250\text{mg}}{9.0\text{L}} = 27.78\text{mg/L}$$

$$= \frac{27.78 \times 1000}{1000}\ \mu\text{g/ml}$$

Ans. 27.78 μg/ml

Example

A patient was given a drug intravenously; after half an hour the plasma concentration was measured and found 0.045mg/ml. The apparent volume of distribution is 20% of the body weight. If the body weight of the patient is 55.5kg, find out the amount of the drug administered.

Solution

Given that, the body weight = 55.5 kg

The apparent volume of distribution, V_d = 20% of body weight

$$= 55.5 \times \frac{20}{100} = 11.1\text{ L}$$

The plasma concentration of the drug, C_p = 0.045 mg/ml

$$V_d = \frac{D}{C_p}$$

Then the total amount of drug administered, $D = V_d \times C_p$

$$= 11.1\text{L} \times 0.045\text{mg/ml}$$

$$= 11.1 \times 1000\text{ ml} \times 0.045\text{mg/ml}$$

Ans. 499.5 mg

Elimination Half-Life and Elimination Rate Constant

After administration the concentration of drug in blood increases initially, the plasma concentration remains within the therapeutic window for some time (duration of time), thereafter the concentration starts falling below the therapeutic window. When the plasma concentration is plotted against time, this phase appears as decline phase indicating elimination of the drug from the body. The *elimination half-life* ($t_{\frac{1}{2}}$) is the time taken for reduction of the plasma drug concentration (as well as the amount of drug in the body) to 50%. For example, if the plasma concentration of a drug falls from 8 to 4 mg/L in 4 hrs, its half-life would be 4 hours. The concentration falls from 4 to 2 mg/L in 4 hours. Similarly, the concentration will fall from 2 to 1mg/L in 4 hours, and so on. Most drugs follow first-order kinetics in their elimination from the body. This means that the rate of drug elimination per unit of time is proportional to the amount present at that time. Similar to biological half life the elimination half-life does not depend on the amount of drug in the body. After five elimination half-lives, about 97% of a drug is eliminated.

When blood level data is plotted against time on regular graph paper an exponential curve is obtained; when it is plotted on semi-logarithmic graph paper a straight line is obtained and the elimination half-life can be determined from the straight line.

The elimination rate constant for a first-order process may be calculated as follows:

$$K_{el} = \frac{0.693}{t_{\frac{1}{2}}}$$

Example

A patient was administered 2 mg of a drug intravenously; at various time intervals the blood samples were drawn and analyzed. The data obtained are given below. Plot the data on semi-logarithmic graph paper and find out the elimination half-life of the drug.

Time (hrs)	1	2	3	4	5	6
Plasma concentration of drug (μg/L)	150	94	56.5	35	20.5	12.2

Solution

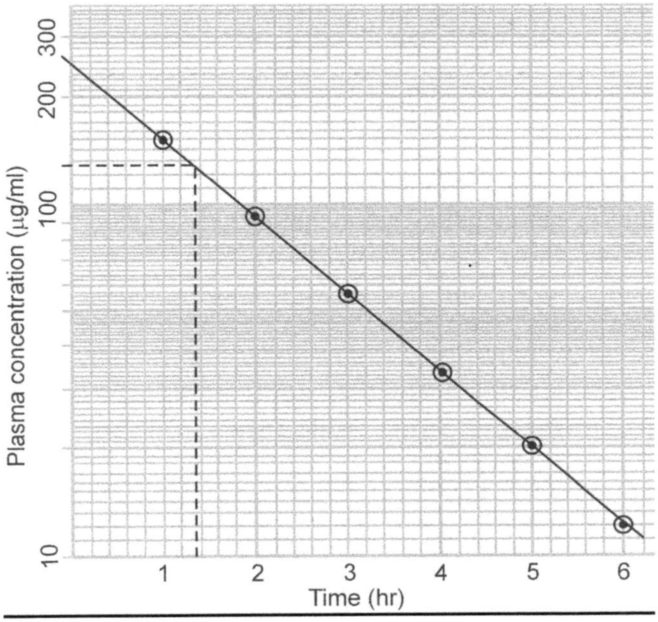

From the plot it is observed that 50% of the drug administered, that is 125mg of the drug was eliminated in 1hr and 18mins.

Thus, the elimination half-life of the drug is

Ans. 1 hr 18 min

Example

If the elimination half life of a drug is 5 hrs, find out the elimination rate constant, K_{el}.

Solution

Given that, elimination half life, $t_{\frac{1}{2}} = 5$ hrs

The elimination rate constant, $K_{el} = \dfrac{0.693}{t_{\frac{1}{2}}}$

$$= \frac{0.693}{5 \text{ hrs}}$$

Ans. $0.126\ \text{hr}^{-1}$

Example

In a formulation development studies three tablet formulations (F_1, F_6, F_8) were selected for further studies. Each tablet contains 250 mg of the drug. The rate and extent of dissolution of drug from the experimental formulations along with the reference formulation (the most popular brand) were estimated for bioequivalence. The results of the dissolution study are given below;

(i) Calculate cumulative % release of drug,

(ii) Plot cumulative % drug release vs. time

iii) Compare the best formulation with the reference one for bioequivalence.

Period (min)	Cumulative amount of drug (mg) dissolved			
	Ref	F_1	F_6	F_8
5	52.2	39.8	36.9	48.5
10	95.7	65.5	68.8	74.2
15	142.5	99.9	100.2	145.6
30	215.8	144.5	140.9	220.6
45	248.9	220.1	210.3	247.3
60	249.7	235.4	220.7	248.7
75	249.9	239.5	225.9	249.0
90	249.9	240.5	237.9	249.0

Solution

Given that, each tablet contains 250 mg of drug

(i) Cumulative % release of the drug

Amount of drug released from ref sample in 5 min = 20.88mg

$$\% \text{ release} = \frac{20.88}{250} \times 100 = 20.88$$

Period (min)	Ref	F_1	F_6	F_8
5	20.88	15.92	14.76	19.40
10	38.28	26.20	27.52	29.68
15	57.00	39.96	40.08	58.24
30	86.32	57.80	56.36	88.24
45	99.56	88.04	84.12	98.92

Table cond....

Period (min)	Ref	F_1	F_6	F_8
60	99.88	94.16	88.28	99.48
75	99.96	95.80	90.36	99.60
90	99.96	96.20	95.16	99.60

(ii) Plot cumulative %drug release vs. time

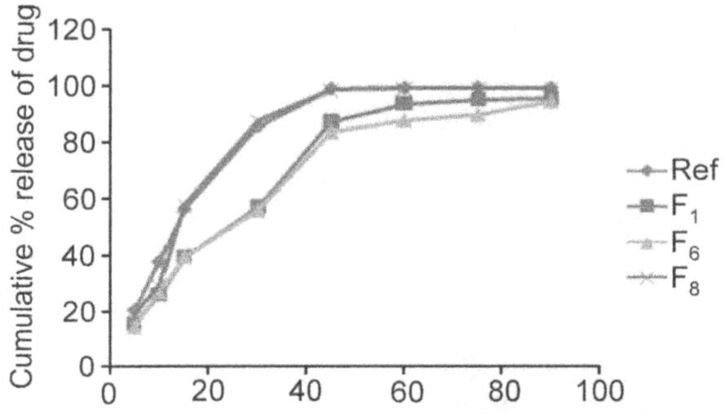

Plot of cumulative % release of drug vs. Time

(iii) The plot shows that the formulation F_8 is the best and bioequivalent to the Ref formulation.

Exercise

1. If the bioavailability factor (F) for a 250mg tablet of a drug is 0.80 compared with the bioavailability factor of 1.0 for an injection of the same drug, how many millilitres of the injection containing 100 mg/mL shall be considered bioequivalent to the tablet?

Ans: 2 ml

2. If 5 mL of an syrup containing 4mg of a drug is bioequivalent to a 15mg tablet having a bioavailability factor of 0.70, what is the bioavailability factor (F) of the syrup?

Ans: 2.625

3. A tablet containing 500 mg of a drug when administered orally, 350 mg are found to be absorbed into the circulation, calculate the bioavailability factor (F).

Ans: 0.7

4. A drug is 60% bioavailable when administered orally and 100% bioavailable when administered through intravenous route. To

replace the injection by tablet what should be the oral dose of the drug?

Ans: 1.67 times of the parenteral dose

5. If a patient has been receiving tablet containing 25mg of drug twice a day which is bioequivalent to 25mg per 5ml elixir. If he wishes to switch to the elixir, how many millilitres of the elixir should be administered to provide the equivalent dose of the drug?

Ans: 5 ml

6. A 2% ointment is 40% bioavailable while a tablet containing the 50mg of same drug is 60% bioavailable. A patient taking 2 tablets a day; if wishes to use ointment in place of tablet, how many grams of ointment he should apply?

Ans: 7.5g

7. An anti-asthmatic drug is 65% bioavailable and its dose is 5mg tablet. When the drug is administered in form of inhalation becomes 87.5% bioavailable. Calculate how many metered 500 µg sprays should be administered every 12 hourly to provide an equivalent dose of the drug?

Ans: 3.71 sprays

8. When a 5-mg dose of a drug is administered intravenously it produces a blood concentration of 0.45 µg/mL. What would be its apparent volume of distribution?

Ans: 11.1 L

9. The volume of distribution for a drug has been found 30 litres. What would be its expected plasma concentration immediately after an intravenous dose of 10 mg (in µg/dL)?

Ans: 33.3 µg/dL

10. If the bioavailability (F) of a drug in a 5 mg tablet is 0.65 compared to the bioavailability (F) of 0.85 in syrup (2mg/5ml), calculate the dose of the syrup equivalent to the tablet.

Ans: 9.56 ml

11. If the bioavailability factor (F) for a 400mg tablet of a drug is 0.70 was compared with the bioavailability factor of 1.0 for an intravenous injection of the same drug. How many millilitres of the injection containing 100 mg/mL would be considered bioequivalent to the tablet?

Ans: 2.8 ml

12. The bioavailability factor (F) for an intravenous injection (50 mg/mL) of a drug is 0.97 and the bioavailability factor was found 0.65 when a 200 mg capsule of the same drug was given. How many millilitres of the injection would be bioequivalent to the capsule?

Ans: 2.68 ml

13. A patient weighing 64 kg was administered 150mg of a drug through intravenous route. If the apparent volume of distribution is 14.7% of the body weight, calculate the plasma concentration of the drug.

Ans: 15.94 μg/ml

14. After intravenous administration of a drug to a patient weighing 59 kg the plasma concentration was measured and found 10.25 μg/mL. The apparent volume of distribution is 12.75% of body weight. Calculate the total amount of drug present in the body fluids after 3 hours of administration of the drug.

Ans: 85.28 mg

15. If the elimination half life of a drug is 4.5 hrs, find out the elimination rate constant, K_{el}.

Ans: 0.154 hr^{-1}

16. If the elimination half life of a drug is 3.75 hrs, find out the elimination rate constant, K_{el}.

Ans: 0.185 hr^{-1}

17. A patient was given a drug intravenously; after half an hour the plasma concentration was measured and found 0.05 mg/ml. The apparent volume of distribution is 15% of the body weight. If the body weight of the patient is 54.5kg, find out the amount of the drug administered.

Ans: 408.5 mg

18. A patient was given a drug intravenously; after half an hour the plasma concentration was measured and found 0.04 mg/ml. The apparent volume of distribution is 12.5% of the body weight. If the body weight of the patient is 49.5 kg, find out the amount of the drug administered.

Ans: 247.6 mg

19. The apparent volume of distribution of a drug is 34.5 litre and 250mg of the drug has been administered intravenously. Find out the expected plasma concentration of the drug.

Ans: 7.25 µg/ml

20. After intravenous administration of a drug to a patient weighing 72 kg the plasma concentration was measured and found 12.5 µg/mL. The apparent volume of distribution is 13.75% of body weight. Calculate the total amount of drug present in the body fluids after 2 hours of administration of the drug.

Ans: 12.37.6 mg

21. A single intravenous dose of 200 mg of a drug was administered and its blood concentration was found 9.75 µg/ml on immediate measurement. What would be the apparent volume of distribution?

Ans: 20.51 L

22. A single intravenous dose of 100 mg of a drug was administered and its blood concentration was found 8.5 µg/ml on immediate measurement. What would be the apparent volume of distribution?

Ans: 11.761 L

23. The bioavailability factor (F) for an intravenous injection (50 mg/mL) of a drug is 1.0 and the bioavailability factor was found 0.62 when a 200mg capsule of the same drug was given. How many millilitres of the injection would be bioequivalent to the capsule?

Ans: 2.48 ml

24. The bioavailability factor (F) for an intravenous injection (40 mg/mL) of a drug is 1.0 and the bioavailability factor was found 0.58 when a 150mg capsule of the same drug was given. How many millilitres of the injection would be bioequivalent to the capsule?

Ans: 1.74 ml

25. If the bioavailability factor (F) for a drug substance in a dosage form is 0.57, how many milligrams of drug would be available for absorption from a 100 mg tablet of the drug?

Ans: 57 mg

10

RADIOPHARMACEUTICALS

There are some elements which possess *isotopes*. Isotopes are chemically identical but physically, in particular their masses may vary slightly. Thus, isotopes may be defined as *atoms of same nuclear charge and same atomic number, but of different masses*. A particular isotope may be physically characterized by the mass number.

Isotopes may be stable and unstable. Stable isotopes never change unless some outside force is applied; while unstable isotopes undergo radioactive transformations. Hence, these are called radioactive isotopes. The radioactive isotope of an element is called *radioisotope* or *radionuclide*. They may be of two types - naturally occurring and artificially produced radionuclides.

Since early twentieth century, the naturally occurring radioisotopes have been used in medicine or pharmacy. The radium was first introduced in radiologic practice. After 1946, the artificially produced radioisotopes were used in hospitals. Since then, radioisotopes have become important tools in medical research. Some radioisotopes have been considered as extremely useful diagnostic and therapeutic agents, and led to develop a separate branch known as *nuclear medicine*.

Pharmacists preparing radioactive pharmaceuticals for use in patient care or for medical practice are called *nuclear pharmacists*.

The United States Pharmacopeia/National Formulary provides a chapter for compounding of radiopharmaceuticals for Positron Emission Tomography (PET). The USP/NF specifies procedures for;

- control of components, materials, and supplies;
- verification of compounding procedures;
- quality control and stability testing;
- Sterilization, sterility assurance and expiration dating.

Appropriate calculations, dilutions, and corrections for radioactive decay are performed by nuclear pharmacists during preparation of products for dosage administration.

Radioactivity

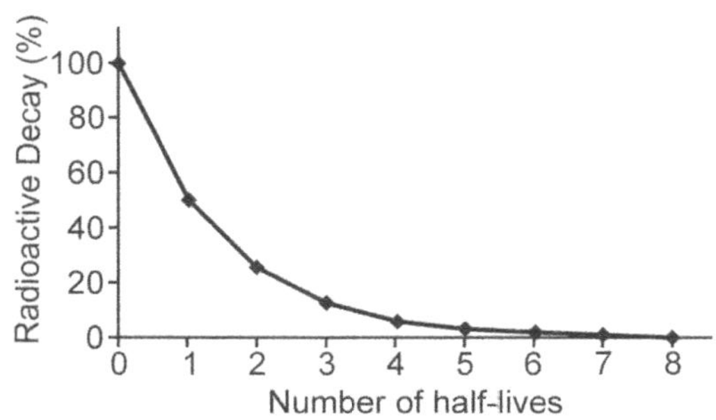

Figure 10.1

When an unstable isotope breaks down the process is called radioactive degradation or radioactive decay; the process of degradation continues till a stable state is reached. During such transforma- tion energy in the form of radiation is emitted. This radiation may consist of *alpha particles, beta particles,* and *gamma rays*. Different radioisotopes differ in the rate of radioactive decay; however in each case, a definite time is required for decaying to half the original atoms. This time is called the *half-life* of the radioisotope. Thus, each radioisotope has a different half-life.

To illustrate the decay rate and half life of radioisotopes a Figure is given below and a list of the half-lives of some commonly used radioisotopes is presented in the Table.

Radioisotope	Half-life	Radioisotope	Half-life
^{14}C (Carbon)	5,700 years	^{198}Au (Gold)	2.70 days
^{45}Ca (Calcium)	180 days	^{42}K (Potassium)	12.4 hours
^{57}Co (Cobalt)	270 days	^{99}Mo (Molybdenum)	2.6 years
^{60}Co (Cobalt)	5.27 years	^{22}Na (Sodium)	2.6 years
^{51}Cr (Chromium)	27.8 days	^{24}Na (Sodium)	15.0 hours
^{59}Fe (Iron)	45.1 days	^{32}P (Phosphorous)	14.3 days
^{203}Hg (Mercury)	46.6 days	^{35}S (Sulphur)	87.2 days
^{123}I (Iodine)	13.2 hours	^{75}Se (Selenium)	120 days
^{125}I (Iodine)	60 days	^{85}Sr (Strontium)	64 days
^{131}I (Iodine)	8.08 days	^{133}Xe (Xenon)	5.24 days

At any time the rate of decay represents a constant fraction of the total number of undecomposed atoms present. Mathematically, the rate of decay may be expressed as follows:

$$= \frac{dN}{dt} = \lambda N \qquad .....(10.1)$$

Where, N = the number of undecomposed atoms at time t and λ is the decay constant or the fraction disintegrating per unit of time.

The constant may be expressed in any unit of time, such as reciprocal seconds, minutes, hours, or days, etc. The equation 1 after integration may be expressed as (the *exponential decay law*),

$$N = N_o e^{-\lambda t} \qquad .....(10.2)$$

ss Where, N is the number of atoms remaining at t (elapsed time), N_o is the initial number of atoms (when t = 0), λ is the decay constant for the unit of time in terms of which the interval t is expressed, and e is the base of the natural logarithm 2.7183.

Because the rate of decay can also be characterized by the half-life ($T_{\frac{1}{2}}$) the value of N in equation 2 at the end

of a half period is $\frac{1}{2}N_o$. The equation then becomes,

$$\frac{1}{2} N_o = N_o^{-\lambda T_{\frac{1}{2}}} \qquad .....(10.3)$$

Or, $\ln 1/2 = -\lambda . T_{\frac{1}{2}}$

Or, $\ln 2 = \lambda . T_{\frac{1}{2}}$

Or, $\lambda . T_{\frac{1}{2}} = 2.303$

$\log 2 = 0.693$

Thus, $$T_{\frac{1}{2}} = \frac{0.693}{\lambda} \qquad .....(10.4)$$

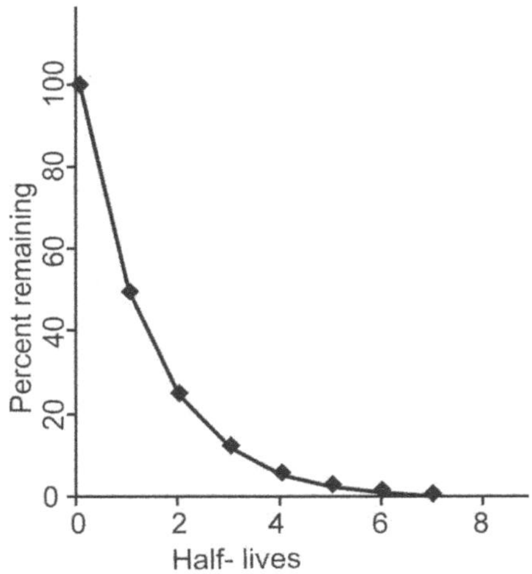

Figure 10.2 Disintegration of decay of radioisotopes.

Therefore, if the half-life ($T_{\frac{1}{2}}$) is known the value of the disintegration constant λ can be determined by using equation 4 and vice versa.

Units of Radioactivity

Earlier the basic unit of radioactive decay has been the *curie* (Ci), which denotes the number of atoms disintegrating in unit time (per second). When in a radioisotope 3.7×10^{10} atoms disintegrate in one second, it is called one Ci. The *milli-curie* (mCi) is one thousandth of a curie, the *micro-curie* (μCi) is one thousandth of a millicurie and the *nano-curie* (nCi) is one thousandth of a microcurie.

According to the International System (SI) unit for radioactivity is the *becquerel* (Bq), which represents one disintegration per second. This unit is so small that the multiples of the unit, such as the *kilo-becquerel* (KBq), *mega-becquerel* (MBq), and *giga-becquerel* (GBq), can be used. One kilo-becquerel represents 1000 disintegrations per second (1 kBq =1000Bq); one mega-becquerel (MBq) is equal to 10^3 kBq (i.e., 10^6disintegrations per second); and one giga-becquerel (GBq), is equal to 10^3MBq (10^9 disintegrations per second). These units have been adopted in the *United States Pharmacopeia*. However, till this date both units are being used to label radioactivity and the doses of many radiopharmaceuticals are expressed in mega-becquerel as well as in milli-curies or micro-curies.

Example

An injection of sodium chromate Cr 51 is administered for the determination of blood volume. The dose is 3.65 MBq. State this dose in terms of microcuries.

Solution

1 MBq = 0.027 mCi

3.65 MBq = 0.027 mCi × 3.65 = 0.09855 mCi

= 0.09855 mCi × 1000

Ans. 98.55μCi

Example

The disintegration or decay constant of a radioisotope is 0.03042 day^{-1}. Find out the half-life of the radio-isotope.

Solution

Given that, $\lambda = 0.03042$ day^{-1}

The disintegration half-life, $T_{\frac{1}{2}} = \frac{0.693}{\lambda}$

$$= \frac{0.693}{0.03042 \text{ day}-1}$$

Ans. 22.78 days

Example

The half-life of ^{60}Co (Cobalt) is 5.27 years. Calculate its disintegration constant.

Solution

Given that, the $T_{\frac{1}{2}}$ = 5.27 years

$$T_{\frac{1}{2}} = \frac{0.693}{\lambda}$$

$$5.27 = \frac{0.693}{\lambda}$$

or, $$\lambda = \frac{0.693}{5.27}$$

Ans. 0.1315 year^{-1}

Example

The initial concentration of a radioisotope was 450μCi per mL. After 20 days the concentration remaining is 115 μCi per mL; calculate (a) the disintegration constant and (b) the half life of the radioisotope.

Solution

Given that, initial concentration, N_o = 450 μCi/ml

The concentration, N = 115 μCi/ml when t = 20 days

(a) $N = N_o e^{-\lambda t}$

The logarithmic form of the above equation, $\ln \frac{N}{N_o} = -\lambda t$

The disintegration constant, $\lambda = \frac{2.303}{t} \log \frac{N_o}{N}$

$$= \frac{2.303}{20} \log \frac{450\mu Ci}{115\ \mu Ci}$$

$$= 0.1151 \log 3.913$$

$$= 0.1151 \times 0.5925$$

$$= 0.0682 \text{ day}^{-1} \text{ (Answer)}$$

(b) Half-life of the radioisotope, $T_{\frac{1}{2}} = \frac{0.693}{\lambda}$

The disintegration constant, $\lambda = 0.0682 \text{ day}^{-1}$

$$T_{\frac{1}{2}} = \frac{0.693}{0.0682 \text{ day}-1}$$

Ans. 10.16 days

Example

A sample of radioisotope has an initial activity of 205 μCi. Its half-life is 14.3 days. Calculate its activity on 11th day.

Solution

Given that, the initial activity, $N_o = 205\mu Ci$

Half-life, $T_{\frac{1}{2}} = 14.3$ days

Time, t = 10 days

Say, the radioactive activity on 11th day = N

The half-life, $T_{\frac{1}{2}} = 14.3 \text{ days} = \frac{0.693}{\lambda}$

Disintegration constant, $\lambda = \frac{0.693}{14.3 \text{ days}} = 0.0485 \text{ days}^{-1}$

$$\lambda = \frac{2.303}{t} \log \frac{N_o}{N}$$

$$0.0485 = \frac{2.303}{10} \log \frac{205}{N}$$

$$= 0.2303 (\log 2.3118 - \log N)$$

$$\log 2.3118 - \log N = \frac{0.0485}{0.2303} = 0.2106$$

$$\log N = 0.3640 - 0.2106 = 0.1534$$

$$N = \text{antilog } 0.1534$$

Ans. 1.423 μCi

Exercise

1. An injection of radioisotope is administered for the determination of blood volume. The dose is 4.5 MBq. State this dose in terms of microcuries.

   Ans: 121.5 μCi

2. An injection of radioisotope is administered for the determination of blood volume. The dose is 82.15 mCi. State this dose in terms of MBq.

   Ans: 3.04 MBq

3. The disintegration or decay constant of a radioisotope is 0.0402 day^{-1}. Find out the half-life of the radio-isotope.

   Ans: 17.24 days

4. The disintegration or decay constant of a radioisotope is 0.0782 day^{-1}. Find out the half-life of the radio-isotope.

   Ans: 8.86 days

5. The half-life of ^{45}Ca (Calcium) is 180 days. Calculate its disintegration constant.

   Ans: 3.85×10^{-3} min^{-1}

6. The initial concentration of a radioisotope was 425μCi per mL. After 15 days the concentration becomes 95 μCi per mL; calculate the disintegration constant.

   Ans: 0.0998 day^{-1}

7. The disintegration constant of a radio-isotopic degradation is 0.0998 day^{-1}; calculate the half life of the radioisotope.

   Ans: 6.94 days

11

CALCULATIONS RELATED TO PLANT EXTRACTS AND DRUG MOLECULE

At present, the interest in the use of botanicals and dietary supplements has increased among the people. Such products have become widely available to consumers. Even different governmental and non governmental agencies are working to ensure the safety in use of such products. Appropriate quality standards are being set. The *United States Pharmacopeia—National Formulary* (USP/NF) has included official monographs, general tests, assays, and manufacturing practices for a number of botanicals and dietary supplements. Among these echinacea, feverfew, garlic, ginkgo, ginseng, goldenseal, hawthorn, Saint John's wort, saw palmetto, and valerian are some whose official monographs are found. From the dried and pulverized plant parts (*e.g.*, leaves) containing the desired components various dosage forms may be prepared. Other pharmaceutical preparations are prepared by using the process of extraction (removing desired constituents from plant materials by appropriate solvent).

The information provided in this chapter includes:

- Distinguishing between *extracts*, *fluidextracts*, and *tinctures* on the basis of active drug content.
- Calculations related to the concentration and dose of extracted botanicals.
- Calculations related to the concentration and dose of botanic dietary supplements.

The plant materials include seeds, leaves, bark, or other plant parts that contain known or suspected *active therapeutic ingredients* (ATIs) or *active ingredients* (AIs), such as alkaloids, glycosides, or other pharmacologically active complex organic molecules.

There are two major processes used for extraction of active constituents from plant materials - *maceration* and *percolation.*

The term *maceration* originated from the Latin word *macerare,* meaning 'to soak.' In this process, the required crude drug is cut into very small pieces and placed in a suitable vessel, allowed to soak in a solvent or mixture of solvents (called the *menstruum*) for a sufficient period of time. The crude drugs soften and the soluble active constituents dissolve in the solvent. The menstruum is selected on basis of the solubility characteristics of the desired constituents. In most cases hydroalcoholic mixtures are used for extraction.

The dissolved constituents are then separated from the exhausted crude drug (called *marc*) either by straining or by filtration.

The term *percolation* is derived from the Latin word *per,* meaning 'through,' and *colare,* meaning 'to strain.' By this process, the soluble constituents are extracted from the crushed crude drug by the slow passage of a menstruum through a column packed with the plant material. The crushed crude drug is carefully packed in an extraction apparatus (called a *percolator*) and allowed to macerate with the solvent for a prescribed period of time before percolation. The size and material of construction of percolators vary. These may be made of glass or metals.

Small size laboratory percolators are of cone- or cylindrical-shaped. The diameter is several inches, and height is about 12 inches. On the other hand, percolators for industrial use are large in size, made of stainless-steel. Their diameter may range from 6 to 8 ft and height may vary from 12 to 18 feet. At the bottom of the percolator an orifice is there which permits the removal of the extractive (called *percolate*) conveniently.

Whether it is maceration or percolation, the components that are soluble in the menstruum are extracted. These may be therapeutically active as well as inactive, such as, sugars. Thus, an extractive obtained is a mixture of plant constituents.

The plant extractives are primarily extracts, fluid extracts, and tinctures. In general, the active therapeutic ingredient(s) are separated from the primary extractives by physicochemical methods. Then chemically identified, purified, and used as single therapeutic agents in various dosage forms, such as tablets, capsules, elixirs, syrups. In some cases, synthetic replicas or chemical congeners of the active therapeutic ingredients (ATIs) are prepared and used in place of naturally occurring therapeutic agents to make pharmaceutical products.

Extract, Fluidextract and Tincture

The concentrated preparations of vegetable (or animal) drugs are called extracts. Usually most extracts are about 400% concentrated than the crude drug in terms of active constituents; that is 1g of extract is obtained from 4g of crude drug. These are prepared by percolation and concentrated by the evaporation of all or almost all the menstruum. The final product may be either a powder-like or paste-like material. Thus, in an extract the extracted drug remains present in concentrated form. The dry extracts are usually 2 to 6 times more potent than the crude drug on dried basis. In other words, active constituents in one gram of extract may be equivalent to 2 to 6 grams of the crude drug. Some of the official extracts are: B*elladonna Extract, Cascara Sagrada Extract, Powdered Echinacea pallida Extract, Powdered Ginkgo Extract,* and *Powdered Asian Ginseng Extract, etc.*

Fluidextracts

Fluidextracts have fluid consistency and thus, are less potent than the powdered extracts. The drug content in liquid extracts of plant materials adjusted in such a way that each ml of fluid extract contains the active constituents present in 1 gram of the crude drug. Some of the official fluidextracts are: *Cascara Sagrada Fluidextract, Garlic Fluid extract, Licorice Fluid extract,* and *Senna Fluid extract, etc.*

Tinctures

Tinctures are extracts of plant materials. These are alcoholic or hydroalcoholic solutions of active constituents extracted from plant materials. However, hydroalcoholic solutions of some chemical substances, such as iodine are called tincture (Tincture of Iodine). Some of the official tinctures obtained from plant materials are: *Belladonna Tinctures, Compound Cardamom Tincture, Opium Tincture, Sweet Orange Peel Tincture,* and *Tolu Balsam Tincture, etc.*

There is no specified strength for tinctures. Traditionally the tinctures prepared from plant materials have been used have the following strength. Each 100 mL of tincture contains potent drug obtained from10 g crude drug, such as tincture contains essence obtained from 50 g crude drug of fruit or flavor, such as sweet orange peel.

The relative strengths of extracts, fluidextracts, and tinctures are shown below:

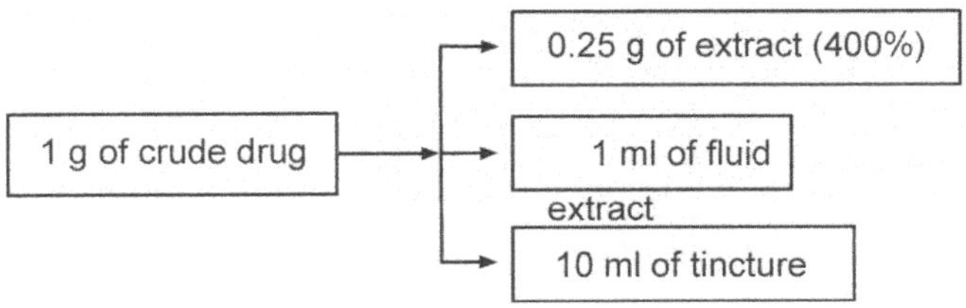

In other words, 1g of crude drug is equivalent to 0.25g of extract (400% extract), is equivalent to 1 ml of fluidextract and is equivalent to 10ml of tincture.

Example

If 5 mg of active ingredient is present in 5g of a crude drug, what would be the concentration, in terms of mg/g or mg/mL, of active ingredient in the corresponding (a) extract (400%), (b) fluidextract, and (c) potent tincture?

Solution

(a) Given that, 5 mg of active ingredient is present in 5g of crude drug.

As per definition, 0.25g of extract is equivalent to 1 g of crude drug in terms of 400% extraction.

Then, $\dfrac{0.25 \text{ g of extract}}{1 \text{ g of crude drug}} = \dfrac{x \text{ g of extract}}{5 \text{ g of crude drug}}$

$x = 1.25$ g of extract shall represent 5 mg of active constituent.

Thus, **250 mg of extract** per g of crude drug would represent 400% extract. (Ans)

(b) By definition, 1 mL of fluidextract is equivalent in active ingredient to 1 g of crude drug,

Since, 5 mg of active ingredient is present in 5 g of crude drug.

When 5 mg of active ingredient is present in 5 ml, it will be called fluidextract,

That is, the concentration would be 1 mg active ingredient/mL, Answer.

(c) 10 ml of a potent tincture represent the active ingredient obtained from each g of crude drug,

Given that, 5 mg of active ingredient is present in 5g of crude drug.

In other words, 5g of crude drug produce 50 ml of tincture

0.1g of crude drug would be needed to prepare 1 mL of tincture.

Thus, $\frac{\text{5g of crude drug}}{\text{0.1g of crude drug}} = \frac{\text{5 mg of active ingredient}}{x \text{ mg of active ingredient}}$

x = 0.1 mg of active ingredient/ml of tincture/g of crude drug. Answer

Example

If the dose of Nux Vomica tincture is 0.5 mL, what would be the equivalent corresponding dose of (a) Nux Vomica fruit? (b) Nux Vomica fluidextract? (c) An extract (200%) of Nux Vomica?

Solution

(a) A potent tincture contains in each 10 mL, the active constituents from 1 g of crude drug is:

$$\frac{\text{10 ml tincture}}{\text{0.5 ml tincture}} = \frac{\text{1 g crude drug}}{x \text{ g crude drug}}$$

x = 0.05g crude drug. Answer

(b) The active constituents of 1 g of crude drug are present 1 mL of fluid extract; in other words fluid extract is 10 times as concentrated as the potent tincture.

$$\frac{\text{1 g crude drug}}{\text{0.5 g crude drug}} = \frac{\text{1 ml fluid extract}}{x \text{ ml fluid extract}}$$

x = 0.5ml of fluid extract Answer

(c) A "400%" extract refers to 0.25g of extract from each g of crude drug; that is, four times the AI content as the crude drug.

Since the dose of the crude drug is 0.05 g, the dose of the extract would be $\frac{1}{4}$ of the dose:

Or, 0.05 g × $\frac{1}{4}$

Ans. 0.0125 g or 12.5 mg

Determination of Ethanol-Soluble Extractives

The method of extraction may be either maceration or percolation, may be hot or cold extraction. The alcoholic extract obtained is first concentrated over a boiling water bath; then dried under circulating air. The processing condition for extraction depends on the type of compound being extracted. For example, when volatile oil is extracted, heat is not applied. However, after extraction the extractive must be calculated. The crude drug used for extraction should be air-dried and extractive should also be air-dried.

Example

5.0035 g of a crude drug is extracted using method of percolation. The initial weight of the petri dish was 18.2543g and final weight with extractive was 18.3443g. Calculate the ethanol-soluble extractive in terms of percent weight by weight.

Solution

Weight of the sample taken = 5. 0035g ≈ 5.0g

Weight of the petri dish = 18.2543g

Final weight of the petri dish + extract = 18.3443g

Weight of the extract = 18.3443g – 18.2543g = 0.0900g

The content of ethanol-soluble extractive in the crude drug

$$= \frac{0.0900 \times 100}{5}$$

Ans. 1.8%w/w

Example

25 g of a crude drug was subjected to ethanolic extraction by maceration. The weight of petri dish with extractive was found to increase from 18.4523 g to 18.5237g. Calculate the extractive in terms of %w/w.

Solution

Weight of the sample taken = 25 g

Weight of the petri dish = 18.4523 g

Final weight of the petri dish + extract = 18.5237 g

Weight of the extract = 18.5237 g – 18.4523 g = 0.0714 g

The content of ethanol-soluble extractive in the crude drug

$$= \frac{0.0714 \times 100}{25}$$

Ans. 0.2856%w/w

Determination of Water-Soluble Extractives

The method of extraction may be either maceration or percolation, may be hot or cold extraction. The water-soluble extract obtained is first concentrated over a boiling water bath; then dried in hot air oven at 105°C. The processing condition for extraction depends on the type of compound being extracted. However, after extraction the extractive must be calculated. The crude drug used for extraction should be air-dried and extractive should also be calculated on air-dried basis.

Example

20 g of a crude drug was subjected to extraction by maceration using water as the solvent. After drying the weight of petri dish with extractive was found to increase from 17.9752 g to 18.0773g. Calculate the extractive in terms of %w/w.

Solution

Weight of the sample taken = 20 g

Weight of the petri dish = 17.9752 g

Final weight of the petri dish + extract = 18.0773g

Weight of the extract = 18.0773g – 17.9752 g = 0.1012g

The content of water-soluble extractive in the crude drug

$$= \frac{0.1012 \times 100}{20}$$

Ans. 0.5105%w/w

Determination of Saponification Value

In many organisms fats and oils are the store-house of various forms of energy. These are highly reduced compounds and are derived from fatty acids. Fatty acids are carboxylic acids with hydrocarbon chains of 4 to

36 carbons. These may be saturated or unsaturated. The simplest fatty acids are triacylglycerols or triglycerides. Triacylglycerols are composed of three fatty acids each of which is linked with a glycerol molecule. Since the polar hydroxyl groups of glycerol are bound with the polar carboxyl groups of the fatty acids in ester linkages, triacyl glycerols become non polar, hydrophobic, and insoluble in water.

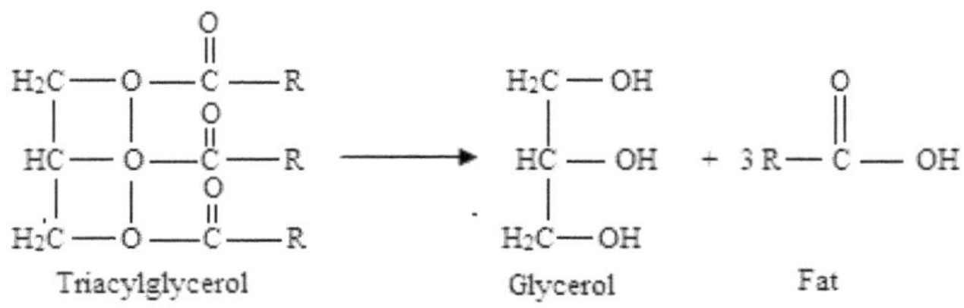

The knowledge about saponification (SAP) value helps in making soap. If the sap value of an oil or fat is high, it requires much of alkali to saponify even though there is soapiness sufficient for cleaning the skin. On the other hand, if the sap value is too less, the soapiness of the fatty acid salts would not be sufficient to remove the dirt or clean the skin. The sap values of some oils along with their effect on skin cleaning are given in tabular form below.

Fat or oil	SAP value	Hard/soft soap	Cleansing property	Lather quality	Skin care
Castor oil	128.6	Soft	Fair	Fluffy & stable	Good
Coconut oil	191.1	Hard	Good	Fluffy & non-stable	Fair
Jojoba oil	69.5	Soft	Fair	Stable, but not fluffy	Good
Kukui nut oil	135.5	Soft	Good	Stable, but not fluffy	Good
Lard	138.7	Hard	Good	Stable, but not fluffy	Fair
Olive oil	135.3	Soft	Good	Unstable & not fluffy	Good
Palm oil	142	Hard	Good	Stable, but not fluffy	Fair
Peanut oil	137	Soft	Fair	Stable, but not fluffy	Good
Soybean oil	135.9	Soft	Good	Stable, but not fluffy	Fair
Sweet almond oil	137.3	Soft	Good	Stable, but not fluffy	Excellent
Tallow	140.5	Hard	Good	Stable, but	Fair

				not fluffy	

Saponification value is the number of milligrams of potassium hydroxide required to neutralize the free acids and to saponify esters present in 1g of oil.

Adequate sample (say, x g) is taken in a standard joint flask; 25 ml of 0.5M ethanolic-KOH is added. Reflux condenser is fitted and put over a boiling water-bath for 45 – 60 min; allowed to cool, the condenser is removed and the content in the flask is titrated against 0.5M HCl using phenolphthalein solution as indicator (z ml). In a separate flask 2 ml of water and 25 ml of 0.5M ethanolic-KOH is taken; refluxed for same time, cooled to room temperature and titrated against 0.5M HCl using same indicator (Blank titration, say y ml). The difference in the titer value represents the amount of KOH consumed by the sample.

Then the saponification value $= \dfrac{(y-z \text{ ml}) \times 28.05}{x \text{ g}}$

Example

2.0541 g of oil was subjected to determination of saponification value. It was refluxed for 50 min with 25 ml of 0.498 M ethanolic-KOH; when titrated against 0.504 M HCl, the titer value was 17.95ml. 25 ml of 0.498 M ethanolic-KOH was equivalent to 24.70ml of 0.504 M HCl. Calculate the saponification value of the sample.

Solution

Given that, 25 ml of 0.498 M ethanolic-KOH

$\approx$ 24.70ml of 0.504 M HCl (y).

The titer value = 17.95 ml of 0.504 M HCl (z).

The difference in titer values = 6.75 ml ($y - z$).

The volume of 0.498 M ethanolic-KOH consumed by the sample

$$= \frac{6.75 \times 0.504}{0.5} = 6.80\text{ml}$$

[Each ml of 1M ethanolic-KOH is equivalent to 56.10 mg of KOH

Each ml of 0.5M ethanolic-KOH is equivalent to 28.05 mg of KOH]

Saponification value of the sample is the milligrams of KOH consumed by 1g of sample

$$= \frac{6.8 \text{ mg} \times 28.05}{2.0541\text{g}}$$

Ans. 92.86

Example

For determination of saponification value 5.0 g of a sample was taken for refluxing with 15 ml of 1M Ethanolic-potassium hydroxide solution. After refluxing the solution was titrated with 1.004M hydrochloric acid and 13.75 ml was the titer value. In blank titration 15 ml of 1M ethanolic-potassium hydroxide solution was found equivalent to 15.20 ml of 1.004 M HCl; calculate the saponification value.

Solution

Given that, the strength of 1M hydrochloric acid = 1.004

Sample taken = 5.0 g

15.00 ml of ethanolic-potassium hydroxide solution

$\approx$ 15.20 ml of 1.004 M HCl

Volume of 15.20 ml of 1.004 M HCl required in titration = 13.75 ml

The difference in titer values = 15.20 – 13.75 ml = 1.45 ml$(y - z)$.

Each ml of 0.5 M ethanolic-KOH is equivalent to 28.05 mg of KOH

Each ml of 1 M ethanolic-KOH is equivalent to 56.10 mg of KOH

Saponification value of the sample is the milligrams of KOH consumed by 1g of sample

$$= \frac{1.45 \text{ mg} \times 56.10}{5.0\text{g}}$$

Ans. 16.27

Determination of Iodine Value

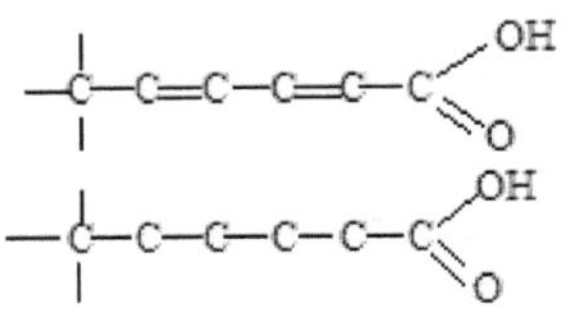

Unsaturated fatty acid

Saturated fatty acid

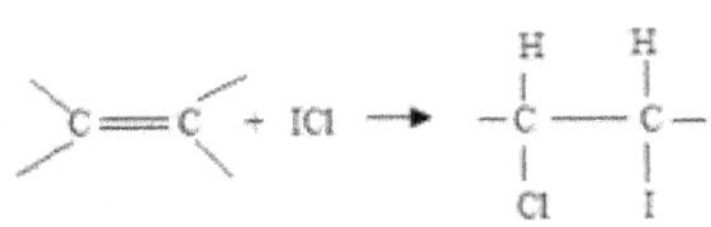

Fats and oils are a mixture of triglycerides. When three fatty acids are attached to glycerol by fatty acyl esters trigly cerides are formed. Fatty acids are long chain hydrocarbons containing carboxyl groups (COOH groups). Based on the number of double bonds present in the fatty acid these are classified into saturated or unsaturated fatty acids. If the fatty acids contain only single bond between the carbon atoms these are called saturated fatty acids and these are solids at room temperature. While in unsaturated fatty acids the carbon atoms are joined with double bonds in addition to the single bonds present in the fatty acid chain. At room temperature these are found to exist as liquids. Fatty acids react with a halogen such as iodine and form addition products. Addition of the halogen takes place at the site of C=C double bond. The iodine monochloride reacts with fatty acid and produce a di-halogenated compound. One carbon of the double bond is linked to chlorine and the other to iodine. After completion of the reaction, the amount of iodine reacted is determined by adding a solution of potassium iodide to the reaction product. The unreacted iodine monochloride (ICl) remaining in the sample form molecular iodine. The liberated iodine (I_2) is then titrated with a standard solution of 0.1M sodium thiosulphate. Saturated fatty acids do not take part in the halogenation reaction. In case of fats the iodine number is within 0 to 70, and in case of oil the value is more than 70. Starch is used as the indicator for this reaction; the liberated iodine reacts with starch and produce purple colored starch-iodide. At the endpoint the solution becomes colorless.

$$ICl + KI \longrightarrow KCl + I_2$$

$$I_2 + 2\,Na_2S_2O_3 \longrightarrow 2\,NaI + Na_2S_2O_4$$

Iodine value of a substance is defined by the numbers of grams of halogen calculated as iodine absorbed by 100g of the substance.

The quantity of sample to be taken for determination of iodine value depends on expected/presumed iodine value of the sample; it varies from 0.1g to 1.0g. If the iodine value is less than 20 the sample quantity should be about 1.0 g; if the iodine value is more than 100 the least amount (0.1g) of sample to be taken. In general, for addition of halogen 20 – 25 ml of iodine monochloride solution is added to sample and the unreacted iodine is determined with 0.1M sodium thiosulphate standard solution.

Calculation: Iodine value $= 0.01269 \dfrac{(a-b)s}{x} \times 100$

$$= 1.269 \frac{(a-b)s}{x}$$

Where, a = the volume of 0.1M Sodium thiosulphate standard solution equivalent to 20 ml of iodine monochloride solution (Blank titer value)

b = the volume of 0.1 M Sodium thiosulphate standard solution equivalent to unreacted iodine monochloride solution (sample titer value)

s = strength of Sodium thiosulphate standard solution, and

x = the amount of sample taken.

0.01269g of iodine equivalent to 1 ml of 0.1 M Sodium thiosulphate solution

---

Example

A sample of 0.5056g was taken for iodine value determination. 20 ml of Iodine monochloride solution was added which was equivalent to 22.15 ml of 0.1 M solution of Sodium thiosulphate. After completion of reaction unreacted iodine consumed 15.75 ml of 0.1 M solution of Sodium thiosulphate. If the strength of Sodium thiosulphate solution was 1.0015 M, calculate the iodine value of the sample.

Solution

The strength of Sodium thiosulphate solution is 1.001M (s)

The volume of 0.1M Sodium thiosulphate standard solution equivalent to 20 ml of iodine monochloride solution (blank titer value, a) = 22.15 ml

The volume of 0.1M Sodium thiosulphate standard solution equivalent to unreacted iodine monochloride solution (sample titer value, b) = 15.75 ml

Amount of sample taken (x) = 0.5056g

Then, Iodine value = $1.269 \frac{(22.15-15.75) \times 1.001\text{ml}}{0.5056\text{g}}$

Ans. 12.67

Determination of Acid Value

One of the common parameter in the specification of fats and oils is the acid value. It is defined as the milligrams of KOH required to neutralize the organic acids present in 1 g of fat. It is a measure of the free fatty acids (FFA) present in the fat or oil. Sometimes the amount of free fatty acids in a sample of oil or fat may increase; this is due to hydrolysis of triglycerides. The enzyme, lipase is responsible for such reaction (hydrolysis) and it indicates inadequate processing and storage conditions, such as high temperature, relative humidity, and tissue damage. The source of the enzyme may be the tissue from which the oil or fat has been extracted or it can be a contaminant from other cells including microorganisms. Hydrolysis of triglycerides produces glycerol in addition to free fatty acids.

Free fatty acids are a source of flavors and aromas. There are short chain free fatty acids which tend to be water soluble and volatile with characteristic odor; and the long chain saturated and unsaturated fatty acids. The long chain saturated and unsaturated fatty acids are more prone to oxidation in their free form and their breakdown products (aldehydes, ketones, alcohols, and organic acids) provide characteristic flavors and aromas. In most cases these flavors and aromas are unwanted in oils, fats, and foods in which these are present. However, in some cases hydrolysis of triglycerides and oxidation of free fatty acids are necessary for the development of desirable flavor and aroma in foods; for example in case of aged cheeses and some processed meats.

The acid value is defined as the number of milligrams of potassium hydroxide required to neutralize the free acids present in 1g of a substance.

Usually 10 g of sample is dissolved in 50ml of alcohol (95%) and ether mixture (1:1). The solvent is previously neutralized with 0.1M KOH solution using phenolphthalein as indicator. If the sample does not go into solution in cold solvent, the mixture of sample and solvent may be refluxed at warm temperature for dissolution with occasional shaking until the substance goes into solution. Cooled to room temperature and then titrated against 0.1M KOH solution using phenolphthalein as indicator.

Calculation: Acid value $= 5.61 \times \frac{a \times s}{x}$;

where, a = volume of 0.1M KOH solution required for neutralization,

s = strength of 0.1M KOH solution

x = weight of substance taken

Example

For determination of acid value 10.1405g of oil was taken and 2.45 ml of 0.1M KOH solution were required for neutralization. Calculate the acid value of the oil. The strength of the 0.1M KOH solution was 1.01 2M.

Solution

Given that, a = 2.45 ml

$s = 1.012\text{M}$ and $x = 10.1405$ g

$$\text{Acid value of the oil} = 5.61\text{mg} \times \frac{2.45 \text{ ml} \times 1.012}{10.012\text{g}}$$

Ans. 0.25 mg/g

Determination of Acetyl Value

It is a measure of the free hydroxyl groups in a substance, such as a fat or oil, determined by acetylation. It is defined as *the number of milligrams of potassium hydroxide required for neutralization of the acetic acid formed by hydrolysis of one gram of the acetylated substance.*

In general the substance under investigation is mixed with acetic anhydride and boiled for specified hours as per the official method. After cooling, water is added to the mixture and boiled again. The acetylated product is separated from the other substances present in aqueous layer and purified by washing with water and saline solution as described in the official method. Then the acetylated product is mixed with anhydrous sodium sulphate and filtered through a dry pleated filter. Finally the product is saponified as per the standard method. The saponification value of substance is determined as such (without acetylation) and acetyl value is calculated as follows.

$$\text{Acetyl value} = \frac{1335\,(b-a)}{1335-a}$$

where, a = saponification value of the substance and

b = saponification value of the acetylated substance

Example

The saponification value of a substance is 12.89 and after acetylation when acetylated product is saponified it is found to be 1.25. Calculate the acetyl value of the substance.

Solution

Given that, $a = 12.89$ and $b = 1.25$

$$\text{Acetyl value} = \frac{1335\,(b-a)}{1335-a}$$

$$= \frac{1335\,(12.89-1.25)}{1335-12.89}$$

Ans. 11.75

Calculation of Retention Factors (R_f) for Thin Layer Chromatography

Thin Layer Chromatography (TLC) is a simple technique for quick screening of active constituents obtained from plant extractives or synthesis. It is inexpensive and does not require well equipped laboratory. A standard or developed TLC method can be useful for rapid screening by comparing the sample solution with different concentrations of reference material.

Conventional TLC requires thick glass tanks, beakers, or other glass containers for development of the chromatograms, Development bag, Saturation pads, thin layer support, plastic bag for visualizing solution, and positioning rod. For spotting 3 positions at the bottom 1.5, 2.5, and 3.5 cm from the edge of the sheet or plate are to be marked with pencil. The sample solution, expected to be equivalent to 100% in the center position, about 85% reference at the left position and the 115% reference (120% reference for antibiotics) at the right position are to be spotted. The eluting solvent or solvent mixture is allowed to separate the components present in the sample spotted. According to the solubility the components are eluted on the adsorbent plate. As shown in the figure the solvent moves upward and carries the component. Once the solvent reaches the desired height the plate is withdrawn carefully and dried. Then the distance travelled by the solvent and the distance travelled by the component are measured and the R_f-value is calculated and compared with that of sample.

Retention factors are numbers between zero and one, representing the position of the spot on the TLC plate.

The distance travelled by the solvent (solvent front) = b and the distance travelled by the component = a; then $R_f = \frac{a}{b}$.

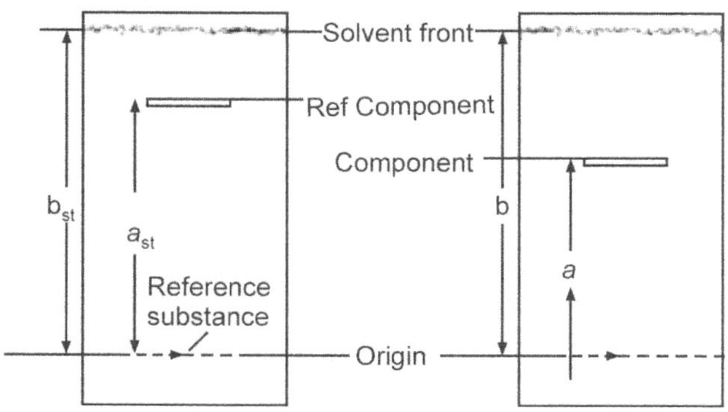

In case of reference substance or standard a_{st} and b_{st} stand for a and b respectively.

Example

In a TLC experiment the distance travelled by the eluting solvent is 10cm and the distance travelled by the component is 6cm. Calculate the R_f value for the component.

Solution

Given that, a = 6cm and b = 10cm

$$R_f = \frac{a}{b} = \frac{6}{10}$$

Ans. 0.6

Calculation of Chemical Moiety and Equivalency

Sometimes it is necessary to calculate the pharmacologically active drug (chemical) moiety when present in plant, herb, or in chemical form as salt, ester, hydrated, or complex. Such calculations become essential when products of the same drug moiety but differing in chemical form are to be compared quantitatively.

The calculations involve application of atomic and molecular weights. Most chemical problems involve the use of atomic or combining weights of the elements, and the validity of their solutions depends on the law of Definite Proportions.

The atomic weight of an element is considered as the ratio of the weight of its atom to the weight of an atom of another element taken as a standard. Earlier hydrogen was used as the standard. Thereafter for many years oxygen, has been used as standard element. Since 1961, the International Union of Pure and Applied Chemistry released the most up-to-date table of atomic weights based on carbon, taking 12 (the mass of the isotope ^{12}C).

Example

Calculate the percentage composition of sucrose.

Solution

The molecular formula of sucrose is $C_{12}H_{22}O_{11}$

The molecular weight of sucrose = 12 × C + 22 × H + 11 × O

$$= 12 \times 12.01 + 22 \times 1.008 + 11 \times 16$$

$= 144.12 + 22.176 + 176$

$= 342.188$

Percent content of carbon $= \frac{144.12 \times 100}{342.188} = 42.117 \approx 42.12$ (Answer)

Percent content of hydrogen $= \frac{22.176 \times 100}{342.188} = 6.48$ (Answer)

Percent content of oxygen $= \frac{176 \times 100}{342.188} = 51.43$ (Answer)

[Verification: 42.12 + 6.48 + 51.43 = 100.03]

Example

Calculate the percentage content of oxygen in potassium permanganate.

Solution

The molecular formula of potassium permanganate is $KMnO_4$

The molecular weight $= 1 \times K + 1 \times Mn + 4 \times O$

$= 1 \times 39.09 + 1 \times 54.94 + 4 \times 16$

$= 39.09 + 54.94 + 64$

$= 158.03$

Percent content of oxygen $= \frac{64 \times 100}{158.03}$

Ans. 40.50

Example

Each tablet of Ferrous Sulphate tablets contains an amount of $FeSO_4$ equivalent to 300 mg of $FeSO_4$ $7H_2O$. Find out the amount of FeSO4 per tablet.

Solution

Molecular weight of $FeSO_4,7H_2O$

$= 1\times55.85 + 1\times32.06 + 4\times16 + 7(2\times1.008 + 1\times16)$

$= 55.85 + 32.066 + 64 + 7(18.016)$

$= 278.026 \approx 278.03$

Molecular weight of $FeSO_4 = 1\times55.85 + 1\times32.06 + 4\times16$

$= 55.85 + 32.066 + 64$

$= 151.91$

$$= 55.85 + 32.066 + 64$$

$$= 151.91$$

Chemically 1 mole of $FeSO_4,7H_2O \approx$ 1 mole of $FeSO_4$

That is, 278.03 g of $FeSO_4,7H_2O \approx 151.91$g of $FeSO_4$

$$1 \text{ mg of } FeSO_4,7H_2O \approx \frac{151.91}{278.03} \text{ mg of } FeSO_4$$

$$300 \text{ mg of } FeSO_4,7H_2O \approx \frac{151.91}{278.03} \times 300 \text{ mg of } FeSO_4$$

$$= 163.91 \text{ mg of } FeSO_4$$

Hence, each tablet should contain

Ans. 163.91 mg of $FeSO_4$

Example

Meclizine Hydrochloride, $C_{25}H_{27}ClN_2$, 2HCl.H_2O contains one molecule of water of crystallization. Each tablet contains 25 mg of $C_{25}H_{27}ClN_2$, 2HCl.H_2O. Calculate the amount of $C_{25}H_{27}ClN_2$, 2HCl per tablet.

Solution

Molecular weight of hydrous Meclizine hydrochloride, $C_{25}H_{27}ClN_2$, 2HCl.H_2O

$$= 25\times12 + 27\times1.008 + 1\times35.457 + 2\times14.008$$

$$+ 2(1.008 + 35.457) + 2\times1.008 + 16$$

$$= 300 + 27.216 + 35.457 + 28.016 + 72.93 + 18.016$$

$$= 481.635$$

Molecular weight of anhydrous Meclizine hydrochloride, $C_{25}H_{27}ClN_2$, 2HCl

$$= 25\times12 + 27\times1.008 + 1\times35.457 + 2\times14.008$$

$$+ 2(1.008 + 35.457)$$

$$= 300 + 27.216 + 35.457 + 28.016 + 72.93$$

$$= 463.619$$

Functionally 1 mole of $C_{25}H_{27}ClN_2$, 2HCl.$H_2O \approx$ 1 mole of $C_{25}H_{27}ClN_2$, 2HCl.

That is, 481.635 g of $C_{25}H_{27}ClN_2$, 2HCl.H_2O ≈ 463.619 g of $C_{25}H_{27}ClN_2$, 2HCl

Or, 481.635 mg of $C_{25}H_{27}ClN_2$, 2HCl.H_2O ≈ 463.619 mg of $C_{25}H_{27}ClN_2$, 2HCl

1 mg of $C_{25}H_{27}ClN_2$, 2HCl.$H_2O \approx \frac{463.619}{481.635}$ mg of $C_{25}H_{27}ClN_2$, 2HCl

25 mg of $C_{25}H_{27}ClN_2$, 2HCl.$H_2O \approx \frac{463.619}{481.635} \times 25$ mg of $C_{25}H_{27}ClN_2$, 2HCl

= 24.06 mg of $C_{25}H_{27}ClN_2$, 2HCl

Hence, each tablet contains

Ans. 24.06 mg of $C_{25}H_{27}ClN_2$, 2HCl

Example

Each capsule contains Ampicillin Trihydrate equivalent to 500mg of Ampicillin. The molecular weight of Ampicillin is 349.41. Calculate how many milligrams of Ampicillin Trihydrate should be filled in each capsule.

Solution

The molecular weight of Ampicillin,

$C_{16}H_{19}N_3O_4S$ is 349.41

$(16 \times 12 + 19 \times 1.008 + 3 \times 14.008 + 4\times 16 + 1 \times 32.006$

$= 192 + 19.152 + 42.024 + 64 + 32.006 = 349.18)$

The molecular weight of Ampicillin trihydrate, $C_{16}H_{19}N_3O_4S,3H_2O$ would be $349.41+3\times18.016 = 403.458$

Chemically 1 mole of Ampicillin ≈ 1 mole of Ampicillin trihydrate

That is, 349.41g of Ampicillin ≈ 403.458 g of Ampicillin trihydrate

Or, 1mg of Ampicillin $\approx \frac{403.46}{349.41}$ mg of Ampicillin trihydrate

500 mg of Ampicillin $\approx \frac{403.46}{349.41} \times 500$ mg of Ampicillin trihydrate

= 577.34 mg of Ampicillin trihydrate

Hence, each capsule should be filled with 577.34 mg of Ampicillin trihydrate. Answer

Example

Each 5 ml of an oral suspension contains erythromycin stearate ($C_{37}H_{67}NO_{13}.C_{18}H_{36}O_2$) equivalent to 100mg of erythromycin ($C_{37}H_{67}NO_{13}$). Calculate the quantity of erythromycin stearate to be contained in 5 ml.

Solution

Molecular weight of erythromycin stearate:

$$C_{37}H_{67}NO_{13}.C_{18}H_{36}O_2 = 37\times C + 67\times H + 1\times N + 13\times O + 18\times C + 36\times H + 2\times O$$

$$= 37\times 12 + 67\times 1.008 + 1\times 14.008 + 13\times 16 + 18\times 12 + 36\times 1.008 + 2\times 16$$

$$= 444 + 67.536 + 14.008 + 208 + 216 + 36.288 + 32$$

$$= 1017.83$$

Molecular weight of erythromycin:

$$C_{37}H_{67}NO_{13} = 37\times C + 67\times H + 1\times N + 13\times O$$

$$= 37 \times 12 + 67 \times 1.008 + 1 \times 14.008 + 13 \times 16$$

$$= 444 + 67.536 + 14.008 + 208$$

$$= 733.54$$

Functionally 1 mole of erythromycin ≈ 1 mole of erythromycin stearate

That is, 733.54g of erythromycin ≈ 1017.83g of erythromycin stearate

$$1 \text{ mg of erythromycin} \approx \frac{1017.83}{733.54} \text{ mg of erythromycin stearate}$$

$$100 \text{ mg of erythromycin} \approx \frac{1017.83}{733.54} \times 100 \text{ mg of erythromycin stearate}$$

$$= 138.75 \text{ mg of Erythromycin stearate.}$$

Thus, each 5ml of suspension should contain 138.75 mg of erythromycin stearate. (Answer)

Example

On test the drug content of a sample of tablet was found to be 97.98% on 'as is' basis and loss on drying was 2.05%. According to the pharmacopoeial monograph the assay value should be not less than

99% on dried basis. Express the assay value as per the pharmacopoeial standard.

Solution

Given that the assay value = 97.98%

Loss on drying = 2.05%

Assay value on dried basis $= \frac{97.98 \times 100}{100-2.05} = \frac{97.98 \times 100}{97.95}$

Ans. 100.03%

Example

A tablet was prepared from ferrous sulphate to provide 100mg of elemental iron per tablet. Calculate how many kilo grams of ferrous sulphate (heptahydrate) was used to prepare 2.0 lakh tablets.

Solution

Given that, each tablet contains 100mg of elemental iron (Fe)

Lot size or number of tablets = 200 000

Now, molecular weight of ferrous sulphate (heptahydrate) $FeSO_4,7H_2O$

$= 56 + 32 + 4\times16 + 7\times18$

$= 56 + 32 + 64 + 126$

$= 278$

Atomic weight of iron = 56

Thus, each molecule of $FeSO_4,7H_2O$ provides one Fe atom

Or, 56 mg of Fe can be obtained from 278mg of $FeSO_4,7H_2O$

100 mg of Fe can be obtained from $\frac{278 \times 100}{56}$ mg of $FeSO_4,7H_2O$

= 496.43mg of $FeSO_4,7H_2O$

Hence, to prepare 1 tablet 496.43mg of $FeSO_4,7H_2O$ was required

To prepare 200 000 tablets 200000 × 496.43mg of $FeSO_4,7H_2O$ was required

= 99286000mg of $FeSO_4,7H_2O$ was required

Ans. 99.286 kg

Example

An antacid suspension contains 250mg of aluminium hydroxide, calculated as Al_2O_3, per 10ml. The suspension was prepared using colloidal aluminium hydroxide containing 4.2% w/w of Al_2O_3. Calculate the amount of colloidal aluminium hydroxide required for one liter of suspension.

Solution

Given that, each 10 ml of suspension contain 250 mg of Al_2O_3

Colloidal aluminium hydroxide contains 4.2%w/w of Al_2O_3

Volume of suspension prepared = 1 liter = 1000 ml

4.2 g of Al_2O_3 is present in 100 g of Colloidal aluminium hydroxide

Or, 4.2 mg of Al_2O_3 is present in 100 mg of Colloidal aluminium hydroxide

250 mg of Al_2O_3 is present in $\frac{100 \times 250}{4.2}$ mg = 5952.4 mg of Colloidal aluminium hydroxide

= 5.95 g of Colloidal aluminium hydroxide

Thus, 10 ml of suspension contains 5.95g of Colloidal aluminium hydroxide

So, 1000ml of suspension contains $\frac{5.95 \times 1000}{10}$ g = 595 g of Colloidal aluminium hydroxide

Hence, for 1 liter 595 g of Colloidal aluminium hydroxide would be required. (Answer)

Exercise

1. If 25 mg of active constituent is present in 10 gram of a crude drug, what would be the concentration, in terms of mg/g or mg/mL, of active ingredient in the corresponding (a) extract (400%), (b) fluid extract, and (b) potent tincture?

Ans: (a) 10 mg of active constituent per g of extract represent 400% extract.

(b) 2.5 mg of active ingredient/mL.

(c) 0.25 mg of active ingredient/ml of tincture.

2. If the dose of Belladonna tincture is 0.25 mL, what would be the equivalent corresponding dose of (a) Belladonna fruit? (b) Belladonna fluidextract? (c) An extract (200%) of Belladonna?

Ans: (a) 0.025g crude drug

(b) 0.5ml of fluidextract

(c) 0.00625 g or 6.25 mg

3. If 30 mg of active ingredient is present in 5 g of a crude drug, what would be the concentration, in terms of mg/g or mg/mL, of active ingredient in the corresponding (a) 400% extract, (b) fluidextract, and (c) potent tincture?

Ans: (a) 24 mg of active constituent/g of extract per 5 g of crude drug

(b) 6 mg active ingredient/mL of fluidextract

(c) 0.6 mg of active ingredient/ml of tincture

4. If the dose of a tincture is 0.5 mL, what would be the equivalent corresponding dose of (a) fruit extract? (b) Fluid extract? (c) An extract (200%)?

Ans: (a) 0.05g crude drug

(b) 0.5ml of fluid extract

(c) 0.0125 g or 12.5 mg

5. 10.0 g of a crude drug was extracted by the method of percolation. The concentrated ethanolic extract was finally taken in a 25 ml glass cylinder and dried. The initial weight of the cylinder was 28.5543 g and final weight with extractive was 28.5815 g. Calculate the ethanol-soluble extractive in terms of percent weight by weight.

Ans: 0.272%w/w

6. Erythromycin tablet contains 100mg of $C_{3}7H_{67}NO_{13}$ present in the form of erythromycin stearate ($C_{37}H_{67}NO_{13}$, $C_{18}H_{36}O_2$). How much erythromycin stearate is present in each tablet?

Ans: 138.76 mg

7. Calculate the percentage composition of glucose.

Ans: Carbon content = 40%,
Hydrogen content = 6.67%,
Oxygen content = 53.3%

8. Calculate the percentage composition of erythromycin, $C_{37}H_{67}NO_{13}$.

Ans: Carbon content = 60.53%,
Hydrogen content = 9.21%,
Nitrogen content = 1.91%
Oxygen content = 28.35%

9. As per label each ml of Atropine Sulphate injection contains 0.5mg of Atropine Sulphate and as per the monograph the content of $(C_{17}H_{23}ON_3)_2.H_2SO_4.H_2O$ must be within 93% to 107%. Calculate the minimum quantity of Atropine Sulphate should be in each milliliter of the injection.

Ans: 0.465 g per ml

10. In a test 9.5 g of belladonna leaf was taken for assay and 5.65 ml of 0.02 N NaOH were consumed in the titration. If 1 ml of 0.02 N NaOH solution is equivalent to 5.788mg of the belladonna alkaloids calculate the drug content in the sample (%w/w).

Ans: 0.344%w/w

11. In a TLC experiment the distance travelled by the eluting solvent is 10 cm and the distance travelled by the component is 7.5 cm. Calculate the R_f value for the component.

Ans: 0.75

12. The saponification value of a substance is 9.85 and after acetylation when acetylated product is saponified it is found to be 1.05. Calculate the acetyl value of the substance.

Ans: 8.86

13. The saponification value of a substance is 16.12 and after acetylation when acetylated product is saponified it is found to be 2.35. Calculate the acetyl value of the substance.

Ans: 13.94

14. 18.5 g of a crude drug was subjected to extraction by maceration using water as the solvent. After drying the weight of petri dish with extractive was found to increase from 17.9558 g to 19.0773 g. Calculate the extractive in terms of %w/w.

Ans: 6.06%

15. 2.0074g of oil was taken for determination of saponification value. After refluxing with 25 ml of 0.5001 M ethanolic-KOH for 50 min when titrated against 0.4998 M HCl; the titer value was 14.75 ml. 25 ml of 0.5001 M ethanolic-KOH was equivalent to 25.01 ml of 0.4998 M HCl. Calculate the saponification value of the sample.

Ans: 143.37

16. 0.4986g of a sample was taken for iodine value determination. 20 ml of Iodine monochloride solution was added which was equivalent to 20.25 ml of 0.1M solution of Sodium thiosulphate. After completion of reaction the sample was titrated with 0.1M solution of Sodium thiosulphate. The sample consumed 14.55ml of 0.1M solution of Sodium thiosulphate. If the strength of Sodium thiosulphate solution was 1.005M, calculate the iodine value of the sample.

Ans: 11.49

17. To determine acid value 10.0507g of oil was taken; 1.65 ml of 0.1M KOH solution was required for neutralization. Calculate the acid value of the oil. The strength of the 0.1M KOH solution was 1.009M.

Ans: 0.16

18. The saponification value of a substance is 10.9 and after acetylation when acetylated product is saponified it is found to be 1.15. Calculate the acetyl value of the substance.

Ans: 9.82

19. The saponification values of a substance are13.09 and 1.02 before and after acetylation respectively. Calculate the acetyl value of the substance.

Ans: 12.19

20. For determination of acid value 9.5405g of oil was taken and 4.85ml of 0.1M KOH solution was required for neutralization. Calculate the acid value of the oil. The strength of the 0.1M KOH solution was 1.007M.

Ans: 0.51

12

BIOSTATISTICS

Statistics can be defined in various ways. In simple words it can be defined according to King as *the science which deals with methods of collecting, classifying, presenting, comparing and interpreting numerical data collected to throw some light on any sphere of enquiry*. The statistical methods are *devices, rules of procedure and general principles which are applicable to all kinds or groups of data*. When *the statistical tools or principles are applied to study living organisms or numerical data obtained from biological sources, it is called biostatistics*.

Mean, Median and Mode

Mean, median and mode are three types of average and most commonly used. The *mean* is calculated by adding up all the numbers and then divided by the number of numbers. In the list of numbers the middle value is called *median*. To find the median, the numbers are listed in numerical order, so the first list is rewritten. The *mode* is the value that occurs most often. If no number is repeated, then there is no mode for the list. The *range* is the difference between the largest and smallest values.

Example

Find out the mean, median, mode and range for the listed values.

(a) 8, 5, 5, 3, 11, 12, 7, 9, 5, 13

(b) 12, 18, 19, 23, 22, 35, 43, 21, 24

Solution

(a) There are 10 numbers in the list.

The sum of the numbers is 8+5+5+3+11+12+7+9+5+13 = 78

$$Mean = \frac{78}{10} = 7.8$$

The numbers after orderly arrangement become

3, 5, 5, 5, 7, 8, 9, 11, 12, 13

Since there are even numbers of values, there is no middle value, the average of two middle numbers 7 and 8 would be the median

Thus, $$Median = \frac{7+8}{2} = 7.5$$

Mode is the value repeated more in the list. Among the numbers the number 5 is repeated three times; hence, 5 is the mode for the list given.

Range = largest number – lowest number = 13 – 3 = **10**

Mean, $$\bar{x} = \frac{\Sigma x}{n}$$

$$\bar{x} = \frac{\Sigma fx}{\Sigma f}$$

$$\bar{x} = \frac{\Sigma fm}{\Sigma f}$$

[x is the variables and n is the number of occurrence, f is the frequency, m is the mid value of class interval]

Variance, $$s^2 = \frac{\Sigma(x - \bar{x})^2}{n-1}$$

Standard deviation, $$s = \sqrt{\frac{\Sigma(x - \bar{x})^2}{n-1}}$$

Coefficient of variation, C.V. (%) = $\frac{s}{\bar{x}} \times 100$

$$Mode = L + \frac{\Delta_1}{\Delta_1 + \Delta_2} \times i$$

(*Where:* Δ_1= Frequency of modal class – frequency before model class; Δ_2= Frequency of modal class – frequency after model class; L = Lower value of modal class; i = class interval)

(b) There are 9 numbers in the list.

The sum of the numbers is

12 + 18 + 19 + 23 + 22 + 35 + 43 + 21 + 24 = 217

$$Mean = \frac{217}{9} = 24.1$$

The numbers after orderly arrangement become

= 12, 18, 19, 21, 22, 23, 24, 35, 43

Since there are odd numbers of values, there is a middle value, 22 which would be the median

Thus, *Median* is **22**

Mode is the value repeated more in the list. Among the numbers no number is repeated; hence, there is no mode for the list given.

Range = largest number – lowest number = 43 – 12 = **31**

Example

Calculate the mean, variance, standard deviation, and coefficient of variation from the following data collected on weight of 10 children of 2 years old.

Weights (x kg) of 10 children are 7.5, 7.9, 8.0, 8.2, 8.5, 8.3, 8.1, 7.9, 7.8, 6.9

Solution

The data collected are tabulated in form of ascending order as follows:

x	$(x - \bar{x})$	$(x - \bar{x})^2$
6.9	- 1.01	1.020
7.5	- 0.41	0.168
7.8	- 0.11	0.012
7.9	- 0.01	0.0001
7.9	- 0.01	0.0001
8.0	+ 0.09	0.008
8.1	+ 0.19	0.036
8.2	+ 0.29	0.084
8.3	+ 0.39	0.152
8.5	+ 0.59	0.348
$\sum x = 79.1$		$\sum(x - \bar{x})^2 = 1.828$

$$\text{Mean, } \bar{x} = \frac{\sum x}{n} = \frac{79.1}{10} = 7.91$$

$$\text{Variance, } s^2 = \frac{\sum(x - \bar{x})^2}{n-1} = \frac{1.828}{10-1} = \frac{1.828}{9} = 0.203$$

Standard deviation, s = $\sqrt{\frac{\Sigma(x-\bar{x})^2}{n-1}} = \sqrt{0.203} = 0.451$

Coefficient of variation, C.V.(%) = $\frac{s}{\bar{x}} \times 100 = \frac{0.451}{7.91} \times 100$

Ans. 5.70

Example

There are two sets of observation on hemoglobin (Hb) content of 10 male persons (sample A and B). Calculate the mean, variance, standard deviation, and coefficient of variation from the following data collected. Comment on the variation of two data.

Sample A (Hb content, *x*)	11.5, 10.9, 12.0, 12.2, 12.5, 11.3, 13.1, 11.9, 10.8, 12.9
Sample B (Hb content, *x*)	10.3, 10.5, 12.8, 12.5, 12.5, 11.7, 12.1, 11.9, 11.8, 11.9

Solution

The data of Sample A are tabulated in ascending order as follows:

x	$(x - \bar{x})$	$(x - \bar{x})^2$
10.8	–1.11	1.232
10.9	–1.01	1.020
11.3	–0.61	0.372
11.5	–0.41	0.168
11.9	–0.01	0.0001
12.0	+ 0.09	0.008
12.2	+ 0.29	0.084
12.5	+ 0.59	0.348
12.9	+ 0.99	0.980
13.1	+ 1.19	1.416
$\sum x = 119.1$		$\Sigma(x - \bar{x})^2 = 5.628$

Mean, $\bar{x} = \frac{\sum x}{n} = \frac{119.1}{10} = 11.91$

Variance, $s^2 = \frac{\Sigma(x-\bar{x})^2}{n-1} = \frac{5.628}{10-1} = \frac{5.628}{9} = 0.625$

Standard deviation, $s = \sqrt{\frac{\Sigma(x-\bar{x})^2}{n-1}} = \sqrt{0.625} = 0.790$

Coefficient of variation, C.V.(%) $= \frac{s}{\bar{x}} \times 100 = \frac{0.790}{11.91} \times 100$

Ans. 6.63

The data of Sample B are tabulated in ascending order as follows:

x	$(x - \bar{x})$	$(x - \bar{x})^2$
10.3	- 1.50	2.25
10.5	- 1.30	1.69
11.7	- 0.10	0.01
11.8	0.00	0.00
11.9	0.10	0.01
11.9	0.10	0.01
12.1	0.30	0.09
12.5	0.70	0.49
12.5	0.70	0.49
12.8	1.00	1.00
$\sum x = 118.0$		$\Sigma(x - \bar{x})^2 =$ 6.04

Mean, $\bar{x} = \frac{\Sigma x}{n} = \frac{118.0}{10} = 11.80$

Variance, $s^2 = \frac{\Sigma(x-\bar{x})^2}{n-1} = \frac{6.04}{10-1} = \frac{6.04}{9} = 0.671$

Standard deviation, $s = \sqrt{\frac{\Sigma(x-\bar{x})^2}{n-1}} = \sqrt{0.671} = 0.819$

Coefficient of variation, C.V.(%) $= \frac{s}{\bar{x}} \times 100 = \frac{0.819}{11.80} \times 100$

Ans. 6.94

Comment: The Coefficient of variation in sample ‘A’ is less than that of sample ‘B’; although there is narrow variation. Still sample ‘A’ shows more consistency than sample ‘B’.

Example

The blood sugar (x) of 150 persons (male) was determined at fasting condition. The data collected have been classifies in terms of frequency (f) and shown in the table below. Calculate the mean, variance, standard deviation, and coefficient of variation from the following data collected.

x	80	81	82	83	84	85	86	87	88	89	90
f	12	10	14	17	13	19	15	13	18	9	10

Solution

The data shown above may be further classified and tabulated as below:

x	x^2	f	$f \times x$	$f \times x^2$
80	6400	12	960	76800
81	6561	10	810	65610
82	6724	14	1148	94136
83	6889	17	1411	117113
84	7056	13	1092	91728
85	7225	19	1615	137275
86	7396	15	1290	110940
87	7569	13	1131	98397
88	7744	18	1584	139392
89	7921	9	801	71289
90	8100	10	900	81000
$\sum x = 935$		$\sum f = 150$	$\sum f.x = 12742$	$\sum f.x^2 = 1083680$

$$\text{Mean, } \bar{x} = \frac{\sum fx}{\sum f} = \frac{12742}{150} = 84.94666\ (\approx 84.95)$$

$$\text{Variance, } s^2 = \frac{\sum f.x^2 - \frac{(\sum fx)^2}{\sum f}}{\sum f} = \frac{1083680 - \frac{(12742)^2}{150}}{150}$$

$$= \frac{1083680 - 1082390.43}{150} = \frac{1289.57}{150} = 8.597$$

$$\text{Standard deviation, } s = \sqrt{\frac{\sum f.x^2 - \frac{(\sum f.\ x)^2}{\sum f}}{\sum f}} = \sqrt{\frac{1083680 - \frac{(12742)^2}{150}}{150}}$$

$$= \sqrt{\frac{1083680-1082390.43}{150}} = \sqrt{\frac{1289.57}{150}}$$

$$= \sqrt{8.597} = 2.932$$

Coefficient of variation, C.V.(%) = $\frac{s}{\bar{x}} \times 100 = \frac{2.932}{84.95} \times 100 = 3.45$

Or,

By using *short-cut method*

Solution

x	f	dx = (x – A*)	f.dx	dx^2	f. dx^2
80	12	- 5	– 60	25	300
81	10	- 4	– 40	16	160
82	14	- 3	– 42	9	126
83	17	- 2	– 34	4	68
84	13	- 1	– 13	1	13
85	19	0	0	0	0
86	15	1	15	1	15
87	13	2	26	4	52
88	18	3	54	9	162
89	9	4	36	16	144
90	10	5	50	25	250
	$\sum f = 150$		- 8		1290

A* is the assumed mean = 85

Standard deviation, s = $\sqrt{\frac{\sum f.dx^2}{\sum f} - \frac{(\sum f.dx)^2}{\sum f}}$

$$= \sqrt{\frac{1290-(-8)^2}{150}} = \sqrt{\frac{1226}{150}} = 2.85$$

Mean, $\bar{x} = A + \frac{\sum f.dx}{\sum f} = 85 + \frac{-8}{150} = 85 - 0.053 = 84.95$

Coefficient of variation, C.V.(%) = $\frac{s}{\bar{x}} \times 100 = \frac{2.85}{84.95} \times 100 = 3.35$

Example

The weight of 60 men have been measured and grouped under different classes. The table below shows the classes and frequency of occurrence. Calculate the mean, variance, standard deviation, and coefficient of variation from the following data collected.

x Class	51 - 55	56 - 60	61 - 65	66 - 70	71 - 75	76 - 80	81 - 85	86 - 90
f	5	7	8	9	11	6	8	6

Solution

The data given in the table are arranged in different categories as shown below:

x	m	f	$f \times m$	m^2	$f \times m^2$
51 – 55	53	5	265	2809	14045
56 – 60	58	7	406	3364	23548
61 – 65	63	8	504	3969	31752
66 – 70	68	9	612	4624	41616
71 – 75	73	11	803	5329	58619
76 – 80	78	6	468	6084	36504
81 – 85	83	8	664	6889	55112
86 – 90	88	6	528	7744	46464
		$\Sigma f = 60$	$\Sigma f \times m = 4250$		$\Sigma f \times m^2 = 307660$

Mean, $\bar{x} = \dfrac{\Sigma fm}{\Sigma f} = \dfrac{4250}{60} = 70.83$

$$\text{Variance, } s^2 = \frac{\Sigma f.m^2 - \frac{(\Sigma f.m)^2}{\Sigma f}}{\Sigma f} = \frac{307660 - \frac{(4250)^2}{60}}{60}$$

$$= \frac{307660 - 301041.67}{60} = \frac{6618.33}{60}$$

$$= 110.30$$

$$\text{Standard deviation, } s = \sqrt{\frac{\Sigma f.m^2 - \frac{(\Sigma fm)^2}{\Sigma f}}{\Sigma f}} = \sqrt{\frac{307660 - \frac{(4250)^2}{60}}{60}}$$

$$= \sqrt{\frac{307660 - 301041.67}{60}} = \sqrt{\frac{6618.33}{60}}$$

$$= \sqrt{110.30}$$

$$= 10.5$$

$$\text{Coefficient of variation, C.V.(\%)} = \frac{s}{\bar{x}} \times 100 = \frac{10.5}{70.83} \times 100$$

Ans. 14.82

Coefficient of Skewness

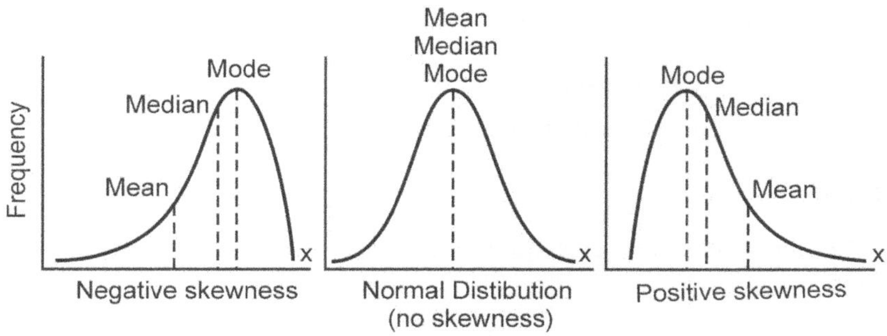

Figure 12.1

Absolute measures of skewness, S_k = Mean – Mode

A relative measure of skewness is determined by dividing the absolute skewness by standard deviation. Relative measures of skewness is alternatively called coefficient of skewness.

Absolute measures of skewness, S_k = Mean – Mode

$$\text{Coefficient of skewness,} = \frac{\text{Mean} - \text{Mode}}{\text{Standard deviation}}$$

$$\text{or,} \quad = \frac{\text{Mean} - \text{Median}}{\text{Standard deviation}}$$

$$\text{or,} \quad = \frac{\text{Median} - \text{Mode}}{\text{Standard deviation}}$$

(Karl Pearson's Coefficient of skewness, Sk_p)

$$Sk_p = \frac{\text{Mean} - \text{Mode}}{\text{Standard deviation}}$$

when $Sk_p = 0$, the distribution is normal

$Sk_p > 0$, the distribution is positively skewed

$Sk_p < 0$, the distribution is negatively skewed

(Mean – Mode) = 3(Mean – Median)

Thus, $$Sk_p = \frac{\text{(Mean -Median)}}{\text{Standard deviation}}$$

Example

During a survey in 32 hospitals (*f*) the patients (*x*) suffering from hypertension have been recorded and the data have been tabulated below. Calculate the Coefficient of skewness.

No of patients (*x*)	7	10	15	16	19	21
No of hospitals (*f*)	2	5	7	8	6	4

Solution

The above data are classified into different categories and tabulated below:

x	x^2	f	$f.x$	$f.x^2$
7	49	2	14	98
10	100	5	50	500
15	225	7	105	1575
16	256	8	128	2048
19	361	6	114	2166
21	441	4	84	1764
		$\Sigma f = 32$	$\Sigma f.x = 495$	$\Sigma f.x^2 = 8151$

$$\text{Mean, } \bar{x} = \frac{\Sigma fx}{\Sigma f} = \frac{495}{32} = 15.47$$

$$\text{Standard deviation, s} = \sqrt{\frac{\Sigma f.x^2 - \frac{(\Sigma f.\,x)^2}{\Sigma f}}{\Sigma f}} = \sqrt{\frac{8151 - \frac{(495)^2}{32}}{32}}$$

$$= \sqrt{\frac{8151-7657.03}{32}} = \sqrt{\frac{493.97}{32}}$$

$$= \sqrt{15.44} = \mathbf{3.93}$$

Modal value = 16 (by inspection)

$$\text{Coefficient of skewness, } Sk_p = \frac{\text{Mean}-\text{Mode}}{\text{Standard deviation}}$$

$$= \frac{15.44-16}{3.93} = \frac{-0.56}{3.93}$$

Ans. – 0.142

Example

In a study the height of 100 children of 12 years old have been measured and grouped under different classes as indicated below. The numbers of children fall in particular group (f) are noted. Calculate the coefficient of skewness from the given data.

Classes (height, ft)	3.00 – 3.25	3.25 – 3.50	3.50 – 3.75	3.75 – 4.00	4.00 – 4.25	4.25 – 4.50	4.50 – 4.75	4.75 – 5.00
Frequency (*f*)	7	25	36	19	5	4	2	2

Solution

The given data has been further grouped and tabulated below:

Class	**Mid-point *m***	***f***	***f.m***	***m*²**	***f.m*²**
3.00 – 3.25	3.125	7	21.875	9.765	68.359
3.25 – 3.50	3.375	25	84.375	11.390	284.75
3.50 – 3.75	3.625	36	130.55	13.140	473.04
3.75 – 4.00	3.875	19	73.625	15.015	285.297
4.00 – 4.25	4.125	5	20.625	17.015	85.078
4.25 – 4.50	4.375	4	17.5	19.140	76.562
4.50 – 4.75	4.675	2	9.35	21.855	43.711
4.75 – 5.00	4.875	2	9.75	23.765	47.531
		Σf = 100	$\Sigma f.m$ = 364.8		$\sum f.m^2$ = 1364.32

$$\text{Mean, } \bar{x} = \frac{\Sigma fm}{\Sigma f} = \frac{364.8}{100} = 3.648 \ (\approx \mathbf{3.65})$$

$$\text{Mode} = L + \frac{\Delta_1}{\Delta_1 + \Delta_2} \times i$$

(*where:* Δ_1= Frequency of model class- frequency before model class; Δ_2= Frequency of modal class- frequency after model class; L= Lower value of modal class; i = class interval)

$$= 3.50 + \frac{(36-25)}{(36-25)+(36-19)} \times 0.25$$

$$= 3.50 + \frac{11}{11+17} \times 0.25$$

$$= 3.50 + 0.098 = 3.598\ (\approx \mathbf{3.60})$$

Standard deviation, $s = \sqrt{\dfrac{\sum f.m^2 - \dfrac{(\sum fm)^2}{\sum f}}{\sum f}} = \sqrt{\dfrac{1364.32 - \dfrac{(364.8)^2}{100}}{100}}$

$$= \sqrt{\frac{1364.32 - 1330.79}{100}} = \sqrt{\frac{33.53}{100}}$$

$$= \sqrt{0.335}$$

$$= \mathbf{0.579}$$

Coefficient of skewness, $Sk_p = \dfrac{\text{Mean} - \text{Mode}}{\text{Standard deviation}}$

$$= \frac{3.65 - 3.60}{0.579} = \frac{0.05}{0.579}$$

Ans. 0.086

Probability

Probability is commonly defined as the chance of occurrence of an event among all possibilities. For example, it may happen. In a coin toss experiment getting the head is one out of two possibilities (head and tail). When an activity can produce well-defined outcomes is called experiment. When all the possible outcomes of an experiment are predictable but the exact output cannot be predicted in advance, the experiment is called a *random experiment.*

In statistics, the term probability (p) is expressed as:

$$p = \frac{a}{a+b} = \frac{\text{Number of events occurring}}{\text{Total number of trials}}$$

Where, p is the probability of 'happening', a is the number of ways for an event to happen and b is the number of ways for an event not to happen. Similarly if q is the probability of 'not happening', then $q = \dfrac{a}{a+b}$

Example

In a survey it is noticed that 100 patients out of 500 cancer patients recovered on treatment. Calculate the probability of survival and non survival.

Solution

Let us assume that the probability of survival is p and that of non survival is q; then

$$\text{The probability of survival, } p = \frac{\text{No. of patients survived}}{\text{Total no. of cancer patients}}$$

$$= \frac{100}{500} = \frac{1}{5}$$

Similarly the probability of non survival,

$$q = \frac{\text{No. of patients not survived}}{\text{Total no. of cancer patients}} = \frac{400}{500} = \frac{4}{5}$$

> When two events A and B are mutually exclusive; then
>
> $$p(\text{A or B}) = p(\text{A}) + p(\text{B})$$

Example

In 100 people there are 4 persons suffering from hypertension and 4 suffering from diabetes. Find out the probability of patient of diabetes or hypertension.

Solution

The events are mutually exclusive. There are 4 p ersons suffering from hypertension and 4 suffering from diabetes out of 100 people.

So, the probability of getting a person with diabetes is 4/100 and the probability of getting a person with hypertension is 4/100.

The probability of getting a person with either diabetes (D) or hypertension (H)

$$\text{p(D or H)} = \text{p(D)} + \text{p(H)}$$

$$= \frac{4}{100} + \frac{4}{100} = \frac{8}{100} = \frac{2}{25}$$

When two events A and B are not mutually exclusive; then

$$p(\text{A or B}) = p(\text{A}) + p(\text{B}) - p(\text{A and B})$$

Example

A set of 52 cards there are 13 hearts cards and 4 kings. The set of cards are well shuffled and one is drawn. What would be probability that the card would be either heart (H) or king (K)?

Solution

The probability of a heart card = $p(H) = \frac{13}{52} = \frac{1}{4}$

The probability of a king = $p(H) = \frac{4}{52} = \frac{1}{13}$

The desired probability = p(H or K)

$$= p(H) + p(K) - p(H \text{ and } K)$$

$$= \frac{1}{4} + \frac{1}{13} - (\frac{1}{4} \times \frac{1}{13})$$

$$= \frac{1}{4} + \frac{1}{13} - \frac{1}{52} = \frac{16}{52} = \frac{4}{13}$$

When two events A and B are independent the probability of joint occurrence would be

$$p(\text{A and B}) = p(\text{A}) \times p(\text{B})$$

Example

A coin is tossed twice. What would be the probability of getting tail on two or three successive tosses?

Solution

Let us assume that the probability of getting tail in first toss

$$= p(\text{A}) = \frac{1}{2} = 0.5$$

The probability of getting tail in second toss = $p(\text{B}) = \frac{1}{2} = 0.5$

The probability of getting tail in both tosses

$$= p(\text{A and B}) = p(\text{A}) \times p(\text{B})$$

$$= \frac{1}{2} \times \frac{1}{2} = 0.25$$

Example

A coin is tossed thrice. What would be the probability of getting tail on three successive tosses?

Solution

Let us assume that the probability of getting tail in first toss

$$= p(\text{A}) = \frac{1}{2} = 0.5$$

The probability of getting tail in second toss $= p(\text{B})$

$$= \frac{1}{2} = 0.5, \text{ and}$$

The probability of getting tail in second toss $= p(\text{C})$

$$= \frac{1}{2} = 0.5, \text{ and}$$

The probability of getting tail in three tosses $= p(\text{A, B and C})$

$$= p(\text{A}) \times p(\text{B}) \times p(\text{C})$$

$$= \frac{1}{2} \times \frac{1}{2} \times \frac{1}{2} = 0.125$$

When two events A and B are dependent the probability of occurrence of one event would depend on the occurrence of the other event; then

$$p(\text{A and B}) = p(\text{A}) \times p(\text{A/B})$$

or

$$p(\text{A, B and C}) = p(\text{A}) \times p(\text{A/B}) \times p(\text{C/AB})$$

Example

In a box there are 7 marble balls and 3 glass balls. If two balls are drawn randomly one after the other; what would be the probability that both the balls are of glass?

Solution

Probability of drawing glass ball $p\left(\frac{A}{B}\right) = \frac{3}{7+3} = \frac{3}{10}$

Probability of drawing second glass ball $p\left(\frac{A}{B}\right) = \frac{2}{7+2} = \frac{2}{9}$

The probability that both the balls are of glass

$$p\,(AB) = p(A) \times \left(\frac{A}{B}\right) = \frac{3}{10} \times \frac{2}{9}$$

$$= \frac{1}{15}$$

Conditional Probability

When an event A happens on the condition that the event B has already happened, is called conditional probability and it is denoted by the symbol $p(B/A)$

$$p(B/A) = p(B) \times p(A/B) \quad \text{or,} \; p(A/B) = \frac{p(B \cap A)}{p(B)}$$

When the event B is dependent on A;

$$p(A/B) = p(A) \times p(B/A) \quad \text{or,} \; p(B/A) = \frac{p(A \cap B)}{p(A)}$$

Example

There are two tablet press machines. Machine 1 produces 30% and machine 2 produces 70% of the total tablets produced. Percent of rejects 5% in case of machine 1 and 1% in case of machine 2. On random sampling one defective tablet is drawn.

What would be the probability that the defective tablet has been produced by machine 1 or machine 2?

Solution

Let us assume that A_1 = machine 1,

A_2 = machine 2, and

B = machine 1 or machine 2

Then, $p(A_1) = 30\% = 0.30$ and $p(A_2) = 70\% = 0.70$

$p(B/A_1) = 5\% = 0.05$, and $p(B/A_2) = 1\% = 0.01$

	Prior Probability $p(A_1)$	Conditional Probability $p(B/A_1)$	Joint Probability $p(A_1 \text{ and } B)$	Post Probability $p(A_1/B)$
A_1	0.3	0.05	$0.3 \times 0.5 = 0.015$	$\frac{0.015}{0.022} = 0.682$
A_2	0.7	0.01	$0.7 \times 0.1 = 0.007$	$\frac{0.007}{0.022} = 0.318$
Total	1.0		$p(B) = 0.022$	1.000

$p(A_1) = 30\%$ is less than $p(A_2) = 70\%$

Defective tablets produced by

Machine 1 = 0.681 or 68.2% and

Machine 2 = 0.318 or 31.8%

Thus, the defective tablet drawn was produced by the Machine 1.

Example

There are three tableting machines. Machine 1 produces 3.0 lac, machine 2 produces 5 lac, and machine 3 produces 6 lac of the tablets. as per records percent of rejects 0.05% in case of machine 1, 0.01% in case of machine 2, and 0.03% in case of machine 3. On random sampling one defective tablet is drawn.

(a) What would be the probability that the defective tablet has been produced by machine 1, 2 or 3?

(b) What would be probability that the defective has been produced by machine 1?

Solution

(a) Which machine produced the defective tablet

According to the Bayes' theorem

A_1 = production capacity of the machine 1 = 3.0 lac tablets

A_2 = production capacity of the machine 2 = 5.0 lac tablets

A_3 = production capacity of the machine 3 = 6.0 lac tablets

E = defective tablet

Therefore, $p(A/E) = p(A \cap E)$

(i) Prior probability

$$p(A_1) = \frac{3}{3+5+6} = \frac{3}{14}$$

$$p(A_2) = \frac{5}{3+5+6} = \frac{5}{14}$$

(ii) Likelihood

$p(E/A_1) = 0.05\%$, $p(E/A_2) = 0.01\%$, and $p(E/A_3) = 0.03\%$,

(iii) Joint probabilities

$$p(A_1 \cap E) = p(A_1) \times p(E/A_1) = \frac{3}{14} \times 0.05 = \frac{0.15}{14}$$

$$p(A_2 \cap E) = p(A_2) \times p(E/A_2) = \frac{5}{14} \times 0.01 = \frac{0.05}{14}$$

$$p(A_3 \cap E) = p(A_3) \times p(E/A_3) = \frac{6}{14} \times 0.03 = \frac{0.18}{14}$$

$$p(E) = p(A_i) \times p(E/A_i) = p(A_1) \times p(E/A_1) + p(A_2) \times p(E/A_2) + p(A_3) \times p(E/A_3) = \frac{0.09}{14}$$

(iv) Posterior probability

$$p(A_1/E) = \frac{p(A_1 \cap E)}{p(E)} = \frac{\frac{0.15}{14}}{\frac{0.09}{14}} = \frac{15}{9}$$

$$p(A_2/E) = \frac{p(A_2 \cap E)}{p(E)} = \frac{\frac{0.05}{14}}{\frac{0.09}{14}} = \frac{5}{9}$$

$$p(A_3/E) = \frac{p(A_3 \cap E)}{p(E)} = \frac{\frac{0.18}{14}}{\frac{0.09}{14}} = \frac{18}{9}$$

(b) Probability of being produced by machine1 =

$$\frac{\frac{3}{14} \times 0.05}{\left(\frac{3}{14} \times 0.05\right) + \left(\frac{5}{14} \times 0.01\right) + \left(\frac{6}{14} \times 0.03\right)}$$

$$= \frac{0.15}{0.15+0.05+0.18}$$

$$= \frac{0.15}{0.38} = \mathbf{0.395}$$

Probability Distribution

Mainly there are three types of probability distributions:

(a) Binomial distribution: Discrete probability distributions
(b) Poisson distribution: Discrete probability distributions
(c) Normal distribution: Continuous probability distributions

(a) Binomial distribution: It is a discrete probability distribution. There are two assumptions of Binomial distribution. which are:

1. Each trial has only two possible outcomes – success and failure.
2. The probability of success expressed as p is constant for all trials. Similarly the probability of failure expressed as q is constant for all trials.

Say, the number of trials is 'n' and the number of success is 'r':

Then the number of failure would be (n – r).

Then the probability of r for n trials, $p(\text{r}) = \frac{n'}{r'(n-r)'} p^r q^{n-r}$

Where the symbol 'stands for factorial, such as 0' is 1

2' is 2 × 1 = 2,

4' is 4 × 3 × 2 × 1 = 24, etc.

Example

What would be the probability of getting 1, 2, 3 and 4 heads when a coin is tossed four times?

Solution

(a) $p(1) = \frac{n'}{r'(n-r)'} p^r q^{n-r}$

$$= \frac{4'}{1'(4-1)'} \left(\frac{1}{2}\right)^1 \left(\frac{1}{2}\right)^{4-1}$$

$$= \frac{4'}{1'3'} \left(\frac{1}{2}\right) \left(\frac{1}{2}\right)^3$$

$$= \frac{4 \times 3 \times 2 \times 1}{1 \times 3 \times 2 \times 1} \left(\frac{1}{2}\right)\left(\frac{1}{2}\right)\left(\frac{1}{2}\right)\left(\frac{1}{2}\right)$$

$$= \frac{24}{6} \times \frac{1}{16} = \frac{4}{16}$$

$$= \mathbf{0.25}$$

(b) $$p(2) = \frac{n'}{r'(n-r)'} p^r q^{n-r}$$

$$= \frac{4'}{2'(4-2)'} \left(\frac{1}{2}\right)^2 \left(\frac{1}{2}\right)^{4-2}$$

$$= \frac{4'}{2'2'} \left(\frac{1}{2}\right)^2 \left(\frac{1}{2}\right)^2$$

$$= \frac{4 \times 3 \times 2 \times 1}{2 \times 1 \times 2 \times 1} \left(\frac{1}{2}\right)\left(\frac{1}{2}\right)\left(\frac{1}{2}\right)\left(\frac{1}{2}\right)$$

$$= \frac{24}{4} \times \frac{1}{16} = \frac{6}{16}$$

$$= \mathbf{0.375}$$

(c) $$p(3) = \frac{n'}{r'(n-r)'} p^r q^{n-r}$$

$$= \frac{4'}{3'(4-3)'} \left(\frac{1}{2}\right)^3 \left(\frac{1}{2}\right)^{4-3}$$

$$= \frac{4'}{3'1'} \left(\frac{1}{2}\right)^3 \left(\frac{1}{2}\right)^1$$

$$= \frac{4 \times 3 \times 2 \times 1}{3 \times 2 \times 1 \times 1} \left(\frac{1}{2}\right)\left(\frac{1}{2}\right)\left(\frac{1}{2}\right)\left(\frac{1}{2}\right)$$

$$= \frac{24}{6} \times \frac{1}{16} = \frac{4}{16}$$

$$= \mathbf{0.250}$$

(d) $$p(4) = \frac{n'}{r'(n-r)'} p^r q^{n-r}$$

$$= \frac{4'}{4'(4-4)'} \left(\frac{1}{2}\right)^4 \left(\frac{1}{2}\right)^{4-4}$$

$$= \frac{4'}{4'0'} \left(\frac{1}{2}\right)^4 \left(\frac{1}{2}\right)^0$$

$$= \frac{4 \times 3 \times 2 \times 1}{4 \times 3 \times 2 \times 1 \times 1} \left(\frac{1}{2}\right)\left(\frac{1}{2}\right)\left(\frac{1}{2}\right)\left(\frac{1}{2}\right)$$

$$= \frac{24}{24} \times \frac{1}{16} = \frac{6}{16}$$

= **0.0625**

(b) ***Poisson distribution:***

Poisson distribution may be obtained as a limiting case of binomial distribution under following circumstances;

- This is also a discrete probability distribution.
- It has a single parameter which is the mean of the distribution and is defined by *m*.
- $np = m$ which remains constant

> If the probability of success is r, then
>
> $$p(\mathrm{r}) = \frac{e^{-m} \times m^{r}}{r'}$$
>
> where, p = probability
>
> r = 0, 1, 2, 3 ....n successes
>
> e = 2.7183 (constant)

Example

At a traffic point an average of 5 cars reach every minute. What would be the probability that exactly 0, 1, 2, 3 and 4 cars reach in one minute? Assume that this is a poisson distribution.

Solution

(a) Probability of 0 cars, $\mathrm{p}(0) = \frac{e^{-m} \times m^{r}}{r'}$

$$= \frac{e^{-5} \times 5^{0}}{0'} = \frac{0.0067 \times 1}{1}$$

= **0.0067**

(b) Probability of one car, p(1) = $\dfrac{e^{-m} \times m^r}{r'}$

$$= \frac{e^{-5} \times 5^1}{1'} = \frac{0.0067 \times 5}{1}$$

$$= 0.0335$$

(c) Probability of two cars, p(2) = $\dfrac{e^{-m} \times m^r}{r'}$

$$= \frac{e^{-5} \times 5^2}{2'} = \frac{0.0067 \times 25}{2}$$

$$= \frac{0.0067 \times 25}{2 \times 1}$$

$$= 0.0838$$

(d) Probability of three cars, p(3) = $\dfrac{e^{-m} \times m^r}{r'}$

$$= \frac{e^{-5} \times 5^3}{3'}$$

$$= \frac{0.0067 \times 125}{3 \times 2 \times 1}$$

$$= \frac{0.0067 \times 125}{3 \times 2 \times 1} = \frac{0.838}{6}$$

$$= \mathbf{0.1396}$$

(e) Probability of four cars, p(4) = $\dfrac{e^{-m} \times m^r}{r'}$

$$= \frac{e^{-5} \times 5^4}{4'} = \frac{0.0067 \times 625}{4 \times 3 \times 2 \times 1}$$

$$= \frac{0.0067 \times 625}{24}$$

$$= \frac{4.1875}{24}$$

$$= 0.1745$$

(c) ***Normal Distribution*:** Normal distribution is useful for probability distribution for continuous variables. The characteristics of a normal distribution curve are:

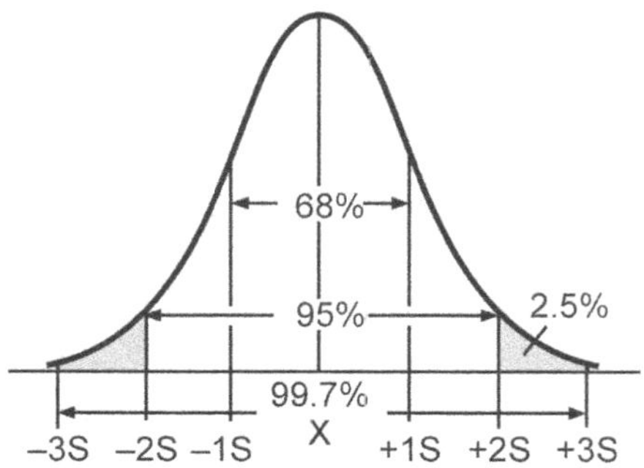

- The curve is "bell-shaped", usually looks symmetrical with a single peak.
- At the centre of a curve the mean exists. At centre of the mean the peak shows maximum height and it divides the curve in almost two equal parts.
- In a normal distribution mean, median and mode are all equal.
- Two tails of the curve never touch the base line; hence the curve is asymptotic.
- The area under the curve is distributed as – 68.27% of the population (values) remain within $\overline{x} \pm$ 1s, 95.45% of the population remain within $\overline{x} \pm$ 2s, and 99.73% of the population remain within $\overline{x} \pm$ 3s; where $\overline{x}$ is the mean and s is the standard deviation.

On sample basis: Normal distribution, $z = \frac{x - \bar{x}}{s}$

where, z is the number of standard deviations

x is the random variable

$\overline{x}$ is mean

s is standard deviation

On population basis: Normal distribution, $z = \frac{x - \mu}{\sigma}$

where, z is the number of standard deviations

x is the random variable

μ is mean

σ is standard deviation

Example

The usual shelf-life of a type of drug product is 3 years and standard deviation is 3 months. What is the probability that a similar drug product will have 3.5 years shelf-life?

Solution

Given that,

$x = 3.5$ years

$\bar{x}$ = 3 years

s = 3 months = $\frac{3}{12}$ year = 0.25 year

$$z = \frac{x - \bar{x}}{s} = \frac{3.5 - 3.0}{0.25}$$

$$= \frac{0.50}{0.25}$$

Ans. 2

Example

There are 40 capsules of red color, 30 of blue color and 50 of pink color in a box. What would the probability of getting red or pink color capsule at random drawl of a single capsule?

Solution

The probability of getting a red color capsule = $\frac{40}{120} = \frac{4}{12}$

The probability of getting a blue color capsule = $\frac{30}{120} = \frac{3}{12}$

The probability of getting a pink color capsule = $\frac{50}{120} = \frac{5}{12}$

The probability of getting a red or pink color capsule = $\frac{4}{12} + \frac{5}{12} = \frac{9}{12}$

Or, $\frac{9}{12} \times 100$

Ans. 75%

Example

The compliance of disintegration test of paracetamol tablets has been found to occur in 4 out of 5 lots. In another situation compliance has been found in 3 out of 4 lots. What would be the probability of compliance when both the situations are tried?

Solution

The probability of paracetamol tablet meeting disintegration test in first situation

$$(A) = \frac{4}{5}$$

The probability of complying disintegration test in second situation

$$(B) = \frac{3}{4}$$

The events are not mutually exclusive because all the tablets can comply the test.

Therefore, the required probability

$$p(\text{A or B}) = p(\text{A}) + p(\text{B}) - p(\text{A and B})$$

$$= \frac{4}{5} + \frac{3}{4} - (\frac{4}{5} \times \frac{3}{4})$$

$$= \frac{4}{5} + \frac{3}{4} - \frac{12}{20}$$

$$= \frac{31}{20} - \frac{12}{20} = \mathbf{\frac{19}{20}}$$

Example 21

The Rh factor and sex of birth are independent events and occur in any child. What would be the probability of a child being male and Rh^+, and female and Rh^+?

Solution

Probability of a child being male, $p_1 = \frac{1}{2}$

Probability of a child being Rh^+, $p_2 = \frac{9}{10}$

Probability of single birth, $p_3 = \frac{79}{80}$

Thus, Probability of a child being male and Rh^+

$$= p_1 \times p_2 = \frac{1}{2} \times \frac{9}{10} = \frac{9}{20} = \frac{9 \times 80}{20 \times 80} = \mathbf{\frac{720}{1600}}$$

The probability of a child being female, Rh^+ and single child

$$= p_1 \times p_2 \times p_3$$

$$= \frac{1}{2} \times \frac{9}{10} \times \frac{79}{80}$$

Ans. $\mathbf{\frac{711}{1600}}$

Example

Two samples of a same product A_1 and A_2 are produced for selection of one. The probability of selection of sample A_1 is 1/7; while that of A_2 is 1/5. What is the probability that

(i) both the samples would be selected,

(ii) only one would be selected,

(iii) both the samples would be rejected?

Solution

The probability of selection of sample A_1, $p_1 = \frac{1}{7}$ and

The probability of rejection of sample A_1, $q_1 = \frac{6}{7}$

The probability of selection of sample A_2, $p_2 = \frac{1}{5}$

The probability of rejection of sample A_2, $q_2 = \frac{4}{5}$

(i) Probability that both the samples would be selected would be $p(A_1 \text{ and } A_2)$

$$= p_1 \times p_2 = \frac{1}{7} \times \frac{1}{5}$$

$$= \frac{1}{35}$$

(ii) Probability that only one would be selected,

(a) A_1 would be selected and A_2 would be rejected, then

$$p_1 \times q_2 = \frac{1}{7} \times \frac{4}{5}$$

$$= \frac{4}{35}$$

(b) A_2 would be selected and A_1 would be rejected, then

$$p_2 \times q_1 = \frac{1}{5} \times \frac{6}{7}$$

$$= \frac{6}{35}$$

Above two events (a) and (b) are mutually exclusive; so the combined probability would be: $\frac{4}{35}+\frac{6}{35}=\frac{10}{35}$

(iii) Probability that both the samples would be rejected

$$q(A_1 \text{ and } A_2) = q(A_1) \times q(A_2)$$

$$= q_1 \times q_2$$

$$= \frac{6}{7} \times \frac{4}{5} = \frac{24}{35}$$

Example

A manufacturer prepares corrugated boxes of which 1% is defective. The boxes are packed and supplied. Each packet contains 5 boxes. Calculate the probability of packets which do not contain any defective boxes.

Solution

Given that; p = 0.99, q = 0.01, r = 5, n = 5

The probability of success, r in n trials $= \frac{n'}{r'\,(n-r)'} p^r q^{n-r}$

$$= \frac{5'}{5'\,(5-5)'} (0.99)^5 (0.01)^{(5-5)}$$

$$= \frac{5'}{5'\,(5-5)'} (0.99)^5 (0.01)^{(5-5)}$$

$$= \frac{5'}{5'\,(0)'} (0.99)^5 (0.01)^{(0)}$$

$$= \frac{5'}{5'} (0.951)(0.01)$$

$$= 0.00951$$

Correlation and Regression

Correlation: Correlation can be explained in terms of casual connection existing between two series or groups of data. In other words, if a group of items are recorded with respect to the values of two distinct variables and the pairs of values are found to be associated, the two variables are considered to be correlated.

Correlation and causation: Correlation refers to the degree of relationship between two or more variables. It does not speak about cause and effect of the relationship. The reasons for correlation may be due to –

- Pure chance
- Influence of some external factors
- Mutual influence (influence of one variable on the other and vice versa)

Correlation may be of different types:

- Positive and negative correlation; e.g. one variable increases and other also increases (positive); one variable increases and other decreases (negative).
- Simple, partial or multiple correlation; if only two variables out of 5/6 are studied it is simple, relation between a dependable variable and 2/3 independent variables is multiple correlation; relation between two variables excluding some other variable is partial correlation.
- Linear or non-linear correlation

Methods to measure correlation

- Scatter diagram method
- Graphic method
- Coefficient of correlation
- Coefficient of correlation by rank difference
- Coefficient of concurrent deviation

Coefficient of correlation, $r = \frac{\sum(x-\bar{x})(y-\bar{y})}{\sqrt{\sum(x-\bar{x})^2 \sum(y-\bar{y})^2}}$

$$= \frac{\sum d_x\, d_y}{\sum d_x^2 \times \sum d_y^2}$$

$$= \frac{\sum xy - \frac{\sum x . \sum y}{n}}{\sqrt{\left[\sum x^2 - \frac{(\sum x)^2}{n}\right]\left[\sum y^2 - \frac{(\sum y)^2}{n}\right]}}$$

Note: The value of r shall remain within +1 and – 1.

- Positive value indicates that if one variable increases, the other also increases and vice versa.
- Negative value indicates that if one variable increases, the other decreases and vice versa.
- When the value of r is zero, it indicates that there is no correlation between two variables.

Example

The sale values of two products (variable A and B) are tabulated below. Check whether there is any correlation between two variables:

Sale values (lac) (variables)	Jan	Mar	June	Sept	Dec	Jan
Product A	4.50	5.40	6.75	8.775	11.85	14.22
Product B	5.20	6.24	7.80	10.14	13.69	16.43

Solution

Graphic method

The graphs show that two variables are closely related. The correlation is positive since these are moving in the same direction.

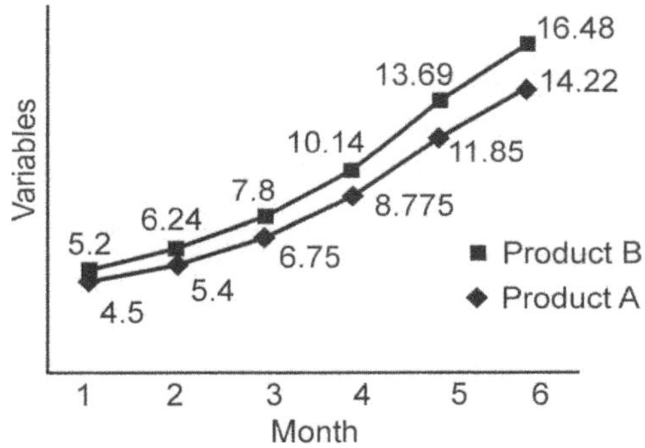

Figure 12.2

Degree of Correlation

According to Karl Pearson the degree of correlation is given in the table below:

Degree of correlation	Positive	Negative
Perfect	+1	- 1
Very high	+0.9 and >	- 0.9 and >
Sufficiently high	+0.75 to + 0.90	- 0.75 to – 0.90
Moderate	+0.6 to + 0.75	- 0.6 to – 0.75
Possibility of correlation	+0.3 to + 0.6	- 0.3 to – 0.6
Possibility of no correlation	Less than + 0.3	Less than – 0.3
Absence of correlation	0	0

Significance Test of Coefficient of Correlation

This test speaks whether a correlation coefficient (r) between paired values in the population is sufficiently large, or whether the derived 'r' can be attributed to chance. To test the significance of deviation of the estimated correlation coefficient (r) from, the 't' test can be applied with n-2 degree of freedom. The formula of the 't' test is:

$$t = \frac{r\sqrt{(n-2)}}{\sqrt{1-(r)^2}}$$

Example

The height and weight of 10 young persons were measured and tabulated. Calculate the test of significance of the correlation coefficient (r) and the value of 't' for the data presented in the table below:

Variables										
Height (inches)	32.5	34	31	35	32.5	36	33.5	33	34	35.5
Weight (lbs)	64	70	60	76	68.5	80	67.5	65	62.5	82.5

Solution

Height x (inches)	Weight y (lbs)	x^2	y^2	xy
32.5	64	1056.25	4096	2080
34	70	1156	4900	2380
31	60	961	3600	1860
35	76	1225	5776	2660
32.5	68.5	1056.25	4692.25	2226.25
36	80	1296	6400	2880
33.5	67.5	1122.25	4556.25	2261.25
33	65	1089	4225	2145
34	62.5	1156	3906.25	2125
36.5	82.5	1332.25	6806.25	3011.25
$\sum x = 338$	$\sum y = 696$	$\sum x^2 = 11450$	$\sum y^2 = 48958$	$\sum xy = 23628.75$

$$\text{Correlation coefficient, } r = \frac{\sum xy - \frac{\sum x . \sum y}{n}}{\sqrt{\left[\sum x^2 - \frac{(\sum x)^2}{n}\right]\left[\sum y^2 - \frac{(\sum y)^2}{n}\right]}}$$

$$= \frac{23628.75 - \frac{338 \times 696}{10}}{\sqrt{\left[11450 - \frac{(338)^2}{10}\right]\left[48958 - \frac{(696)^2}{10}\right]}}$$

$$= \frac{23628.75 - \frac{23524.80}{10}}{\sqrt{\left(11450 - \frac{114244}{10}\right)\left(48958 - \frac{484416}{10}\right)}}$$

$$= \frac{23628.75 - 23524.80}{\sqrt{(11450 - 11424.4)(48958 - 48441.6)}}$$

$$= \frac{103.15}{\sqrt{(25.6 \times 516.4)}}$$

$$= \frac{103.95}{\sqrt{13219.84}}$$

$$= \frac{103.95}{114.98} = 0.904$$

Significance test, $t = \frac{r\sqrt{(n-2)}}{\sqrt{1-(r)^2}} = \frac{0.904\sqrt{(10-2)}}{\sqrt{1-(0.904)^2}}$

$$= \frac{0.904 \times \sqrt{8}}{\sqrt{1-0.817}}$$

$$= \frac{0.904 \times 2.828}{\sqrt{1-0.817}}$$

$$= \frac{2.556}{\sqrt{0.183}}$$

$$= \frac{2.556}{0.428} = 5.97$$

***Interpretation*:** Since the calculated t value is higher than the tabulated value both at 5% (3.35) and at 1% (4.5) levels of probability of significance with n – 2 = 8 degree of freedom; the correlation coefficient between height and weight of population of 10 young persons is highly correlated.

Regression Analysis

The correlation coefficient indicates the degree of relationship between two variables; while regression analysis indicates the cause and effect between two variables. The co-variation of the two variables is expressed through correlation coefficient; while the nature of relationship between two variables is expressed by regression analysis.

Table 12.1 t - distribution critical values

	Upper-tail probability *p*											
df	**.25**	**.20**	**.15**	**.10**	**.05**	**.025**	**.02**	**.01**	**.005**	**.0025**	**.001**	**.0005**
1	1.000	1.376	1.963	3.078	6.314	12.71	15.89	31.82	63.66	127.3	318.3	636.6
2	0.816	1.061	1.386	1.886	2.920	4.303	4.849	6.965	9.925	14.09	22.33	31.60
3	0.765	0.978	1.250	1.638	2.353	3.182	3.482	4.541	5.841	7.453	10.21	12.92
4	0.741	0.941	1.190	1.533	2.132	2.776	2.999	3.747	4.604	5.598	7.173	8.610
5	0.727	0.920	1.156	1.476	2.015	2.571	2.757	3.365	4.032	4.773	5.893	6.869
6	0.718	0.906	1.134	1.440	1.943	2.447	2.612	3.143	3.707	4.317	5.208	5.959
7	0.711	0.896	1.119	1.415	1.895	2.365	2.517	2.998	3.499	4.029	4.785	5.408
8	0.706	0.889	1.108	1.397	1.860	2.306	2.449	2.896	3.355	3.833	4.501	5.041
9	0.703	0.883	1.100	1.383	1.833	2.262	2.398	2.821	3.250	3.690	4.297	4.781
10	0.700	0.879	1.093	1.372	1.812	2.228	2.359	2.764	3.169	3.581	4.144	4.587
11	0.697	0.876	1.088	1.363	1.796	2.201	2.328	2.718	3.106	3.497	4.025	4.437
12	0.695	0.873	1.083	1.356	1.782	2.179	2.303	2.681	3.055	3.428	3.930	4.318
13	0.694	0.870	1.079	1.350	1.771	2.160	2.282	2.650	3.012	3.372	3.852	4.221
14	0.692	0.868	1.076	1.345	1.761	2.145	2.264	2.624	2.977	3.326	3.787	4.140
15	0.691	0.866	1.074	1.341	1.753	2.131	2.249	2.602	2.947	3.286	3.733	4.073
16	0.690	0.865	1.071	1.337	1.746	2.120	2.235	2.583	2.921	3.252	3.686	4.015
17	0.689	0.863	1.069	1.333	1.740	2.110	2.224	2.567	2.898	3.222	3.646	3.965
18	0.688	0.862	1.067	1.330	1.734	2.101	2.214	2.552	2.878	3.197	3.611	3.922
19	0.688	0.861	1.066	1.328	1.729	2.093	2.205	2.539	2.861	3.174	3.579	3.883
20	0.687	0.960	1.064	1.325	1.725	2.086	2.197	2.528	2.845	3.153	3.552	3.850
21	0.686	0.859	1.063	1.323	1.721	2.080	2.189	2.518	2.831	3.135	3.527	3.819
22	0.686	0.858	1.061	1.321	1.717	2.074	2.183	2.508	2.819	3.119	3.505	3.792
23	0.685	0.858	1.060	1.319	1.714	2.069	2.177	2.500	2.807	3.104	3.485	3.768
24	0.685	0.857	1.059	1.318	1.711	2.064	2.172	2.492	2.797	3.091	3.467	3.745
25	0.684	0.856	1.058	1.316	1.708	2.060	2.167	2.485	2.787	3.078	3.450	3.725
26	0.684	0.856	1.058	1.315	1.706	2.056	2.162	2.479	2.779	3.067	3.435	3.707
27	0.684	0.855	1.057	1.314	1.703	2.052	2.158	2.473	2.771	3.057	3.421	3.690
28	0.683	0.855	1.056	1.313	1.701	2.048	2.154	2.467	2.763	3.047	3.408	3.674
29	0.683	0.854	1.055	1.311	1.699	2.045	2.150	2.462	2.756	3.038	3.396	3.659
30	0.683	0.854	1.055	1.310	1.697	2.042	2.147	2.457	2.750	3.030	3.385	3.646
40	0.681	0.851	1.050	1.303	1.684	2.021	2.123	2.423	2.704	2.971	3.307	3.551
50	0.679	0.849	1.047	1.299	1.676	2.009	2.109	2.403	2.678	2.937	3.261	3.496
60	0.679	0.848	1.045	1.296	1.671	2.000	2.099	2.390	2.660	2.915	3.232	3.460

Table contd....

Upper-tail probability *p*												
df	**.25**	**.20**	**.15**	**.10**	**.05**	**.025**	**.02**	**.01**	**.005**	**.0025**	**.001**	**.0005**
100	0.677	0.845	1.042	1.290	1.660	1.984	2.081	2.364	2.626	2.871	3.174	3.390
1000	0.675	0.842	1.037	1.282	1.646	1.962	2.056	2.330	2.581	2.813	3.098	3.300
Z*	0.674	0.841	1.036	1.282	1.645	1.960	2.054	2.326	2.576	2.807	3.091	3.291
	50%	60%	70%	80%	90%	95%	96%	98%	99%	99.5%	99.8%	99.9%
	Confidence level C											

In simple regression analysis there is only one independent variable; but in multiple regressions there are dependent and independent variables. Regression may be linear and non-linear. The simple or linear regression is represented graphically by a straight line; while non-linear or multiple regressions are represented by a curve. Hence, the later one is called curvilinear regression.

Regression equation

The linear regression equation y on x and x on y are given below.

> Regression equation of x on y, $x_y = a + by$
>
> Regression equation of y on x, $y_x = a + bx$
>
> x and y are the variables, a and b are intercept and slope (constants) of the line

The figure represents the equation

$$y_x = 4 + 2x \; (y_x = a + bx);$$

where, x = 0, 1, 2, 3, 4, 5 and

$$y = 4, 6, 8, 10, 12$$

The constant b is also called regression coefficient. This indicates that for every one unit change in x, there shall be two units change in y. The following formula can be used to calculate the values of a and b;

$$b = \frac{\sum d_x d_y}{\sum d_x^2} = \frac{\sum xy - \frac{\sum x.\sum y}{n}}{\sum x^2 - \frac{(\sum x)^2}{n}} \quad \text{and } a = \bar{y} - b\bar{x}$$

where, $d_x = (x - \bar{x})$ and $d_y = (y - \bar{y})$, $\bar{x}$ and $\bar{y}$ are the respective means.

$$b = \frac{\sum d_x d_y}{\sum d_x^2} = \frac{\sum xy - \frac{\sum x . \sum y}{n}}{\sum x^2 - \frac{(\sum x)^2}{n}} \quad \text{and } a = \bar{y} - b\bar{x}$$

where, $d_x = (x - \bar{x})$ and $d_y = (y - \bar{y})$, $\bar{x}$ and $\bar{y}$ are the respective means.

Example

The values of x are 0, 2, 4, 6, 8, 10, 12, 14, 16, 18 and those of y are 3.2, 4.5, 5.8, 7.1, 8.4, 9.7, 11, 12.3, 13.6, 14.9. Find out the values of a and b.

Solution

The given data and their derived data are put in tabular form below:

x	x^2	y	y^2	xy	x	x^2	y	y^2	xy
0	0	3.2	10.24	0	10	100	9.7	94.09	97
2	4	4.5	20.25	9	12	144	11	121	132
4	16	5.8	33.64	23.2	14	196	12.3	151.29	172.2
6	36	7.1	50.41	42.6	16	256	13.6	184.96	217.6
8	64	8.4	70.56	67.2	18	324	14.9	222.01	268.2

$\sum x = 90$, $\sum x^2 = 1140$, $\bar{x} = 9$, $\sum y = 90.5$, $\sum y^2$

$= 958.45$, $\bar{y} = 9.05$, $\sum xy = 1029$, $n = 10$

$$r = \frac{\sum xy - \frac{\sum x . \sum y}{n}}{\sqrt{\left[\sum x^2 - \frac{(\sum x)^2}{n}\right]\left[\sum y^2 - \frac{(\sum y)^2}{n}\right]}} = \frac{1027.4 - \frac{90 \times 90.5}{10}}{\sqrt{\left[1140 - \frac{(90)^2}{10}\right]\left[958.45 - \frac{(90.5)^2}{10}\right]}}$$

$$= \frac{1029 - \frac{8145}{10}}{\sqrt{\left[1140 - \frac{8100}{10}\right]\left[958.45 - \frac{8190.25}{10}\right]}}$$

$$= \frac{1029 - 814.5}{\sqrt{[1140 - 810]\,[958.45 - 819.02]}}$$

$$= \frac{2145}{\sqrt{330 \times 139.43}}$$

$$= \frac{214.5}{\sqrt{46011.9}}$$

$$= \frac{214.5}{214.5} = 1.0$$

Now, the regression equation of y on x; y = a + bx

$$b = \frac{\sum d_x d_y}{\sum d_x^2} = \frac{\sum xy - \frac{\sum x . \sum y}{n}}{\sum x^2 - \frac{(\sum x)^2}{n}} = \frac{1029 - \frac{90 \times 90.5}{10}}{1140 - \frac{(90)^2}{10}}$$

$$= \frac{1029 - 814.5}{1140 - 810}$$

$$= \frac{214.5}{330} = \mathbf{0.65}$$

and $a = \bar{y} - b\bar{x} = 9.05 - 0.65 \times 9.0 = 9.05 - 5.805 = \mathbf{3.245}$

Then, y = a + bx = 3.245 + 0.65x

Significance Test for Regression Coefficient

There are two tests used to determine whether the estimated value of regression coefficient, b deviates significantly from zero:

- **'t' test**

  The 't' can be calculated by using the following equation:

$$t = \frac{b}{\text{SE of b}}$$ where b is the regression coefficient, and

$$\text{SE of b} = \sqrt{\frac{\frac{1}{n-2}\left[\sum d_y^2 - \frac{(\sum d_x d_y)^2}{\sum d_x^2}\right]}{\sum d_x^2}} \quad \text{or,} \quad t = \frac{b}{\sqrt{\frac{\frac{1}{n-2}\left[\sum d_y^2 - \frac{(\sum d_x d_y)^2}{\sum d_x^2}\right]}{\sqrt{\sum d_x^2}}}}$$

Degree of freedom = n – 2

- **Analysis of variance (F test)**

  The degree of variance or F test can be calculated by using following equation:

$$F = \frac{\text{Regression mean square}}{\text{Residual mean square}}$$

Degree of freedom $n_1 = n - 1$ and $n_2 = n - 2$

Source of variation	Degree of freedom	S.S.	M.S.
Regression	1	$SSR = \frac{(\Sigma d_x d_y)^2}{\Sigma d_x^2}$	$\frac{\frac{(\Sigma d_x d_y)^2}{\Sigma d_x^2}}{1}$
Residual	n – 2	$SSE = \Sigma d_y^2 - \frac{(\Sigma d_x d_y)^2}{\Sigma d_x^2}$	$\frac{\Sigma d_y^2 - \frac{(\Sigma d_x d_y)^2}{\Sigma d_x^2}}{n-2}$
Total	n – 2	$SST = \Sigma d_y^2$	

Example

Fifty samples of a crude drug were collected and extracted. The results obtained are classified below. Find out the

(i) correlation coefficient, r

(ii) regression coefficient, b and

(iii) test the level of significance.

Extractive value, (%w/v) x	4.5	4.0	5.2	4.6	5.2	5.2	4.3	4.0	4.5	5.5
No. of samples, y	5	5	6	6	6	7	4	4	5	6

Solution

x	y	x^2	y^2	xy
4.5	5	20.25	25	22.5
4.0	5	16.00	25	20.0
5.2	6	27.04	36	31.2
4.6	6	21.16	36	27.6
5.2	6	27.04	36	31.2
5.2	7	27.04	49	36.4
4.3	4	18.49	16	17.2
4.0	4	16.00	16	16.0
4.5	5	20.25	25	22.5
5.5	6	30.25	36	33.0
$\sum x = 47$	$\sum y = 54$	$\sum x^2 = 223.52$	$\sum y^2 = 300$	$\sum xy = 257.6$

$$\sum d_x^2 = \sum x^2 - \frac{(\Sigma x)^2}{n} = 223.52 - \frac{(47)^2}{10} = 223.52 - \frac{2209}{10}$$

$$= 223.52 - 220.9$$

$$= 2.62$$

$$\sum d_y^2 = \sum y^2 - \frac{(\Sigma y)^2}{n} = 300 - \frac{(54)^2}{10} = 300 - \frac{2916}{10}$$

$$= 300 - 291.6$$

$$= 8.4$$

$$\sum d_x\, d_y = \sum xy - \frac{\Sigma x \times \Sigma y}{n} = 257.6 - \frac{47 \times 54}{10} = 257.6 - \frac{2538}{10}$$

$$= 257.6 - 253.8$$

$$= 3.8$$

$$\bar{x} = \frac{47}{10} = 4.7 \quad \text{and} \quad \bar{y} = \frac{54}{10} = 5.4$$

Correlation coefficient, $r = \dfrac{\sum xy - \frac{\Sigma x . \Sigma y}{n}}{\sqrt{\left[\Sigma x^2 - \frac{(\Sigma x)^2}{n}\right]\left[\Sigma y^2 - \frac{(\Sigma y)^2}{n}\right]}}$

$$= \frac{\sum d_x d_y}{\sqrt{\Sigma d_x^2 . \Sigma d_y^2}}$$

$$= \frac{3.8}{\sqrt{2.62 \times 8.4}}$$

$$= \frac{3.8}{\sqrt{22.01}}$$

$$= \frac{3.8}{4.69} = 0.81$$

Significance test, $t = \dfrac{r\sqrt{(n-2)}}{\sqrt{1-(r)^2}} = \dfrac{0.81\sqrt{(10-2)}}{\sqrt{1-(0.81)^2}}$

$$= \frac{0.81\sqrt{8}}{\sqrt{1-0.6561}} = \frac{0.81 \times 2.828}{\sqrt{0.3439}}$$

$$= \frac{2.29}{0.586} = 3.9$$

$$\text{Regression coefficient, b} = \sqrt{\frac{\frac{1}{n-2}\left[\sum d_y^2 - \frac{(\sum d_x d_y)^2}{\sum d_x^2}\right]}{\sum d_x^2}} = \frac{\sum d_x . \sum d_y}{\sum d_x^2}$$

$$= \frac{\sum xy - \frac{\sum x \sum y}{n}}{\sum x^2 - \frac{(\sum x)^2}{n}}$$

$$= \frac{257.6 - \frac{47 \times 54}{10}}{223.52 - \frac{(47)^2}{10}}$$

$$= \frac{257.6 - \frac{2538}{10}}{223.52 - \frac{2209}{10}}$$

$$= \frac{257.6 - 253.8}{223.52 - 220.9} = \frac{3.8}{2.62} = \mathbf{1.45}$$

$$\text{Significance test of b } t = \frac{b}{\text{SE of b}} = \frac{1.35}{\text{SE of b}}$$

$$\text{SE of b} = \sqrt{\frac{\frac{1}{n-2}\left[\sum d_y^2 - \frac{(\sum d_x d_y)^2}{\sum d_x^2}\right]}{\sum d_x^2}} = \sqrt{\frac{\frac{1}{10-2}\left[8.4 - \frac{(3.8)^2}{2.62}\right]}{2.62}}$$

$$= \sqrt{\frac{\frac{1}{8}\left[8.4 - \frac{14.44}{2.62}\right]}{2.62}}$$

$$= \sqrt{\frac{\frac{1}{8}[8.4 - 5.5]}{2.62}}$$

$$= \sqrt{\frac{\frac{1}{8} \times 2.9}{2.62}} = \sqrt{\frac{0.36}{2.62}} = \mathbf{0.37}$$

$$t = \frac{b}{\text{SE of b}} = \frac{1.45}{0.37} = \mathbf{3.92}$$

***Interpretation*:** The calculated value of t is higher than the tabulated value (2.82) at p = 0.01 with degree of freedom of 8. Hence, the correlation coefficient is highly significant.

Example

There are ten samples of freshly collected crude drugs. Each of the samples were weighed (x), dried and weighed after drying (y). The data are presented in tabular form below. Find out the correlation coefficient between x and y, and also find out the level of significance.

Initial weight (g), x	6	10	8	7	5	12	15	14	13	9
Final weight (g), y	4	6	5	4	3	8	10	9	8	6

Solution

Initial wt. x	Final wt. y	x^2	y^2	xy
6	4	36	16	24
10	6	100	36	60
8	5	64	25	40
7	4	49	16	28
5	3	25	25	15
12	8	144	64	96
15	10	225	100	150
14	9	196	81	126
13	8	169	64	104
9	6	81	36	54
$\sum x = 99$	$\sum y = 63$	$\sum x^2 = 1089$	$\sum y^2 = 463$	$\sum xy = 697$

Correlation coefficient, $r = \dfrac{\sum xy - \frac{\sum x . \sum y}{n}}{\sqrt{\left[\sum x^2 - \frac{(\sum x)^2}{n}\right]\left[\sum y^2 - \frac{(\sum y)^2}{n}\right]}}$

$$= \frac{697 - \frac{99 \times 63}{10}}{\sqrt{\left[1089 - \frac{(99)^2}{10}\right]\left[463 - \frac{(63)^2}{10}\right]}}$$

$$= \frac{697 - \frac{6237}{10}}{\sqrt{\left[1089 - \frac{9801}{10}\right]\left[463 - \frac{3969}{10}\right]}}$$

$$= \frac{697 - 623.7}{\sqrt{[1089 - 980.1]\,[463 - 369.9]}}$$

$$= \frac{73.3}{\sqrt{108.9 \times 93.1}} = \frac{73.3}{\sqrt{10138.59}} = \frac{73.3}{100.69} = \mathbf{0.728}$$

$$\text{Significance test, } t = \frac{r\sqrt{(n-2)}}{\sqrt{1-(r)^2}} = \frac{0.728\sqrt{(10-2)}}{\sqrt{1-(0.728)^2}}$$

$$= \frac{0.728\sqrt{8}}{\sqrt{1-0.5299}} = \frac{0.728 \times 2.828}{\sqrt{0.4701}}$$

$$= \frac{2.059}{0.685} = \mathbf{3.00}$$

Test of Significance

In research when samples are investigated the results obtained are used to make decisions. Hence samples investigated represent a population. Two samples drawn from same population may not produce exactly same results. Hence, statistical test of hypotheses have great importance to interpret the results properly. Usually in statistical test two hypotheses are used;

- ***Null hypothesis*:** It is denoted by H_o. To test the significance of the difference between the values of the sample and the population, or between the values of two samples the Null hypothesis is set up. It is usually used to ascertain that the difference in two results *is not significant* and to *test for acceptance or rejection*. The difference in result may be due to sample fluctuations.

$H_o : \mu = \bar{x}$ where μ is the mean value of the population $\bar{x}$ is the mean value of the sample

- ***Alternative hypothesis*:** It is a complementary to the null hypothesis. When H_o is rejected, alternative hypothesis, H_1 is accepted.

  For example, H_o: μ = 15 (Null hypothesis); while H_o: $\mu \neq 15$ (Alternative hypothesis).

There are two types of error:

Type I *error:* rejection of null hypothesis which is true

Type II *error:* acceptance of null hypothesis which is false

In other words,

(a) Reject H_o when it is true (Type I error) = α

(b) Accept H_o when it is false (Type II error) = β

(c) Accept H_o when it is true (correct decision)

(d) Reject H_o when it is false (correct decision)

When an inference is drawn on null hypothesis, type II error (β) should be minimized even with certain risk of type I error.

One and Two-tailed Test of Hypothesis

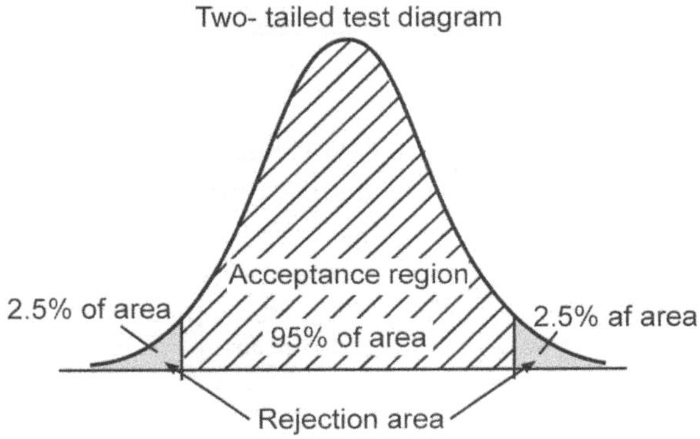

Figure 12.2

The area under the probability curve is divided into two regions – acceptance region and rejection or critical region. If the sample statistics falls in critical (rejection) region, the hypothesis is rejected; because it may lead to the false decision. The rejection region is always on the tail of the distribution curve which represents the level of significance α. If the rejection region lies on both the sides it is called two-tailed test; if it falls on either left side or right side of the curve it is called one-tailed test.

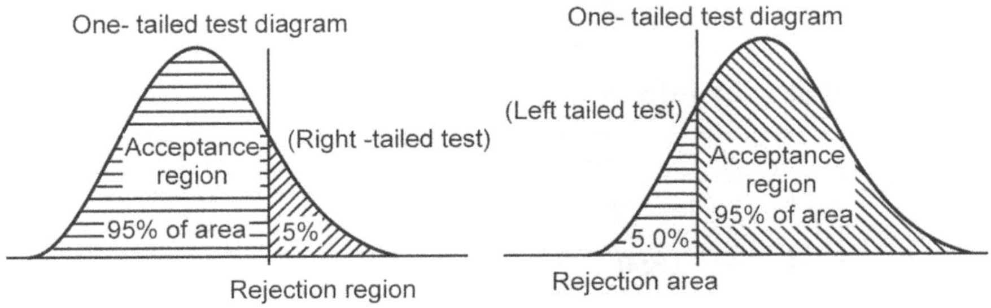

Figure 12.3

Comparison of Means of Two Large Samples (The Sample are Independent)

From a sample population when two samples are drawn randomly, it is assumed that the sample means are normally distributed and independent.

The means of the two large samples ($\bar{x}_1$ and $\bar{x}_2$) are compared and null hypothesis is applied.

$$t = \frac{\text{Difference of means of two samples}}{\text{Standard error of difference}} = \frac{\bar{x}_1 - \bar{x}_2}{s_d}$$

$$s_d = \sqrt{\frac{s_1^2}{n_1} + \frac{s_2^2}{n_2}}$$

Example

The following data relate to the sample A and B. Find out whether the two means are significantly different.

	Sample A	Sample B
n	25	28
mean	30	34
variance	8.72	10.54

Solution

Null hypothesis: H_o: There is no significant difference between the two samples.

Pooled variance, $s_d^2 = \frac{s_1^2}{n_1} + \frac{s_2^2}{n_2} = \frac{8.72}{25} + \frac{10.54}{28} = 0.348 + 0.376 =$ 0.724

Standard error of difference,

$$s_d = \sqrt{\frac{s_1^2}{n_1} + \frac{s_2^2}{n_2}} = \sqrt{\frac{8.72}{25} + \frac{10.54}{28}} = \sqrt{0.348 + 0.376}$$

$$= \sqrt{0.724} = \mathbf{0.850}$$

Difference between means $= \bar{x}_1 - \bar{x}_2 = 34 - 30 = 4$

$$t = \frac{\text{Difference of means of two samples}}{\text{Standard error of difference}} = \frac{\bar{x}_1 - \bar{x}_2}{s_d} = \frac{4}{0.85} = 4.70$$

Degree of freedom $= (n_1 + n_2 - 2) = 25 + 28 - 2 = \mathbf{51}$

Interpretation: The calculated value of t (4.70) is greater than the tabulated value of t (2.67) for 51 (nearest to 50) degree of freedom at 1%.

Hence, the two means are very much different. Null hypothesis stating that there is no significant difference between the two samples – is rejected at $p = 0.01$.

Example

The table shows the results of microbiological assay of a sample using Gentamycin as reference drug. The zones of inhibition for sample and reference standard are tabulated below. Analyze the data using t-test and comment on the antimicrobial activity of the sample.

Reference	1.78	1.82	1.93	1.89	1.79	1.69	1.81	1.80	1.75	1.67
Sample	1.69	1.71	1.78	1.74	1.60	1.48	1.65	1.59	1.60	1.69

Solution

***Null hypothesis*: H_0:** There is no significant difference between the means of two test results.

Reference		**Sample**	
x_1(cm)	**x_1^2(cm^2)**	**x_2(cm)**	**x_2^2(cm^2)**
1.78	3.17	1.69	2.86
1.82	3.31	1.71	2.92
1.93	3.72	1.78	3.17
1.89	3.57	1.74	3.03
1.79	3.20	1.60	2.56
1.69	2.86	1.48	2.19
1.81	3.28	1.65	2.72
1.80	3.24	1.59	2.53
1.75	3.06	1.60	2.56
1.67	2.79	1.69	2.86
$\sum x_1 = 17.93$	$\sum x_1^2 = 32.2$	$\sum x_2 = 16.53$	$\sum x_2^2 = 27.4$

$$\bar{x}_1 = \frac{\sum x_1}{n_1} = \frac{17.93}{10} = 1.79 \qquad \bar{x}_2 = \frac{\sum x_2}{n_2} = \frac{16.53}{10} = 1.65$$

$$\sum x_1^2 - \frac{(\sum x_1)^2}{n_1} = 32.2 - \frac{(17.93)^2}{10} = 32.2 - \frac{321.48}{10}$$

$$= 32.2 - 32.15 = 0.05$$

$$\sum X_2^2 - \frac{(\sum x_2)^2}{n_2} = 27.4 - \frac{(16.53)^2}{10} = 27.4 - \frac{273.2}{10}$$

$$= 27.4 - 27.32 = 0.08$$

Degree of freedom = $(n_1 + n_2 - 2) = 10+10-2 = 20 - 2 = 18$

Pooled variance, $s_d^2 = \frac{0.05+0.08}{18} = \frac{0.13}{2} = 0.0072$

Pooled standard deviation, $s_d = \sqrt{s_d^2} = \sqrt{0.0072} = 0.0848$

$$t = \frac{\text{Difference of means of two samples}}{\text{Standard error of difference}} = \frac{\bar{x}_1 - \bar{x}_2}{s_d} = \frac{17.93-16.53}{0.255}$$

$$= \frac{1.4}{0.255} = 5.49$$

Interpretation: Calculated value of t = 5.49, degree of freedom = 18

Tabulated value of t at $p = 0.01 = 2.878$ and at $p = 0.05, = 2.101$

Since the calculated value of t is greater than the tabulated value at 5% level of probability with 18 d.f., the difference between the two sample means is significant.

The null hypothesis stating that there is no significant difference between the means is rejected at p=0.05 and p=0.01.

Hence, antimicrobial activity of the sample is significant.

t-test for Paired Samples

Previous examples demonstrate that the samples are independent. There are cases where the samples are dependent. Such samples are called paired samples. The purpose of comparing paired samples is to eliminate maximum number of sources of irrelevant variations by making the pairs similar with respect to as many variables as possible.

When the null hypothesis is applied to paired comparison, it is assumed that the mean of the difference between the pairs is zero.

$$t = \frac{\bar{d}\sqrt{n}}{s_d} \quad \text{or,} \quad t = \frac{\bar{d}}{SE_d}$$

where, $\bar{d}$ is the mean of difference between the paired values $= \frac{\sum d}{n}$

SE_d = standard error of the difference $= \frac{s_d}{\sqrt{n}}$

S_d = standard deviation of the difference = $\sqrt{\dfrac{\sum d^2 - \dfrac{(\sum d)^2}{n}}{n-1}}$

Example

During 1991 to 2000 the sales turnover in Lakhs of rupees of product A (paracetamol tablet) and product B (paracetamol syrup) have been tabulated below. Analyze the data and find out whether the two products have the same mean.

year	Turnover of Product A	Turnover of Product B	Year	Turnover of Product A	Turnover of Product B
1991	16.89	15.24	1996	20.00	17.90
1992	17.45	15.80	1997	20.25	18.40
1993	17.90	16.25	1998	20.80	18.95
1994	18.20	16.95	1999	21.35	19.65
1995	18.95	17.10	2000	21.90	20.85

Solution

Null hypothesis: H_o: There is no significant difference between the means of turnover of two products A and B.

Since A and B are of the same drug, paracetamol, it may be assumed that turnovers are not independent; these are paired samples.

Years	Turnover of Product A (x_1)	Turnover of Product B(x_2)	Difference $d = x_1 - x_2$	$d^2 = (x_1 - x_2)^2$
1991	16.89	15.24	1.65	2.72
1992	17.45	15.80	1.65	2.72
1993	17.90	16.25	1.65	2.72
1994	18.20	16.95	1.25	1.56
1995	18.95	17.10	1.85	3.42
1996	20.00	17.90	2.1	4.41
1997	20.25	18.40	1.85	3.42
1998	20.80	18.95	1.85	3.42
1999	21.35	19.65	1.7	2.89
2000	21.90	20.85	1.05	1.10
			$\sum d = 16.6$	$\sum d^2 = 28.38$

$$\bar{d} = \frac{\sum d}{n} = \frac{16.6}{10} = 1.66$$

$$s_d^2 = \frac{\sum d^2 - \frac{(\sum d)^2}{n}}{n-1} = \frac{28.38 - \frac{(16.6)^2}{10}}{10-1} = \frac{28.38 - \frac{275.56}{10}}{9} = \frac{28.38 - 27.55}{9}$$

$$= \frac{0.83}{9} = 0.092$$

$$s_d = \sqrt{s_d^2} = \sqrt{0.092} = 0.303$$

$$SE_d = \frac{s_d}{\sqrt{n}} = \frac{0.303}{\sqrt{10}} = \frac{0.303}{3.16} = 0.096$$

$$t = \bar{d}/SE_d = \frac{1.66}{0.096} = 17.29$$

Interpretation: Calculated t value = 17.29, Tabulated t value = 2.26 ($p = 0.05$), d.f. = 10 – 1 = 9

Since the calculated value of t is much greater than the tabulated value at 5% level of probability with 9 d.f.; the difference between the two sample means is significant.

The null hypothesis stating that there is no significant difference between the means is rejected at $p = 0.05$ and $p = 0.01$.

Hence, the null hypothesis is rejected.

Chi-Square Test

In all genetical studies, it is necessary to test the significance of overall deviation between the observed and expected frequencies. The significance test of such deviation is known as chi-square test or χ^2 test. It is used to examine whether the recoded data are in agreement or not with the hypothesis. It is defined as;

$$\chi^2 = \sum \frac{(fo - fe)^2}{fe}$$

where '*fo*' is the observed frequency and '*fe*' is the expected frequency.

The degree of freedom (d.f.) = d.f. = (r – 1)(c – 1)

where 'r' is the number of rows in a contingency table, and 'c' is the number of columns in the table.

It the $fo = fe$, then the value of χ^2 would be zero and the possible value of χ^2 becomes greater than zero.

If the degree of freedom is less than 5, the corrected formula should be used to calculate the value of χ^2. The corrected formula is:

$$\chi^2 \text{ (corrected)} = \sum \frac{[(f_o - f_e) - 0.5]^2}{f_e} + \sum \frac{[(f_o - f_e) - 0.5]^2}{f_e}$$

$$\text{or,} \quad = \sum \frac{(|f_o - f_e| - 0.5)^2}{f_e}$$

Where expected value (fe) is to be calculated:

- *Determination of hypotheses*

  Null hypothesis (H_o): Two variables are independent

  Alternative hypothesis (H_1): Two variables are dependent.

- *Determination of the expected value* (fe)

  Expected value (fe) $= \frac{\text{(row total)} \times \text{(column total)}}{\text{sample size}}$ [Chi-Square test would be valid when 'fe' is = 5 or more]

- *Determination of the Chi-Square value, χ^2*

  $$\chi^2 = \frac{\Sigma(\text{Observed value} - \text{Expected value})^2}{\text{Expected value}} = \sum \frac{(fo - fe)^2}{fe}$$

- *Determination of Degree of Freedom*

  d.f. = (rows – 1) × (columns – 1)

- *Comparison of calculated value and tabulated Chi-Square value at $\chi^2_{0.05}$:*

  1. If the calculated value of χ^2 is less than the tabulated value (critical value), the null hypothesis is accepted (i.e., the variables are independent)
  2. If the calculated value of χ^2 is more than the tabulated value (critical value), the null hypothesis is rejected and the alternate hypothesis is accepted (i.e., the variables are not independent).

Example

According to a report one third of population are suffering from diabetes. In a study 900 people have been examined for having diabetes. Out of 900 persons 200 are found to suffer from diabetes and 700 are normal. Examine whether they deviate from the ratio of 1:3.

Solution

Null hypothesis: Ho: it is presumed that the ratio of normal persons and persons having diabetes is 3:1. The data are put in the table below:

	Normal persons	Persons with diabetes	Total
Observed frequency (*fo*)	700	200	900
Expected frequency (*fe*)	675	225	900
Deviation (*fo - fe*)	25	-25	

$$\chi^2 = \sum \frac{(fo-fe)^2}{fe} = \frac{(25)^2}{675} + \frac{(-25)^2}{225} = \frac{625}{675} + \frac{625}{225} = 0.925 + 2.777 = \mathbf{3.702}$$

The calculated value of χ^2 is less than the tabulated value which is 3.84 at probability level of 5% with single degree of freedom (since, there are two phenotypes; so, the d. f. = 2 – 1 = 1).

Therefore, the corrected formula is used to calculate the value of χ^2.

$$\chi^2 \text{ (corrected)} = \sum \frac{(|f_o - f_e| - 0.5)^2}{f_e} = \frac{(15-0.5)^2}{675} + \frac{(-15-0.5)^2}{225}$$

$$= \frac{(14.5)^2}{675} + \frac{(-15.5)^2}{225}$$

$$= 0.311 + 1.067 = \mathbf{1.378}$$

***Interpretation*:** Since the calculated and corrected value of χ^2 is much less than the tabulated value, the null hypothesis is accepted.

Example

Persons affected with poliomyelitis were surveyed. Some were vaccinated and some were not. The report is given below.

Vaccinated	Affected (fo’)	Not affected (fo”)	Total
Yes	56	44	**100**
No	78	47	**125**
Total	**134**	**91**	**225**

Solution

Assuming null hypothesis (Ho) that there is positive effect of vaccination.

Let us calculate the expected values on the basis of given data

$$\text{Expected value (fe)} = \frac{\text{(rows total)×(columns total)}}{\text{sample size}}$$

Vaccinated	Affected (fo')	Expected value (fe')	Not affected (fo")	Expected vaalue (fe")	Total
Yes	56	$\frac{100\times134}{225} = 59.55$	44	$\frac{100\times91}{225} = 40.44$	**100**
No	78	$\frac{125\times134}{225} = 74.44$	47	$\frac{125\times91}{225} = 50.55$	**125**
Total	**134**		**91**		**225**

Determination of the Chi-Square value, χ^2

Vaccinated	Affected χ^2 value	Not affected χ^2 value
Yes	$\frac{(fo-fe)^2}{fe} = \frac{(56-59.55)^2}{59.55} = \frac{(-3.55)^2}{59.55} = \frac{12.60}{59.55} = 0.211$	$\frac{(fo-fe)^2}{fe} = \frac{(44-40.44)^2}{44} = \frac{(3.56)^2}{44} = \frac{12.67}{44} = 0.288$
No	$\frac{(fo-fe)^2}{fe} = \frac{(78-74.44)^2}{78} = \frac{(3.56)^2}{74.44} = \frac{12.60}{59.55} = 0.170$	$\frac{(fo-fe)^2}{fe} = \frac{(47-50.55)^2}{50.55} = \frac{(-3.55)^2}{50.55} = \frac{12.60}{50.55} = 0.249$

$$\chi^2 = \sum\frac{(fo-fe)^2}{fe} = 0.211 + 0.288 + 0.170 + 0.249$$

$$= 0.918$$

Determination of degree of freedom, d.f. = (rows – 1) × (columns – 1)

$$= (2-1)(2-1) = 1\times1 = 1$$

Comparison between calculated χ^2 value with tabulated value, $\chi^2_{0.05}$

Calculated χ^2 value = **0.918**

Tabulated value, $\chi^2_{0.05}$ (with d.f. = 1) = 3.84

***Interpretation*:** Since the Calculated χ^2 value is less than the Tabulated value, $\chi^2_{0.05}$ (with d.f. = 1), the null hypothesis is accepted. The variables are independent.

Table 12.2 Chi square (χ^2) Distribution

d.f.	$x^2_{0.995}$	$x^2_{0.990}$	$x^2_{0.975}$	$x^2_{0.950}$	$x^2_{0.900}$	$x^2_{0.100}$	$x^2_{0.050}$	$x^2_{0.025}$	$x^2_{0.010}$	$x^2_{0.005}$
1	0.000	0.000	0.001	0.004	0.016	2.706	3.841	5.024	6.635	7.879
2	0.010	0.020	0.051	0.103	0.211	4.605	5.991	7.378	9.210	10.597
3	0.072	0.115	0.216	0.352	0.584	6.251	7.815	9.348	11.345	12.838
4	0.207	0.297	0.484	0.711	1.064	7.779	9.488	11.143	13.277	14.860
5	0.412	0.554	0.831	1.145	1.610	9.236	11.070	12.833	15.086	16.750
6	0.676	0.872	1.237	1.635	2.204	10.645	12.592	14.449	16.812	18.548
7	0.989	1.239	1.690	2.167	2.833	12.017	14.067	16.013	18.475	20.278
8	1.344	1.646	2.180	2.733	3.490	13.362	15.507	17.535	20.090	21.955
9	1.735	2.088	2.700	3.325	4.168	14.684	16.919	19.023	21.666	23.589
10	2.156	2.558	3.247	3.940	4.865	15.987	18.307	20.483	23.209	25.188
11	2.603	3.053	3.816	4.575	5.578	17.275	19.675	21.920	24.725	26.757
12	3.074	3.571	4.404	5.226	6.304	18.549	21.026	23.337	26.217	28.300
13	3.565	4.107	5.009	5.892	7.042	19.812	22.362	24.736	27.688	29.819
14	4.075	4.660	5.629	6.571	7.790	21.064	23.685	26.119	29.141	31.319
15	4.601	5.229	6.262	7.261	8.547	22.307	24.996	27.448	30.578	32.801
16	5.142	5.812	6.908	7.962	9.312	23.542	26.296	28.845	32.000	34.267
17	5.697	6.408	7.564	8.672	10.085	24.769	27.587	30.191	33.409	35.718
18	6.265	7.015	8.231	9.390	10.865	25.989	28.869	31.526	34.805	37.156
19	6.844	7.633	8.907	10.117	11.651	27.204	30.144	32.852	36.191	38.582
20	7.434	8.260	9.591	10.851	12.443	28.412	31.410	34.170	37.566	39.997
21	8.034	8.897	10.283	11.591	13.240	29.615	32.671	35.479	38.932	41.401
22	8.643	9.542	10.982	12.338	14.041	30.813	33.924	36.781	40.289	42.796
23	9.260	10.196	11.689	13.091	14.848	32.007	25.172	38.076	41.638	44.181
24	9.886	10.856	12.401	13.848	15.659	33.196	36.415	39.364	42.980	45.559
25	10.520	11.524	13.120	14.611	16.473	34.382	37.652	40.646	44.314	46.928
26	11.160	12.198	13.844	15.379	17.292	35.563	38.885	41.923	45.642	48.290
27	11.808	12.879	14.573	16.151	18.114	36.741	40.113	43.195	46.963	49.645
28	12.461	13.565	15.308	16.928	18.939	37.916	41.337	44.461	48.278	50.993
29	13.121	14.256	16.047	17.708	19.768	39.087	42.557	45.722	49.588	52.336
30	13.787	14.953	16.791	18.493	20.599	40.256	43.773	46.797	50.892	53.672
40	20.707	22.164	24.433	26.509	29.051	51.805	55.758	59.342	63.691	66.766
50	27.991	29.707	32.357	34.764	37.689	63.167	67.505	71.420	76.154	79.490
60	35.534	37.485	40.482	43.188	46.459	74.397	79.082	83.298	88.379	91.952
70	43.275	45.442	48.758	51.739	55.329	85.527	90.531	95.023	100.425	104.215
80	51.172	53.540	57.153	60.391	64.278	96.578	101.879	106.629	112.329	116.321
90	59.196	61.754	65.647	69.126	73.291	107.565	113.145	118.136	124.116	128.299
100	67.328	70.065	74.222	77.929	82.358	118.498	124.342	129.561	135.807	140.169

Analysis of Variance

Analysis of variance is used to test for the significance of the difference among sample means. This is done with the help of F-test which indicates the significance of the difference between two variances.

The characteristics of F-values are based on following conditions:

- All populations from which samples have been drawn are normally distributed.
- The variances for the population from which samples have been drawn are equal;

  i.e. $\sigma_1^2 = \sigma_2^2 = \sigma_3^2$

- The individuals being observed have been randomly selected from the populations represented by the samples.

Techniques of Analysis of variance:

- One-way classification, and
- Two-way classification.

One-way Classification

In one-way classification, the data are classified according to only one criterion. The hypothesis is:

1. The null hypothesis (H_o): $\mu_1 = \mu_2 = \mu_3 = \mu_4 \ldots\ldots\ldots\ldots \mu_n$
2. Alternative hypothesis (H_l): All the μ-values are not equal.

The steps involved in calculating variance are:

1. Calculate variance between the samples
2. Calculate variance within the sample
3. Calculate F as follows

$$F = \frac{\text{Variance between the samples}}{\text{Variance within the sample}}$$

4. Compare the calculated value with tabulated value of F.

4.1 If calculated value of F > table value of F; the difference in sample means becomes significant. In other words, the samples are not from same population.

4.2 If calculated value of F < table value of F; the difference in sample means are not significant. In other words, the samples are from same population.

Analysis of variance Table:

Sources of variation	SS (Sum of Square)	V (Degree of freedom)	MS (Mean square)	Variance Ratio of F
Between (column samples)	SSC	V1 = c –1	MSC = SSC/(c–1)	$F = \frac{MSC}{MSE}$
With samples	SSE	V2 = n – c	MSE = SSE/(n–c)	
Total	SST	n – 1		

where,

SSC = Sum of square between samples

SSE = Sum of square within samples

SST = Total sum of square

MSC = Mean square between samples

MSE = Mean square within samples

n = columns × rows = c × r

Determination of SSC

Sample 1 (x1)	Sample 2 (x2)	Sample 3 (x3)
X11	X21	X31
X12	X22	X32
X13	X23	X33
$\overline{x}_1 = \Sigma \frac{x1}{n}$	$\overline{x}_2 = \Sigma \frac{x2}{n}$	$\overline{x}_3 = \Sigma \frac{x3}{n}$

Mean of the means, $X^* = (\overline{x}_1 + \overline{x}_2 + \overline{x}_3)/3$

$(\bar{x}1 - x^*)^2$	$(\bar{x}2 - x^*)^2$	$(\bar{x}3 - x^*)^2$
$(\bar{x}11 - x^*)^2$	$(\bar{x}21 - x^*)^2$	$(\bar{x}31 - x^*)^2$
$(\bar{x}12 - x^*)^2$	$(\bar{x}22 - x^*)^2$	$(\bar{x}32 - x^*)^2$
$(\bar{x}13 - x^*)^2$	$(\bar{x}23 - x^*)^2$	$(\bar{x}33 - x^*)^2$
$\sum(\bar{x}1 - x*)^2$	$\sum(\bar{x}2 - x*)^2$	$\sum(\bar{x}3 - x*)^2$

$$SSC = \sum(\bar{x}1 - x*)^2 + \sum(\bar{x}2 - x*)^2 + \sum(\bar{x}3 - x*)^2$$

Determination of SSE

$(x1 - \bar{x}1)^2$	$(x2 - \bar{x}2)^2$	$(x3 - \bar{x}3)^2$
$(x11 - \bar{x}1)^2$	$(x21 - \bar{x}2)^2$	$(x31 - \bar{x}3)^2$
$(x12 - \bar{x}1)^2$	$(x22 - \bar{x}2)^2$	$(x32 - \bar{x}3)^2$
$(x13 - \bar{x}1)^2$	$(x23 - \bar{x}2)^2$	$(\bar{x}3 - \bar{x}3)^2$
$\sum(x1 - \bar{x}1)^2$	$\sum(x2 - \bar{x}2)^2$	$\sum(x3 - \bar{x}3)^2$

$$SSE = \sum(x1 - \bar{x}1)^2 + \sum(x2 - \bar{x}2)^2 + \sum(x3 - \bar{x}3)^2$$

Example

To assess the significance of variation in the performance in certain test between the convent schools. A common test was given to a number of students taken from 6th class of each school. Concerned results are given below:

School A	School B	School C	School D
8	12	18	13
10	11	12	9
12	9	16	12
8	14	6	16
7	4	8	15

Solution

School A (x1)	School B (x2)	School C (x3)	School D (x4)
8	12	18	13
10	11	12	9
12	9	16	12
8	14	6	16
7	4	8	15
$\sum x1 = 45$	$\sum x2 = 50$	$\sum x3 = 60$	$\sum x4 = 65$
$\bar{x}_1 = \sum \frac{45}{5} = 9$	$\bar{x}_2 = \sum \frac{50}{5} = 10$	$\bar{x}_3 = \sum \frac{60}{5} = 12$	$\bar{x}_4 = \sum \frac{65}{5} = 13$

$X^* = (\bar{x}_1 + \bar{x}_2 + \bar{x}_3 + \bar{x}_4)/4 = (9 + 10 + 12 + 13)/4 = 11$

Variance between the samples

$(\bar{x}_1 - x^*)^2$	$(\bar{x}_2 - x^*)^2$	$(\bar{x}_3 - x^*)^2$	$(\bar{x}_4 - x^*)^2$
$(9 - 11)^2 = 4$	$(10 - 11)^2 = 1$	$(12 - 11)^2 = 1$	$(13 - 11)^2 = 4$
$(9 - 11)^2 = 4$	$(10 - 11)^2 = 1$	$(12 - 11)^2 = 1$	$(13 - 11)^2 = 4$
$(9 - 11)^2 = 4$	$(10 - 11)^2 = 1$	$(12 - 11)^2 = 1$	$(13 - 11)^2 = 4$
$(9 - 11)^2 = 4$	$(10 - 11)^2 = 1$	$(12 - 11)^2 = 1$	$(13 - 11)^2 = 4$
$(9 - 11)^2 = 4$	$(10 - 11)^2 = 1$	$(12 - 11)^2 = 1$	$(13 - 11)^2 = 4$
$\sum(\bar{x}1 - x*)^2 = 20$	$\sum(\bar{x}2 - x*)^2 = 5$	$\sum(\bar{x}3 - x*)^2 = 5$	$\sum(\bar{x}3 - x*)^2 = 20$

SSC = 20 + 5 + 5 + 20 = 50

Variance within the sample

$(x1 - \bar{x}_1)^2$	$(x2 - \bar{x}_2)^2$	$(x3 - \bar{x}_3)^2$	$(x4 - \bar{x}_4 4)^2$
$(8 - 9)^2 = 1$	$(12 - 10)^2 = 4$	$(18 - 12)^2 = 36$	$(13 - 13)^2 = 0$
$(10 - 9)^2 = 1$	$(11 - 10)^2 = 1$	$(12 - 12)^2 = 0$	$(9 - 13)^2 = 16$
$(12 - 9)^2 = 9$	$(9 - 10)^2 = 1$	$(16 - 12)^2 = 16$	$(12 - 13)^2 = 1$
$(8 - 9)^2 = 1$	$(14 - 10)^2 = 16$	$(6 - 12)^2 = 36$	$(16 - 13)^2 = 9$
$(7 - 9)^2 = 4$	$(4 - 10)^2 = 36$	$(8 - 12)^2 = 16$	$(15 - 13)^2 = 4$
$\sum(x1 - \bar{x}1)^2 = 16$	$\sum(x2 - \bar{x}2)^2 = 58$	$\sum(x3 - \bar{x}3)^2 = 104$	$\sum(x3 - \bar{x}3)^2 = 30$

SSE = 16 + 58 + 104 + 30 = 208

Sources of variation	SS (Sum of Square)	V (Degree of freedom)	MS (Mean square)	Variance Ratio of F
Between (column samples)	SSC = 50	V1 = c –1= 4 – 1 = 3	MSC = SSC/ (c – 1) = 50/3 = 16.66	$F = \frac{MSC}{MSE}$ = 16.66/13 = 1.281
With samples	SSE = 208	V2 = n – c = 5 × 4 – 4 = 16	MSE=SSE/ (n – c) = 208/16 = 13	

***Interpretation*:** The calculated value of F (1.285) is less than the table value F0.05; 19, 3 level (3.13). Hence, the difference in sample means is not significant. In other words, the samples are from same population.

Example

From the data given below, find out whether the means of the three samples differ significantly or not.

Sample 1	Sample 2	Sample 3
19	20	14
11	14	13
17	18	11
18	12	14
15	10	8

Solution

Null hypothesis, Ho: There is no significant difference in the means of the three samples.

Sample 1	Sample 2	Sample 3
19	20	14
11	14	13
17	18	11
18	12	14
15	10	8
$\sum S1 = 80 = (x1)$	$\sum S2 = 74 = (x2)$	$\sum S3 = 60 = x3$
$\bar{x}_1 = \sum \frac{80}{5} = 16$	$\bar{x}_2 = \sum \frac{74}{5} = 14.8$	$\bar{x}_3 = \sum \frac{60}{5} = 12$

$X^* = (\bar{x}_1 + \bar{x}_2 + \bar{x}_3)/3 = (16 + 14.8 + 12)/3 = 14.267$

Variance between the samples

$(\bar{x}_1 - x^*)^2$	$(\bar{x}_2 - x^*)^2$	$(\bar{x}_3 - x^*)^2$
$(16 - 14.267)^2 = 3.003$	$(14.8 - 14.267)^2 = 0.284$	$(12 - 14.267)^2 = 5.139$
$(16 - 14.267)^2 = 3.003$	$(14.8 - 14.267)^2 = 0.284$	$(12 - 14.267)^2 = 5.139$
$(16 - 14.267)^2 = 3.003$	$(14.8 - 14.267)^2 = 0.284$	$(12 - 14.267)^2 = 5.139$
$(16 - 14.267)^2 = 3.003$	$(14.8 - 14.267)^2 = 0.284$	$(12 - 14.267)^2 = 5.139$
$(16 - 14.267)^2 = 3.003$	$(14.8 - 14.267)^2 = 0.284$	$(12 - 14.267)^2 = 5.139$
$\Sigma(\bar{x}1 - x*)^2 = 15.015$	$\Sigma(\bar{x}2 - x*)^2 = 1.42$	$\Sigma(\bar{x}3 - x*)^2 = 25.69$

SSC = 15.015 + 1.42 + 25.69 = 42.125

Variance within the sample

$(x1 - \bar{x}_1)^2$	$(x2 - \bar{x}_2)^2$	$(x3 - \bar{x}_3)^2$
$(19 - 16)^2 = 9$	$(20 - 14.8)^2 = 27.04$	$(14 - 12)^2 = 4$
$(11 - 16)^2 = 25$	$(14 - 14.8)^2 = 0.64$	$(13 - 12)^2 = 1$
$(17 - 16)^2 = 1$	$(18 - 14.8)^2 = 10.24$	$(11 - 12)^2 = 1$
$(18 - 16)^2 = 4$	$(12 - 14.8)^2 = 7.84$	$(14 - 12)^2 = 4$
$(15 - 16)^2 = 1$	$(10 - 14.8)^2 = 23.04$	$(8 - 12)^2 = 16$
$\Sigma(x1 - \bar{x}1)^2 = 40$	$\Sigma(x2 - \bar{x}2)^2 = 68.8$	$\Sigma(x3 - \bar{x}3)^2 = 26$

SSE = 40 + 68.8 + 26 = 134.8

Sources of variation	SS (Sum of Square)	V (Degree of freedom)	MS (Mean square)	Variance Ratio of F
Between (column samples)	SSC = 42.125	V1 = c – 1 = 3 – 1 = 2	MSC = SSC/(c - 1) $= \frac{42.125}{2} =$ 21.0625	$F = \frac{MSC}{MSE}$ $= \frac{21.0625}{11.23}$ = 1.875
With samples	SSE =134.8	V2 = n – c = 5×3 –3 = 12	MSE=SSE/(n - c) $= \frac{134.8}{12} = 11.23$	

Interpretation: The calculated value of F (1.285) is less than the table value at F0.05; 2, 12 level (3.89). Hence, the difference in sample means is not significant and null hypothesis is accepted.

Two-Way Classification

In two-way classification the data are classified according to two different criteria or factors. The table below is used to analyze the variance in two-way classification

Sources of variation	Sum of Square	d.f.	Mean Square	Ratio of variance F
Between columns Between rows Residual	SSC SSR SSE	c –1 r –1 (c –1) (r –1)	MSC = SSC/(c –1) MSR = SSR/(r –1) MSE = SSE/(c–1)(r–1)	F = MSC/MSE F = MSR/MSE
Total	SST	N –1		

where, SSC = sum of squares between columns

$$= \frac{x_1^2}{n_1} + \frac{x_2^2}{n_2} + \frac{x_3^2}{n_3} + \ldots\ldots. + \frac{x_n^2}{n_n} - \frac{T^2}{N}$$

[T is the sum of all columns or all rows, N = c × r]

SSR = sum of squares between rows

$$= \frac{y_1^2}{n_1} + \frac{y_2^2}{n_2} + \frac{y_3^2}{n_3} + \ldots\ldots\ldots + \frac{y_n^2}{n_n} - \frac{T^2}{N}$$

SSE = sum of squares for the residual

SST = total sum of square

The total number of degree of freedom (d.f.) = (c × r) – 1 = n –1

Residual (Error or Remainder) = SST – SSC – SSR

Example

In an experiment the effect of nitrogen on production of rice was examined. The mean yield of three varieties of rice and the nitrogen content of the soil are presented in the table below. Analyze the data using the test of analysis of variance to determine whether there is any difference in the mean yield of three varieties of rice (V1, V2, V3) with four nitrogen doses.

Nitrogen Rate, kg/hectare	V1 (ton)	V2 (ton)	V3 (ton)
0	4.00	4.50	5.20
25	4.20	5.30	5.90
50	5.00	5.90	6.50
80	6.10	6.45	7.50

Solution

***Null hypothesis*, Ho:** There is no significant difference in the mean yield of three varieties of rice.

Nitrogen Rate, kg/hectare	V1 (ton)	V2 (ton)	V3 (ton)	Total
0	4.00	4.50	5.20	13.70
25	4.20	5.30	5.90	15.40
50	5.00	5.90	6.70	17.60
80	6.10	6.45	7.50	20.05
Total	19.30	22.15	25.30	66.75

$$\text{Correlation Factor} = \frac{T^2}{N} = \frac{(66.75)^2}{12} = 371.3$$

$$SSC = \frac{x_1^2}{n_1} + \frac{x_2^2}{n_2} + \frac{x_3^2}{n_3} + \ldots\ldots + \frac{x_n^2}{n_n} - \frac{T^2}{N}$$

$$= \frac{(19.3)^2}{4} + \frac{(22.15)^2}{4} + \frac{(25.3)^2}{4} - 371.3$$

$$= 93.12 + 122.65 + 160.02 - 371.3 = 4.49$$

$$SSR = \frac{y_1^2}{n_1} + \frac{y_2^2}{n_2} + \frac{y_3^2}{n_3} + \ldots\ldots + \frac{y_n^2}{n_n} - \frac{T^2}{N}$$

$$= \frac{(13.7)^2}{3} + \frac{(15.4)^2}{3} + \frac{(17.6)^2}{3} + \frac{(20.05)^2}{3} - 371.3$$

$$= 62.56 + 79.05 + 103.25 + 134.00 - 371.3 = 7.56$$

$$SST = (4)^2 + (4.2)^2 + (5)^2 + (6.1)^2 + (4.5)^2 + (5.3)^2 + (5.9)^2 + (6.45)^2 + (5.2)^2 + (5.9)^2 + (6.7)^2 + (7.5)^2 - 371.3$$

$$= 16 + 17.64 + 25 + 37.21 + 20.25 + 28.09 + 34.81 + 41.60 + 27.04 + 34.81 + 44.89 + 56.25 - 371.3$$

$$= 12.29$$

$$SSE = SST - SSR - SSC = 12.29 - 7.53 - 4.49 = 0.27$$

$$MSC = \frac{SSC}{c-1} = \frac{4.49}{3-1} = \frac{4.49}{2} = 2.245$$

$$MSR = \frac{SSR}{r-1} = \frac{7.53}{4-1} = \frac{7.53}{3} = 2.51$$

$$MSE = \frac{SSE}{(c-1)(r-1)} = \frac{0.27}{(3-1)(4-1)} = \frac{0.27}{6} = 0.045$$

$$Fc = \frac{MSC}{MSE} = \frac{2.245}{0.045} = 49.88$$

$$Fr = \frac{MSR}{MSE} = \frac{2.51}{0.045} = 55.78$$

Sources of variation	Sum of Square	d.f.	Mean Square	Ratio of variance F
Between columns	SSC = 4.49	c – 1 = 2	MSC=SSC/(c –1) = 4.49/2 = 2.245	Fc = MSC/MSE = 2.245/0.045 = 49.88
Between rows	SSR = 7.53	r – 1 = 3	MSR=SSR/(r –1) = 7.53/3 = 2.51	Fr = MSR/MSE = 2.51/0.045 = 55.78
Residual	SSE = 0.027	(c –1)(r –1) 2 × 3 = 6	MSE = SSE/(c–1) (r–1) = 0.27/6 = 0.045	
Total	SST = 12.29	N –1 = 3×4 –1 = 11		

***Interpretation*:**

(i) *F for between the rice varieties:* The calculated value of F (49.88) is much greater than the tabulated value of F0.01; (2, 6) which is 10.9; this indicates that the mean yield of the varieties is significant. The null hypothesis (There is no significant difference in the mean yield of three varieties of rice.) is rejected.

(ii) *F for between the nitrogen content:* The calculated value of F (55.78) is much greater than the tabulated value of F0.01; (3, 6) which is 9.78; this indicates that the variation in nitrogen content has significant effect on the mean yield of the rice varieties. The null hypothesis is rejected.

Example

Four samples of Ibuprofen coated tablets were tested for disintegration by three chemists. The results are tabulated below. Analyze the data and comment on the variation in chemists as well as in samples.

Chemists	Sample 1	Sample 2	Sample 3	Sample 4
Chemist A	36 min	36 min	21 min	35 min
Chemist B	28	29	31	32
Chemist C	26	28	29	29

Solution

Chemists	Sample 1	Sample 2	Sample 3	Sample 4	Total
Chemist A	36 min	36 min	21 min	35 min	128 min
Chemist B	28	29	31	32	120
Chemist C	26	28	29	29	112
Total	90 min	93 min	81 min	96 min	360 min

$$\text{Correlation Factor} = \frac{T^2}{N} = \frac{(360)^2}{12} = 10800$$

$$SSC = \frac{x_1^2}{n_1} + \frac{x_2^2}{n_2} + \frac{x_3^2}{n_3} + \ldots\ldots + \frac{x_n^2}{n_n} - \frac{T^2}{N}$$

$$= \frac{(90)^2}{3} + \frac{(93)^2}{3} + \frac{(81)^2}{3} + \frac{(96)^2}{3} - 10800$$

$$= 2700 + 2883 + 2187 + 3072 - 10800 = 42$$

$$SSR = \frac{y_1^2}{n_1} + \frac{y_2^2}{n_2} + \frac{y_3^2}{n_3} + \ldots\ldots\ldots + \frac{y_n^2}{n_n} - \frac{T^2}{N}$$

$$= \frac{(128)^2}{4} + \frac{(120)^2}{4} + \frac{(112)^2}{4} - 10800$$

$$= 4096 + 3600 + 3136 - 10800 = 32$$

$$SST = (36)^2 + (28)^2 + (26)^2 + (36)^2 + (29)^2 + (28)^2 + (21)^2 + (31)^2 + (29)^2 + (35)^2 + (32)^2 + (29)^2 - 10800$$

$$= 1296 + 784 + 676 + 1296 + 841 + 784 + 441 + 961 + 841 + 1225 + 1024 + 841 - 10800$$

$$= 210$$

$$SSE = SST - SSR - SSC$$

$$= 210 - 32 - 42 = 136$$

$$MSC = \frac{SSC}{c-1} = \frac{42}{4-1} = \frac{42}{3} = 14$$

$$MSR = \frac{SSR}{r-1} = \frac{32}{3-1} = \frac{32}{2} = 16$$

$$MSE = \frac{SSE}{(c-1)(r-1)} = \frac{136}{(4-1)(3-1)} = \frac{136}{6} = 22.67$$

$$Fc = \frac{MSC}{MSE} = \frac{14}{22.67} = 0.617$$

$$Fr = \frac{MSR}{MSE} = \frac{16}{22.67} = 0.706$$

Sources of variation	**Sum of Square**	**d.f.**	**Mean Square**	**Ratio of variance F**
Between columns	SSC = 42	c – 1 = 3	MSC = SSC/(c –1) = 42/3 = 14	Fc = MSC/MSE = 14/22.67 = 0.617
Between rows	SSR = 32	r – 1= 2	MSR = SSR/(r –1) = 32/2 = 16	Fr = MSR/MSE = 16/22.67 = 0.706
Residual	SSE = 136	(c –1) (r –1) 3 × 2 = 6	MSE = SSE/(c–1)(r–1) = 136/6 = 22.67	
Total	SST = 210	N –1 = 4×3 –1 = 11		

Interpretation:

(i) *F for between the samples:* The calculated value of Fc (0.617) is much less than the tabulated value of F0.01; (2, 6) which is 10.93; this indicates that the difference in samples is not significant. The null hypothesis is accepted.

(ii) *F for between the chemists:* The calculated value of Fr (0.706) is much less than the tabulated value of F0.01; (3, 6) which is 9.78; this indicates that there is no significant effect on the mean disintegration time of the four varieties of tablets determined by different chemists. The null hypothesis is accepted.

Table 12.3 Critical values of F 0.05(V1,V2) at 5% significance level

d.f	1	2	3	4	5	6	7	8	9	10
1	161.45	199.50	215.71	224.58	230.16	233.99	236.77	238.88	240.54	241.88
2	18.51	19.00	19.16	19.25	19.30	19.33	19.35	19.37	19.39	19.40
3	10.13	9.55	9.28	9.12	9,01	8.94	8.89	8.85	8.81	8.79
4	7.71	6.94	6.59	6.39	6.26	6.16	6.09	6.04	6.00	5.96
5	6.61	5.79	5.41	5.19	5.05	4.95	4.88	4.82	4.77	4.74
6	5.99	5.14	4.76	4.53	4.39	4.28	4.21	4.15	4.10	4.06
7	5.59	4.74	4.35	4.12	3.97	3.87	3.79	3.73	3.68	3.64
8	5.32	4.46	4.07	3.84	3.69	3.58	3.50	3.44	3.39	3.35
9	5.12	4.26	3.86	3.63	3.48	3.37	3.29	3.23	3.18	3.14
10	4.97	4.10	3.71	3.48	3.33	3.22	3.14	3.07	3.02	2.98
11	4.84	3.98	3.59	3.36	3.20	3.10	3.01	2.95	2.90	2.85
12	4.75	3.89	3.49	3.26	3.11	3.00	2.91	2.85	2.80	2.75
13	4.67	3.81	3.41	3.18	3.03	2.92	2.83	2.77	2.71	2.67
14	4.60	3.74	3.34	3.11	2.96	2.85	2.76	2.70	2.65	2.60
15	4.54	3.68	3.29	3.06	2.90	2.79	2.71	2.64	2.59	2.54
16	4.49	3.63	3.24	3.01	2.85	2.74	2.66	2.59	2.54	2.49
17	4.45	3.59	3.20	2.97	2.81	2.70	2.61	2.55	2.49	2.45
18	4.41	3.56	3.16	2.93	2.77	2.66	2.58	2.51	2.46	2.41
19	4.38	3.52	3.13	2.90	2.74	2.63	2.54	2.48	2.42	2.38
20	4.35	3.49	3.10	2.87	2.71	2.60	2.51	2.45	2.39	2.35
21	4.33	3.47	3.07	2.84	2.69	2.57	2.49	2.42	2.37	2.32
22	4.30	3.44	3.05	2.82	2.66	2.55	2.46	2.40	2.34	2.30
23	4.28	3.42	3.03	2.80	2.64	2.53	2.44	2.38	2.32	2.28
24	4.26	3.40	3.01	2.78	2.62	2.51	2.42	2.36	2.30	2.26
25	4.24	3.39	2.99	2.76	2.60	2.49	2.41	2.34	2.28	2.24
26	4.23	3.37	2.98	2.74	2.59	2.47	2.39	2.32	2.27	2.22
27	4.21	3.35	2.96	2.73	2.57	2.46	2.37	2.31	2.25	2.20
28	4.20	3.34	2.95	2.71	2.56	2.45	2.36	2.29	2.24	2.19
29	4.18	3.33	2.93	2.70	2.55	2.43	2.35	2.28	2.22	2.18
30	4.17	3.32	2.92	2.69	2.53	2.42	2.33	2.27	2.21	2.17
31	4.16	3.31	2.91	2.68	2.52	2.41	2.32	2.26	2.20	2.15
32	4.15	3.30	2.90	2.67	2.51	2.40	2.31	2.24	2.19	2.14
33	4.14	3.29	2.89	2.66	2.50	2.39	2.30	2.24	2.18	2.13
34	4.13	3.28	2.88	2.65	2.49	2.38	2.29	2.23	2.17	2.12

Table **12.3** ***contd...***

d.f	1	2	3	4	5	6	7	8	9	10
35	4.12	3.27	2.87	2.64	2.49	2.37	2.29	2.22	2.16	2.11
36	4.11	3.26	2.87	2.63	2.48	2.36	2.28	2.21	2.15	2.11
37	4.11	3.25	2.86	2.63	2.47	2.36	2.27	2.20	2.15	2.10
38	4.10	3.25	2.85	2.62	2.46	2.35	2.26	2.19	2.14	2.09
39	4.09	3.24	2.85	2.61	2.46	2.34	2.26	2.19	2.13	2.08
40	4.09	3.23	2.84	2.61	2.45	2.34	2.25	2.18	2.12	2.08
41	4.08	3.23	2.83	2.60	2.44	2.33	2.24	2.17	2.12	2.07
42	4.07	3.22	2.83	2.59	2.44	2.32	2.24	2.17	2.11	2.07
43	4.07	3.21	2.82	2.59	2.43	2.32	2.23	2.16	2.11	2.06
44	4.06	3.21	2.82	2.58	2.43	2.31	2.23	2.16	2.10	2.05
45	4.06	3.20	2.81	2.58	2.42	2.31	2.22	2.15	2.10	2.05
46	4.05	3.20	2.81	2.57	2.42	2.30	2.22	2.15	2.09	2.04
47	4.05	3.20	2.80	2.57	2.41	2.30	2.21	2.14	2.09	2.04
48	4.04	3.19	2.80	2.57	2.41	2.30	2.21	2.14	2.08	2.04
49	4.04	3.19	2.79	2.56	2.40	2.29	2.20	2.13	2.08	2.03
50	4.03	3.18	2.79	2.56	2.40	2.29	2.20	2.13	2.07	2.03
51	4.03	3.18	2.79	2.55	2.40	2.28	2.20	2.13	2.07	2.02
52	4.03	3.18	2.78	2.55	2.39	2.28	2.19	2.12	2.07	2.02
53	4.02	3.17	2.78	2.55	2.39	2.28	2.19	2.12	2.06	2.02
54	4.02	3.17	2.78	2.54	2.39	2.27	2.19	2.12	2.06	2.01
55	4.02	3.17	2.77	2.54	2.38	2.27	2.18	2.11	2.06	2.01
56	4.01	3.16	2.77	2.54	2.38	2.27	2.18	2.11	2.05	2.01
57	4.01	3.16	2.77	2.53	2.38	2.26	2.18	2.11	2.05	2.00
58	4.01	3.16	2.76	2.53	2.37	2.26	2.17	2.10	2.05	2.00
59	4.00	3.15	2.76	2.53	2.37	2.26	2.17	2.10	2.04	2.00
60	4.00	3.15	2.76	2.53	2.37	2.25	2.17	2.10	2.04	1.99
61	4.00	3.15	2.76	2.52	2.37	2.25	2.17	2.09	2.04	1.99
62	4.00	3.15	2.75	2.52	2.36	2.25	2.16	2.09	2.04	1.99
63	3.99	3.14	2.75	2.52	2.36	2.25	2.16	2.09	2.03	1.99
64	3.99	3.14	2.75	2.52	2.36	2.24	2.16	2.09	2.03	1.98
65	3.99	3.14	2.75	2.51	2.36	2.24	2.15	2.08	2.03	1.98
66	3.99	3.14	2.74	2.51	2.35	2.24	2.15	2.08	2.03	1.98
67	3.98	3.13	2.74	2.51	2.35	2.24	2.15	2.08	2.02	1.98
68	3.98	3.13	2.74	2.51	2.35	2.24	2.15	2.08	2.02	1.97
69	3.98	3.13	2.74	2.51	2.35	2.23	2.15	2.08	2.02	1.97

Table **12.3 *contd...***

d.f	1	2	3	4	5	6	7	8	9	10
70	3.98	3.13	2.74	2.50	2.35	2.23	2.14	2.07	2.02	1.97
71	3.98	3.13	2.73	2.50	2.34	2.23	2.14	2.07	2.02	1.97
72	3.97	3.12	2.73	2.50	2.34	2.23	2.14	2.07	2.01	1.97
73	3.97	3.12	2.73	2.50	2.34	2.23	2.14	2.07	2.01	1.96
74	3.97	3.12	2.73	2.50	2.34	2.22	2.14	2.07	2.01	1.96
75	3.97	3.12	2.73	2.49	2.34	2.22	2.13	2.06	2.01	1.96
76	3.97	3.12	2.73	2.49	2.34	2.22	2.13	2.06	2.01	1.96
77	3.97	3.12	2.72	2.49	2.33	2.22	2.13	2.06	2.00	1.96
78	3.96	3.11	2.72	2.49	2.33	2.22	2.13	2.06	2.00	1.95
79	3.96	3.11	2.72	2.49	2.33	2.22	2.13	2.06	2.00	1.95
80	3.96	3.11	2.72	2.49	2.33	2.21	2.13	2.06	2.00	1.95
81	3.96	3.11	2.72	2.48	2.33	2.21	2.13	2.06	2.00	1.95
82	3.96	3.11	2.72	2.48	2.33	2.21	2.12	2.05	2.00	1.95
83	3.96	3.11	2.72	2.48	2.32	2.21	2.12	2.05	2.00	1.95
84	3.96	3.11	2.71	2.48	2.32	2.21	2.12	2.05	1.99	1.95
85	3.95	3.10	2.71	2.48	2.32	2.21	2.12	2.05	1.99	1.94
86	3.95	3.10	2.71	2.48	2.32	2.21	2.12	2.05	1.99	1.94
87	3.95	3.10	2.71	2.48	2.32	2.21	2.12	2.05	1.99	1.94
88	3.95	3.10	2.71	2.48	2.32	2.20	2.12	2.05	1.99	1.94
89	3.95	3.10	2.71	2.47	2.32	2.20	2.11	2.04	1.99	1.94
90	3.95	3.10	2.71	2.47	2.32	2.20	2.11	2.04	1.99	1.94
91	3.95	3.10	2.71	2.47	2.32	2.20	2.11	2.04	1.98	1.94
92	3.95	3.10	2.70	2.47	2.31	2.20	2.11	2.04	1.98	1.94
93	3.94	3.09	2.70	2.47	2.31	2.20	2.11	2.04	1.98	1.93
94	3.94	3.09	2.70	2.47	2.31	2.20	2.11	2.04	1.98	1.93
95	3.94	3.09	2.70	2.47	2.31	2.20	2.11	2.04	1.98	1.93
96	3.94	3.09	2.70	2.47	2.31	2.20	2.11	2.04	1.98	1.93
97	3.94	3.09	2.70	2.47	2.31	2.19	2.11	2.04	1.98	1.93
98	3.94	3.09	2.70	2.47	2.31	2.19	2.10	2.03	1.98	1.93
99	3.94	3.09	2.70	2.46	2.31	2.19	2.10	2.03	1.98	1.93
100	3.94	3.09	2.70	2.46	2.31	2.19	2.10	2.03	1.98	1.93

Table 12.4 Critical values of F0.01(V1,V2) at 1% significance level

d.f	1	2	3	4	5	6	7	8	9	10
1	4052.19	4999.52	5403.34	5624.62	5763.65	5858.97	5928.33	5981.10	6022.50	6055.85
2	98.50	99.00	99.17	99.25	99.30	99.33	99.36	99.37	99.39	99.40
3	34.12	30.82	29.46	28.71	28.24	27.91	27.67	27.49	27.35	27.23
4	21.20	18.00	16.69	15.98	15.52	15.21	14.98	14.80	14.66	14.55
5	16.26	13.27	12.06	11.39	10.97	10.67	10.46	10.29	10.16	10.05
6	13.75	10.93	9.78	9.15	8.75	8.47	8.26	8.10	7.98	7.87
7	12.25	9.55	8.45	7.85	7.46	7.19	6.99	6.84	6.72	6.62
8	11..26	8.65	7.59	7.01	6.63	6.37	6.18	6.03	5.91	5.81
9	10.56	8.02	6.99	6.42	6.06	5.80	5.61	5.47	5.35	5.26
10	10.04	7.56	6.55	5.99	5.64	5.39	5.20	5.06	4.94	4.85
11	9.65	7.21	6.22	5.67	5.32	5.07	4.89	4.74	4.63	4.54
12	9.33	6.93	5.95	5.41	5.06	4.82	4.64	4,50	4.39	4.30
13	9.07	6.70	5.74	5.21	4.86	4.62	4.44	4.30	4.19	4.10
14	8.86	6.52	5.56	5.04	4.70	4,46	4.28	4.14	4.03	3.94
15	8.68	6.36	5.42	4.89	4.56	4.32	4.14	4.00	3.90	3.81
16	8.53	6.23	5.29	4.77	4.44	4.20	4.03	3.89	3.78	3.69
17	8.40	6.11	5.19	4.67	4.34	4.10	3.93	3.79	3.68	3.59
18	8.29	6.01	5.09	4.58	4.25	4.02	3.84	3.71	3.60	3.51
19	8.19	5.93	5.01	4.50	4.17	3.94	3.77	3.63	3.52	3.43
20	8.10	5.85	4.94	4.43	4.10	3.87	3.70	3.56	3.46	3.37
21	8.02	5.78	4.87	4.37	4.04	3.81	3.64	3.51	3.40	3.31
22	7.95	5.72	4.82	4.31	3.99	3.76	3.59	3.45	3.35	3.26
23	7.88	5.66	4.77	4.26	3.94	3.71	3.54	3.41	3.30	3.21
24	7.82	5.61	4.72	4.22	3.90	3.67	3.50	3.36	3.26	3.17
25	7.77	5.57	4.68	4.18	3.86	3.63	3.46	3.32	3.22	3.13
26	7.72	5.53	4.64	4.14	3.82	3.59	3.42	3.29	3.18	3.09
27	7.68	5.49	4.60	4.11	3.79	3.56	3.39	3.26	3.15	3.06
28	7.64	5.45	4.57	4.07	3.75	3.53	3.36	3.23	3.12	3.03
29	7.60	5.42	4.54	4.05	3.73	3.50	3.33	3.20	3.09	3.01
30	7.56	5.39	4.51	4.02	3.70	3.47	3.31	3.17	3.07	2.98
31	7.53	5.36	4.48	3.99	3.68	3.45	3.28	3.15	3.04	2.96
32	7.50	5.34	4.46	3.97	3.65	3.43	3.26	3.13	3.02	2.93
33	7.47	5.31	4.44	3.95	3.64	3.41	3.24	3.11	3.00	2.91
34	7.44	5.29	4.42	3.93	3.61	3.39	3.22	3.09	2.98	2.89

***Table* 12.4 contd...**

d.f	1	2	3	4	5	6	7	8	9	10
35	7.42	5.27	4.40	3.91	3.59	3.37	3.20	3.07	2.96	2.88
36	7.40	5.25	4.38	3.89	3.57	3.35	3.18	3.05	2.95	2.86
37	7.37	5.23	4.36	3.87	3.56	3.33	3.17	3.04	2.93	2.84
38	7.35	5.21	4.34	3.86	3.54	3.32	3.15	3.02	2.92	2.83
39	7.33	5.19	4.33	3.84	3.53	3.31	3.14	3.01	2.90	2.81
40	7.31	5.18	4.31	3.83	3.51	3.29	3.12	2.99	2.89	2.80
41	7.30	5.16	4.30	3.82	3.50	3.28	3.11	2.98	2.88	2.79
42	7.28	5.15	4.29	3.80	3.49	3.27	3.10	2.97	2.86	2.78
43	7.26	5.14	4.27	3.79	3.48	3.25	3.09	2.96	2.85	2.76
44	7.25	5.12	4.26	3.78	3.47	3.24	3.08	2.95	2.84	2.75
45	7.23	5.11	4.25	3.77	3.45	3.23	3.07	2.94	2.83	2.74
46	7.22	5.10	4.24	3.76	3.44	3.22	3.06	2.93	2.82	2.73
47	7.21	5.09	4.23	3.75	3.43	3.21	3.05	2.92	2.81	2.72
48	7.19	5.08	4.22	3.74	3.43	3.20	3.04	2.91	2.80	2.72
49	7.18	5.07	4.21	3.73	3.42	3.20	3.03	2.90	2.79	2.71
50	7.17	5.06	4.20	3.72	3.41	3.19	3.02	2.89	2.79	2.70
51	7.16	5.05	4.19	3.71	3.40	3.18	3.01	2.88	2.78	2.69
52	7.15	5.04	4.18	3.70	3.39	3.17	3.01	2.87	2.77	2.68
53	7.14	5.03	4.17	3.70	3.38	3.16	3.00	2.87	2.76	2.68
54	7.13	5.02	4.17	3.69	3.38	3.16	2.99	2.86	2.76	2.67
55	7.12	5.01	4.16	3.68	3.37	3.15	2.98	2.85	2.75	2.66
56	7.11	5.01	4.15	3.67	3.36	3.14	2.98	2.85	2.74	2.66
57	7.10	5.00	4.15	3.67	3.36	3.14	2.97	2.84	2.74	2.65
58	7.09	4.99	4.14	3.66	3.35	3.13	2.97	2.84	2.73	2.64
59	7.09	4.98	4.13	3.66	3.35	3.12	2.96	2.83	2.72	2.64
60	7.08	4.98	4.13	3.65	3.34	3.12	2.95	2.82	2.72	2.63
61	7.07	4.97	4.12	3.64	3.33	3.11	2.95	2.82	2.71	2.63
62	7.06	4.97	4.11	3.64	3.33	3.11	2.94	2.81	2.71	2.62
63	7.06	4.96	4.11	3.63	3.32	3.10	2.94	2.81	2.70	2.62
64	7.05	4.95	4.10	3.63	3.32	3.10	2.93	2.80	2.70	2.61
65	7.04	4.95	4.10	3.62	3.31	3.09	2.93	2.80	2.69	2.61
66	7.04	4.94	4.09	3.62	3.31	3.09	2.92	2.79	2.69	2.60
67	7.03	4.94	4.09	3.61	3.30	3.08	2.92	2.79	2.68	2.60
68	7.02	4.93	4.08	3.61	3.30	3.08	2.91	2.79	2.68	2.59
69	7.02	4.93	4.08	3.60	3.30	3.08	2.91	2.78	2.68	2.59

***Table* 12.4 contd....**

d.f	1	2	3	4	5	6	7	8	9	10
70	7.01	4.92	4.07	3.60	3.29	3.07	2.91	2.78	2.67	2.59
71	7.01	4.92	4.07	3.60	3.29	3.07	2.90	2.77	2.67	2.58
72	7.00	4.91	4.07	3.59	3.28	3.06	2.90	2.77	2.66	2.58
73	7.00	4.91	4.06	3.59	3.28	3.06	2.90	2.77	2.66	2.57
74	6.99	4.90	4.06	3.58	3.28	3.06	2.89	2.76	2.66	2.57
75	6.99	4.90	4.05	3.58	3.27	3.05	2.89	2.76	2.65	2.57
76	6.98	4.90	4.05	3.58	3.27	3.05	2.88	2.76	2.65	2.56
77	6.98	4.89	4.05	3.57	3.27	3.05	2.88	2.75	2.65	2.56
78	6.97	4.89	4.04	3.57	3.26	3.04	2.88	2.75	2.64	2.56
79	6.97	4.88	4.04	3.57	3.26	3.04	2.87	2.75	2.64	2.55
80	6.96	4.88	4.04	3.56	3.26	3.04	2.87	2.74	2.64	2.55
81	6.96	4.88	4.03	3.56	3.25	3.03	2.87	2.74	2.63	2.55
82	6.95	4.87	4.03	3.56	3.25	3.03	2.87	2.74	2.63	2.55
83	6.95	4.87	4.03	3.55	3.25	3.03	2.86	2.73	2.63	2.54
84	6.95	4.87	4.02	3.55	3.24	3.03	2.86	2.73	2.63	2.54
85	6.94	4.86	4.02	3.55	3.24	3.02	2.86	2.73	2.62	2.54
86	6.94	4.86	4.02	3.55	3.24	3.02	2.85	2.73	2.62	2.53
87	6.94	4.86	4.02	3.54	3.24	3.02	2.85	2.72	2.62	2.53
88	6.93	4.86	4.01	3.54	3.23	3.01	2.85	2.72	2.62	2.53
89	6.93	4.85	4.01	3.54	3.23	3.01	2.85	2.72	2.61	2.53
90	6.93	4.85	4.01	3.54	3.23	3.01	2.85	2.72	2.61	2.52
91	6.92	4.85	4.00	3.53	3.23	3.01	2.84	2.71	2.61	2.52
92	6.92	4.84	4.00	3.53	3.22	3.00	2.84	2.71	2.61	2.52
93	6.92	4.84	4.00	3.53	3.22	3.00	2.84	2.71	2.60	2.52
94	6.91	4.84	4.00	3.53	3.22	3.00	2.84	2.71	2.60	2.52
95	6.91	4.84	4.00	3.52	3.22	3.00	2.83	2.70	2.60	2.51
96	6.91	4.83	3.99	3.52	3.21	3.00	2.83	2.70	2.60	2.51
97	6.90	4.83	3.99	3.52	3.21	2.99	2.83	2.70	2.60	2.51
98	6.90	4.83	3.99	3.52	3.21	2.99	2.83	2.70	2.59	2.51
99	6.90	4.83	3.99	3.52	3.21	2.99	2.83	2.70	2.59	2.51
100	6.90	4.82	3.98	3.51	3.21	2.99	2.82	2.69	2.59	2.50

Rejection of Data

Two statistical procedures are used to eliminate bad data from a sample. When a data is collected some error or mistake may take place and a data may be outside the expected range of other data.

Before eliminating an unwanted data, the following points are to be considered:

- If there was some clearly identifiable measurement problem, the *outlier* data should be eliminated. For example, the speed of a vehicle is being recorded using a radar gun and the battery charge is low, all values measured using the low battery should be eliminated *even if the measurements seem to be normal.*

Sometimes the *outlier* data points are practically desired. For example, the temperatures in an engine exhaust are being measured and suddenly it rises. Should the reading be eliminated because it is 'out of normal values'? Hence, before elimination of a data the situation or case is to be examined thoroughly.

There are many different outlier-elimination algorithms, and each has its own advantages and disadvantages. Two methods commonly used are Chauvenet's Criterion, and the Thonpson-τ (Thompson's-tau) Method.

Chauvenet's Criterion

Chauvenet's criterion is a method that has gained relatively wide acceptance. According to this criterion the mean value and all points inside a range should be retained. The range is calculated by the values that correspond to a probability of $(1 - \frac{1}{2n})$, where n is the sample size.

The mean and standard deviation of the sample are calculated, x□ and S. then the standardized deviation from the mean for all data values is calculated as;

$$\tau_i = \frac{|x_i - \bar{x}|}{S}$$

Finally, the standardized deviations are compared with tabulated values of Chauvenet's criterion values. Chauvenet's criterion values can be calculated using the following Matlab function. The Matlab function "norminv" is one-sided, the probability of being *less than* $(1 - \frac{1}{4n})$, rather than the probability of being *within* $(1 - \frac{1}{2n})$.

Note: Chauvenet's criterion uses the normal distribution probability values, even for small sample sizes.

Values of Maximum Permissible Ratio of Deviation to Standard Deviation for Chauvenet's Criterion are:

n	τ	n	τ	n	τ	n	τ	n	τ	n	τ
3	1.383	11	2.000	20	2.241	28	2.369	36	2.460	50	2.576
4	1.534	12	2.037	21	2.260	29	2.382	37	2.470	100	2.807
5	1.645	13	2.070	22	2.278	30	2.394	38	2.479	500	3.291
6	1.732	14	2.100	23	2.295	31	2.406	39	2.489	1000	3.481
7	1.803	15	2.128	24	2.311	32	2.418	40	2.498		
8	1.863	16	2.154	25	2.326	33	2.429				
9	1.915	17	2.178	26	2.341	34	2.440				
10	1.960	18	2.200	27	2.355	35	2.450				

Example

While a vehicle was traveling at an essentially constant speed a radar gun was used to measure the following speeds (mph):

58, 60, 61, 62, 61, 57, 63, 62, 61, 58, 61, 60, 60, 50, 53, 64, 61, 55, 55, 56, 61, 58, 67, 47, 62, 68, 57, 63, 72, 58

Using the Chauvenet's criterion, should you reject any measurements from your analysis? If so, which ones?

Solution

There are 30 samples, so the Chauvenet's criterion value is 2.394. The sample mean and standard deviation are

$\bar{x}$ = 59.7 mph

S = 4.998 mph

The following tables shows the measurements, their individual standardized deviations from the mean calculated from $\tau_i = \frac{|x_i - \bar{x}|}{S}$ and an indication of whether this value is greater than Chauvenet's criterion value or not.

Recorded Speed (mph)	Individual Standard Deviations of the Mean $\tau_i = \frac{\lvert x_i - \bar{x} \rvert}{S}$ (mph)	Decision	Recorded Speed (mph	Individual Standard Deviations of the Mean $\tau_i = \frac{\lvert x_i - \bar{x} \rvert}{S}$ (mph)	Decision
58	0.340	Retain	64	0.860	Retain
60	0.060	Retain	61	1.941	Retain
61	0.260	Retain	55	0.940	Retain
62	0.460	Retain	55	0.940	Retain
61	0.260	Retain	56	0.740	Retain
57	0.540	Retain	61	0.260	Retain
63	0.660	Retain	58	0.340	Retain
62	0.460	Retain	67	1.461	Retain
61	0.260	Retain	47	2.541	Eliminate
58	0.340	Retain	62	0.460	Retain
61	0.260	Retain	68	1.661	Retain
60	0.060	Retain	57	0.540	Retain
60	0.060	Retain	63	0.660	Retain
50	1.941	Retain	72	2.461	Eliminate
53	1.341	Retain	58	0.340	Retain

The final data set has 28 samples with: $\bar{x}$ = 59.714 mph; S = 3.905 mph

Thompson-τ Method

The *modified Thompson's-τ* (tau) *technique* is another elimination method that is recommended in *Measurement Uncertainty*.

The mean and standard deviation of the sample, $\bar{x}$ and S are calculated first. The largest or smallest data values (it must be either the first or last data point when the samples are placed in increasing order) are eliminated. For each point the standardized deviation is calculated and which lowest or highest point is the bigger outlier is determined. The standardized deviation for each point is calculated as:

$$\tau_i = \frac{\delta_i}{S} = \frac{\lvert x_i - \bar{x} \rvert}{S}$$

Finally, the largest standardized deviation is compared with tabulated values of Thompson's-τ. If the standardized deviation is larger than Thompson's-τ the associated data point is considered as an outlier and is eliminated from the data set.

The entire process is then repeated on the reduced data set, and is continued until no more values are eliminated.

Note: *At a time only a single data point is eliminated, even if several data points have standardized deviations greater than Thompson's-τ and the entire process is then repeat.*

The values for Thompson's- τ are calculated using following equation,

$$\text{Thompson's-}\tau = \frac{t_{\alpha,n-2}\,(n-1)}{\sqrt{n}\sqrt{n-2+(t_{\alpha,n-2})^2}}$$

where $t\alpha,(n-2)$ is the Student-t statistic at α level of significance and $(n\text{-}2)$ degrees of freedom.

Selected values of Thompson's-τ for 5% significance are shown in the following table. The Thompson's-τ value depends on the number of samples, *n*, in the data set. As you eliminate bad data points, the sample size will reduce by one each time.

Values of Thompson's τ at 5% significance

n	τ	n	τ	n	τ	n	τ	n	τ
3	1.151	11	1.815	19	1.881	27	1.906	35	1.919
4	1.425	12	1.829	20	1.885	28	1.908	36	1.920
5	1.571	13	1.840	21	1.889	29	1.910	37	1.921
6	1.656	14	1.850	22	1.893	30	1.911	38	1.922
7	1.711	15	1.858	23	1.896	31	1.913	39	1.923
8	1.749	16	1.865	24	1.899	32	1.915	40	1.924
9	1.777	17	1.871	25	1.901	33	1.916		
10	1.798	18	1.876	26	1.904	34	1.917		

Example

While a vehicle was traveling at an essentially constant speed and a radar gun was used to measure the speeds (mph) as shown below:

58, 60, 61, 62, 61, 57, 63, 62, 61, 58, 61, 60, 60, 50, 53, 64, 61, 55, 55, 56, 61, 58, 67, 47, 62, 68, 57, 63, 72, 58

Can any measurements be rejected from the analysis by using the Thompson-τ method? If so, which ones?

Solution

Step I: (30 samples)

$\bar{x} = 59.7$ mph,

$S = 4.998$ mph,

$\tau_{30} = 1.911$

Min. data value is 47, gives $\tau_{MIN} = \frac{|x_i - \bar{x}|}{S} = 2.541$

Max. data value is 72, gives $\tau_{MAX} = \frac{|x_i - \bar{x}|}{S} = 2.461$

Min. standardized deviation is larger, and 2.541>1.911, so eliminate 47 mph.

Step II: (29 samples)

$\bar{x} = 60.138$ mph,

$S = 4.462$ mph,

$\tau_{29} = 1.910$

Min. data value is 50, gives $\tau_{MIN} = \frac{|x_i - \bar{x}|}{S} = 2.272$

Max. data value is 72, gives $\tau_{MAX} = \frac{|x_i - \bar{x}|}{S} = 2.659$

Max. standardized deviation is larger, and 2.659 >1.910, so eliminate 72 mph.

Step III: (28 samples)

$\bar{x} = 59.714$ mph,

$S = 3.905$ mph,

$\tau_{28} = 1.908$

Min. data value is 50, gives $\tau_{MIN} = \frac{|x_i - \bar{x}|}{S} = 2.488$

Max. data value is 68, gives $\tau_{MAX} = \frac{|x_i - \bar{x}|}{S} = 2.122$

Min. standardized deviation is larger, and 2.488>1.908, so eliminate 50 mph.

Step IV: (27 samples)

$\bar{x}$ = 60.074 mph

S = 3.474 mph

τ_{27} = 1.906

Min. data value is 53, gives $\tau_{MIN} = \dfrac{|x_i - \bar{x}|}{S} = 2.036$

Max. data value is 68, gives $\tau_{MAX} = \dfrac{|x_i - \bar{x}|}{S} = 2.281$

Max. standardized deviation is larger, and 2.281>1.906, so eliminate 68 mph.

Step V: (26 samples)

$\bar{x}$ = 59.769 mph

S = 3.154 mph

τ_{26} = 1.904

Min. data value is 53, gives $\tau_{MIN} = \dfrac{|x_i - \bar{x}|}{S} = 2.147$

Max. data value is 67, gives $\tau_{MAX} = \dfrac{|x_i - \bar{x}|}{S} = 2.293$

Max. standardized deviation is larger, and 2.293>1.904, so eliminate 67 mph.

Step VI: (25 samples)

$\bar{x}$ = 59.48 mph

S = 2.845 mph

τ_{25} = 1.901

Min. data value is 53, gives $\tau_{MIN} = \dfrac{|x_i - \bar{x}|}{S} = 2.278$

Max. data value is 64, gives $\tau_{MAX} = \dfrac{|x_i - \bar{x}|}{S} = 1.589$

Min. standardized deviation is larger, and 2.278>1.901, so eliminate 53 mph.

Step VII: (24 samples)

$$\bar{x} = 59.75 \text{ mph}$$

$$S = 2.558 \text{ mph}$$

$$\tau_{24} = 1.899$$

Min. data value is 55, gives $\tau_{MIN} = \dfrac{|x_i - \bar{x}|}{S} = 1.857$

Max. data value is 64, gives $\tau_{MAX} = \dfrac{|x_i - \bar{x}|}{S} = 1.661$

Neither standardized deviation is larger than 1.899, so we are done and the final data set has 24 samples with:

$$\bar{x} = 59.75 \text{ mph}$$

$$S = 2.558 \text{ mph}$$

Exercise

1. The marks secured in mathematics by 10 students of B. Pharm, 3rd semester are; 40, 25, 5, 20, 42, 10, 48, 70, and 80 out of 100.

   Calculate the standard deviation.

   Ans: s = 23.07

2. Calculate the variance, standard deviation and the coefficient of variation. The variables (x) are; 32, 35, 40, 33, 35, 42, 37, 40, 41, 42

   Ans: s^2 = 14.23, s = 3.77, C.V. (%) = 10

3. Pulse rate of ten persons have been measured and are 63, 67, 63, 66, 70, 68, 71, 69, 71, 71 per min. Calculate the variance, standard deviation and the coefficient of variation.

   Ans: s^2 = 11.56, s = 3.40, C.V.(%) = 5.7

4. The marks obtained by the students of B. Pharm, 7th semester have been classified and given below:

Classes	51-55	56-60	61-65	66-70	71-75	76-80	81-85
Frequency	4	6	8	10	7	5	2

   Calculate the variance, standard deviation and the coefficient of variation.

   Ans: s^2 = 66.11, s = 8.13, C.V.(%) = 12.15

5. The data collected have been tabulated below in ascending order. Calculate the Pearson's coefficient of skewness

x	12.5	17.5	22.5	27.5	32.5	37.5	42.5	47.5	52.5
y	28	42	54	108	129	61	45	32	25

Ans: $\bar{x}$ = 28.59, Mode = 27.5, s = 8.63,

Coefficient of skewness = +0.13

6. A student appears B. Pharm final examination. If the probability of passing Biopharmaceutics is ¾ and probability of passing Pharmaceutics 2/3 and the probability of passing at least one subject is 2/4; what would be the probability of passing both the subjects?

Ans: 11/12

7. There are 5 red, 3 yellow, and 4 white pills in a bag. What would be the probability of getting a red or white pill on a random single draw?

Ans: 9/12 or 75%

8. In a survey it is found that 20% of the employees working in a corporate office suffer from hypertension. What would be the probability that out of six employees, four or more will suffer from hypertension?

Ans: p = 0.0169

9. There are 100 mistakes in a book of 100 pages. What would be the probability that a page of the book randomly selected will contain at least two mistakes? Assume Poisson distribution.

Ans: 0.264

10. Find out whether there is any significant correlation between the height and weight tabulated below in increasing order.

Height (inches)	55	57	57	58	59	62	63	64	65
Weight (lbs)	111	112	113	116	117	126	126	130	129

Ans: r = 0.98

11. A study was conducted to find out the relationship between rainfall (x) and yield of almond (y). The data collected have been put in

table below. Find out the regression line y on x from the data presented.

Rainfall (x inches)	1	2	3	4	5	5	6	7	8	9
Yield (y ton)	1	3	2	5	5	4	7	6	9	8

Ans: $y = 0.67x + 0.67$

12. Relationship between temperature (°C) and germination time (hr) has been investigated and the results are presented in the table below. Calculate the coefficient correlation.

Temperature (°C)	57	42	40	38	42	42	45	44	40	46	44	43
Germination time (hr)	10	26	30	41	29	27	27	19	18	19	31	29

Ans: r = – 0.73

13. Two samples are drawn randomly from the normal population. Analyze the data of the two samples using t-test and compare the means of the two samples.

Sample I	16	18	19	20	22	23	24	25	26	27
Sample II	33	38	43	27	34	32	28	41	42	35

Ans: t = 6.24

14. The temperatures at two districts' towns were measured during September to June of a year and put in the table below. Find out whether there is any significant difference in the temperatures at two towns. Consider that the samples are independent.

	Sept	Oct	Nov	Dec	Jan	Feb	Mar	Apr	May	June
Town A	40	30	34	39	43	25	49	40	55	45
Town B	39	28	34	35	41	23	45	37	55	43

Ans: t = 0.50

15. For a certain stimulus caused some changes in the blood pressure of twelve persons. The changes in blood pressure are given below;

    5, 2, 8, -1, 3, 0, -2, 1, 5, 0, 4, 6

    Would the stimulus in general be accompanied by an increase in blood pressure?

Ans: t = 2.30

16. Blood group of 100 persons has been determined. The expected and observed frequencies are tabulated below. Find out the value of χ^2 and interpret the result.

	A	B	AB	O
fo	42	9	3	46
fe	23	35	5	37

Ans: χ^2 = 38.00

17. A survey was conducted on 320 families, each has 5 children. The distribution of children is given below.

No. of boys	5	4	3	2	1	0
No. of girls	0	1	2	3	4	5
No. of families	14	56	110	88	40	12

The male and female births are equally probable. Is the result consistent with the hypothesis?

[*Hint*: The data are consistent with the binomial law of equal probability for the male and female births; i.e., p = q = ½. Thus, the binomial distribution is a good fit to the given data.]

Ans: χ^2 = 7.16

18. Treatment of 200 patients suffering from a disease is given below. State whether the new treatment is comparatively superior to the conventional treatment

	Favorable	**Not favorable**	**Total**
New	60	30	90
Conventional	40	70	110
Total	100	100	200

Ans: χ^2 = 18.18

19. In a particular area the numbers of male and female in two age groups were collected. The data obtained is presented below. Examine whether the null hypothesis is correct or not. The null hypothesis is "the male and female populations are independent".

Age group (yr)	**Male**	**Female**
60 – 65	40	48
70 – 75	45	60

Ans: χ^2 = 0.131, Null hypothesis is accepted.

20. In a dissolution test the average amount of drug released from a set of 6 tablets with respect to time have been determined and recorded as shown below: calculate the correlation coefficient.

Drug released (mg) x	0	69.3	117.5	148.1	233.9	246.2	248.8	250
Time (min) y	0	5	10	20	30	40	50	60

Ans: r = 0.915

13

DISSOLUTION TESTS

Solid dosage forms can be divided, with respect to the dissolution test, into the following groups:

1. Solid dosage forms with conventional (unmodified) release of API,
2. Solid dosage forms with prolonged release of API and
3. Solid dosage forms with retarded release of API.

The individual dosage form differs in the dissolution test performance with the change of dissolution medium. The dosage forms must fulfill only one requirement that is to release the minimal specified amount of API in the specified period of time. The calculations involved in dissolution tests include;

- Dissolution rate, the amount of drug released in unit time, total amount released.
- Cumulative dissolution, total amount of drug released during a specified time.
- Drug release characteristics,

Preparation of Standard Calibration Curve

In general before conducting dissolution rate test the standard calibration curve is constructed for ease of calculation. Use of calibration curve for subsequent calculation may appear as a source of error, unless all the glass wares and apparatus used certified and calibrated. However, it is necessary to construct calibration curve using different dissolution medium. Because, dissolution rate test is conducted using various medium of different pH.

Example

The absorbances of five diluted solution of metronidazole in 0.1N Hydrochloric acid solution are given in the table. Calculate their concentrations and construct the standard calibration curve.

Sl. No.	Absorbance
1	0.170
2	0.201
3	0.340
4	0.511
5	0.830

Dilution

- 100mg of a drug dissolved in minimum amount of methanol is diluted to 100ml of with 0.1N HCl solution (stock solution) in a 100ml volumetric flask.
- Pipette out 10ml of the stock solution and dilute to 100ml in a 100ml volumetric flask with 0.1N HCl solution.
- Pipette out 0.20 ml, 0.40ml, 0.60ml, 0.80ml and 1.00ml of the diluted solution, transfer into 10ml volumetric flask, and make up the volume with 0.1N HCl solution, measure the absorbance of each solution at 277mμ.

Solution

(a) Calculation of concentration (μg/ml)

(i) $$\frac{100\text{mg}}{100\text{ml}} \times \frac{10\text{ml}}{100\text{ml}} \times \frac{0.20\text{ml}}{10\text{ml}} = 0.002\text{mg/ml} = 0.002 \times 1000\mu\text{g/ml}$$

$$= 2\ \mu\text{g/ml}$$

(ii) $$\frac{100\text{mg}}{100\text{ml}} \times \frac{10\text{ml}}{100\text{ml}} \times \frac{0.40\text{ml}}{10\text{ml}} = 0.004\text{mg/ml} = 0.004 \times 1000\mu\text{g/ml}$$

$$= 4\ \mu\text{g/ml}$$

(iii) $$\frac{100\text{mg}}{100\text{ml}} \times \frac{10\text{ml}}{100\text{ml}} \times \frac{0.60\text{ml}}{10\text{ml}} = 0.006\text{mg/ml} = 0.006 \times 1000\mu\text{g/ml}$$

$$= 6\ \mu\text{g/ml}$$

(iv) $$\frac{100\text{mg}}{100\text{ml}} \times \frac{10\text{ml}}{100\text{ml}} \times \frac{0.80\text{ml}}{10\text{ml}} = 0.008\text{mg/ml} = 0.008 \times 1000\mu\text{g/ml}$$

$$= 8\ \mu\text{g/ml}$$

(v) $\frac{100\text{mg}}{100\text{ml}} \times \frac{10\text{ml}}{100\text{ml}} \times \frac{1.00}{10\text{ml}} = 0.01\text{mg/ml} = 0.01 \times 1000\mu\text{g/ml}$

$$= 10\ \mu\text{g/ml}$$

Sl. No.	Concentration (μg/ml)	Absorbance
1	2	0.170
2	4	0.201
3	6	0.340
4	8	0.511
5	10	0.830

(b) Construction of standard calibration curve

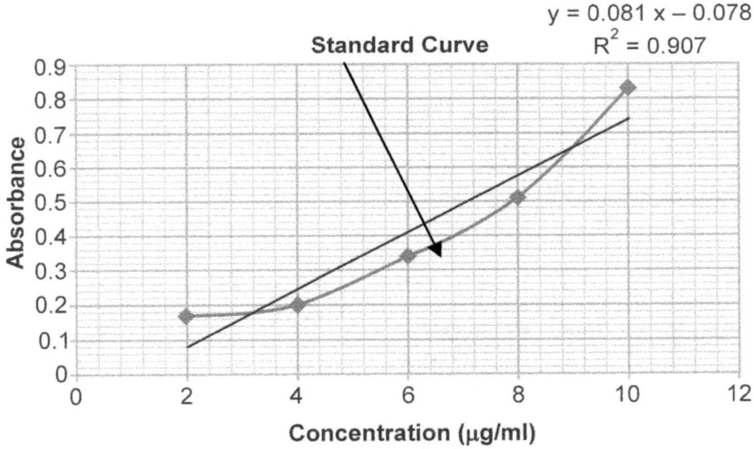

Example

During construction of standard calibration curve the experiment was repeated thrice, the data is shown in the table below. Calculate the standard deviation and construct standard calibration curve.

Sl. No.	Concentration (μg/ml)	Absorbance Set I	Absorbance Set II	Absorbance Set III
1	2	0.175	0.170	0.167
2	4	0.211	0.194	0.205
3	6	0.343	0.347	0.340
4	8	0.503	0.511	0.521
5	10	0.824	0.835	0.830

Solution

Equation for standard deviation,

$s = \sqrt{\frac{\Sigma(x-\bar{x})^2}{n-1}}$ [s = standard deviation, x = each value in the sample,

$\bar{x}$ = mean of x values, n = sample size(nos. of values]

The data given in the table are rearranged as;

Sl. No.	Conc. (µg/ml)	Absorbance Set I (*x*1)	Absorbance Set II (*x*2)	Absorbance Set III (*x*3)	Mean value *x*□
1	2	0.175	0.170	0.167	0.1707
2	4	0.211	0.194	0.205	0.2033
3	6	0.343	0.347	0.340	0.3433
4	8	0.503	0.511	0.521	0.5117
5	10	0.824	0.835	0.830	0.8297

Calculation: $s = \sqrt{\frac{\Sigma(x-\bar{x})^2}{n-1}}$

x	$\bar{x}$	$x-\bar{x}$	$(x-\bar{x})^2$	$\sum(x-\bar{x})^2$	$s = \sqrt{\frac{\Sigma(x-\bar{x})^2}{n-1}}$
0.175 0.170 0.167	0.1707 0.1707 0.1707	0.0043 – 0.0007 – 0.0037	0.0000185 0.00000049 0.0000137	0.00005599	$\sqrt{\frac{0.00005599}{5-1}}$ = **0.00374**
0.211 0.194 0.205	0.2033 0.2033 0.2033	0.0077 – 0.0093 0.0017	0.0000593 0.0000865 0.00000289	0.000149	$\sqrt{\frac{0.000148}{5-1}}$ = **0.00609**
0.343 0.347 0.340	0.3433 0.3433 0.3433	– 0.0003 0.0037 – 0.0033	0.00000009 0.0000137 0.0000109	0.0000247	$\sqrt{\frac{0.0000247}{5-1}}$ = **0.00248**
0.503 0.511 0.521	0.5117 0.5117 0.5117	– 0.0087 – 0.0007 0.0093	0.0000757 0.00000049 0.0000865	0.000163	$\sqrt{\frac{0.000163}{5-1}}$ = **0.00638**
0.824 0.835 0.830	0.8297 0.8297 0.8297	– 0.0057 0.0053 0.0003	0.0000325 0.0000281 0.00000009	0.0000607	$\sqrt{\frac{0.0000607}{5-1}}$ = **0.00389**

Plotting of graph using mean values

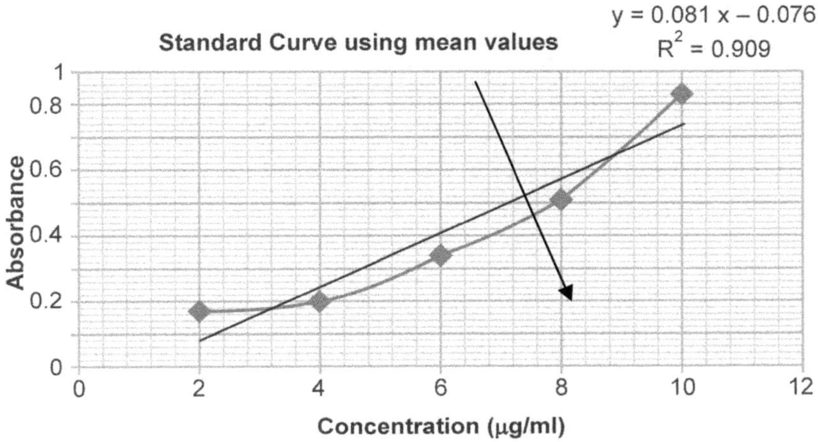

Example

Using the given absorbance data construct standard regressed calibration curve of the drug dissolved in 0.1N Hydrochloric acid.

Sl. No.	Concentration (µg/ml) (x)	Absorbance (y)
1	2	0.055
2	4	0.074
3	6	0.182
4	8	0.313
5	10	0.582

Solution

Equation for regressed curve

$$y = \mathrm{b}\,x + a$$

Where b, the slope = $\dfrac{n\sum xy - \sum x \times \sum y}{n\sum x^2 - (\sum x)^2}$ and

$$a = \bar{y} - \mathrm{b}\bar{x}$$

Sl. No.	x	y	x^2	y^2	xy
1	2	0.055	4	0.0030	0.11
2	4	0.074	16	0.0055	0.296
3	6	0.182	36	0.0331	1.092
4	8	0.313	64	0.0978	2.504
5	10	0.582	100	0.3387	5.82
n = 5	$\sum x = 30$	$\sum y = 1.206$	$\sum x^2 = 220$	$\sum y^2 = 0.4772$	$\sum xy = 9.822$

$$\bar{x} = \frac{30}{5} = 6 \quad \text{and} \quad \bar{y} = \frac{1.206}{5} = 0.2412$$

Equation for regressed curve

$$y = bx + a$$

b, the slope

$$\text{slope} = \frac{n\sum xy - \sum x \times \sum y}{n\sum x^2 - (\sum x)^2} = \frac{5\times9.822 - 30\times1.206}{5\times220 - (30)^2}$$

$$= \frac{49.11 - 36.18}{1100 - 900}$$

$$= \frac{12.93}{200} = 0.0646$$

$$a = \bar{y} - b\bar{x} = 0.2412 - 0.0646 \times 6 = 0.2412 - 0.3876$$

$$= -0.1464$$

Values for standard regressed curve are;

S. No.	*x*	*y*	b	*a*	*y'* = b *x* + *a*	|y' – y|
1	2	0.055	0.0646	– 0.1464	0.0646 × 2 – 0.1464 = – 0.0172	– 0.0722
2	4	0.074	0.0646	– 0.1464	0.0646 × 4 – 0.1464 = 0.1120	0.0380
3	6	0.182	0.0646	– 0.1464	0.0646 × 6 – 0.1464 = 0.2412	0.0592
4	8	0.313	0.0646	– 0.1464	0.0646 × 8 – 0.1464 = 0.3704	0.0574
5	10	0.582	0.0646	– 0.1464	0.0646 × 10 – 0.1464 = 0.4996	– 0.0824

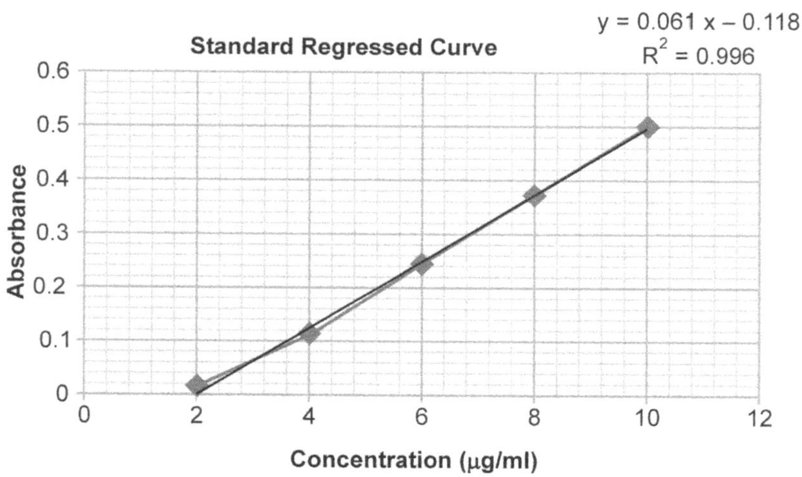

Example

The absorbances of five diluted solution of metronidazole in phosphate buffer solution (pH7.4) solution are given in the table. Calculate their concentrations and construct the standard calibration curve.

Sl. No.	Absorbance
1	0.087
2	0.185
3	0.382
4	0.579
5	0.800

Solution

Dilution

- 50mg of the drug dissolved in minimum amount of methanol is diluted to 50ml of with phosphate buffer solution of pH 7.4 (stock solution) in a 100 ml volumetric flask.
- Pipetted out 10ml of the stock solution and diluted to 100ml in a 100ml volumetric flask with 0.1N HCl solution.
- Pipetted out 1.00 ml, 2.50ml, 5.00ml, 7.50ml and 10.00ml of the diluted solution, transferred into 100ml volumetric flask, and made up the volume with PBS (pH 7.4), measured the absorbance of each solution at 277mμ.

Solution

(a) Calculation of concentration (μg/ml)

(i) $$\frac{50\text{mg}}{50\text{ml}} \times \frac{10\text{ml}}{100\text{ml}} \times \frac{1.00\text{ml}}{100\text{ml}} = 0.001\text{mg/ml} = 0.001 \times 1000\mu\text{g/ml}$$

$$= 1\ \mu\text{g/ml}$$

(ii) $$\frac{50\text{mg}}{50\text{ml}} \times \frac{10\text{ml}}{100\text{ml}} \times \frac{2.50\text{ml}}{100\text{ml}} = 0.0025\text{mg/ml} = 0.0025 \times 1000\mu\text{g/ml}$$

$$= 2.5\ \mu\text{g/ml}$$

(iii) $$\frac{50\text{mg}}{50\text{ml}} \times \frac{10\text{ml}}{100\text{ml}} \times \frac{5.00\text{ml}}{100\text{ml}} = 0.005\text{mg/ml} = 0.005 \times 1000\mu\text{g/ml}$$

$$= 5\ \mu\text{g/ml}$$

(iv) $\frac{50\text{mg}}{100\text{ml}} \times \frac{10\text{ml}}{100\text{ml}} \times \frac{7.50\text{ml}}{100\text{ml}} = 0.0075\text{mg/ml} = 0.0075 \times 1000\mu\text{g/ml}$

$= 7.5\ \mu\text{g/ml}$

(v) $\frac{50\text{mg}}{50\text{ml}} \times \frac{10\text{ml}}{100\text{ml}} \times \frac{10.00}{100\text{ml}} = 0.01\text{mg/ml} = 0.01 \times 1000\mu\text{g/ml}$

$= 10\ \mu\text{g/ml}$

Sl. No.	Concentration (μg/ml)	Absorbance
1	1.00	0.087
2	2.50	0.185
3	5.00	0.382
4	7.50	0.579
5	10.00	0.800

(b) Construction of standard calibration curve.

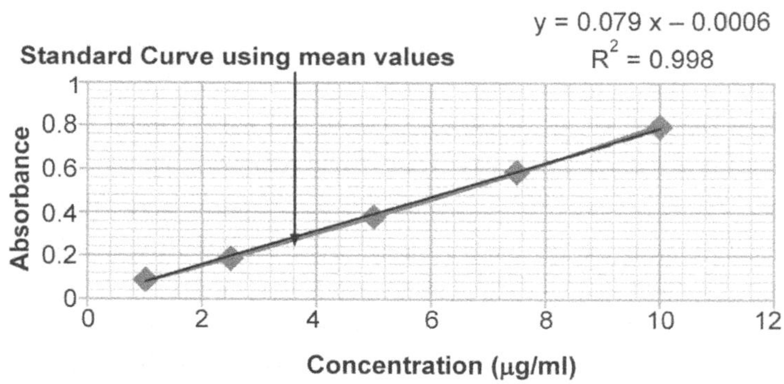

Example

The absorbances values of five diluted solutions of metronidazole in phosphate buffer solution (pH 7.4) solution are given in the table. The experiment has been conducted thrice. Calculate the standard deviation and construct the standard calibration curve.

Sl. No.	Absorbance (I)	Absorbance (II)	Absorbance (III)	Concentration (μg/ml)
1	0.083	0.087	0.080	1.00
2	0.185	0.182	0.186	2.50
3	0.380	0.382	0.382	5.00
4	0.575	0.580	0.580	7.50
5	0.800	0.795	0.800	10.00

Solution

Equation for standard deviation,

$$s = \sqrt{\frac{\Sigma\left(x-\bar{x}\right)^2}{n-1}}$$ [s = standard deviation, x = each value in the sample,

$\bar{x}$ = mean of x values, n = sample size (nos. of values]

The data given in the table are rearranged as;

Sl. No.	Conc. (μg/ml)	Absorbance Set I ($x1$)	Absorbance Set II ($x2$)	Absorbance Set III ($x3$)	Mean value $\bar{x}$
1	1.00	0.083	0.087	0.080	
2	2.50	0.185	0.182	0.186	
3	5.00	0.380	0.382	0.382	
4	7.50	0.575	0.580	0.580	
5	10.00	0.800	0.795	0.800	

Calculation: standard deviation, $s = \sqrt{\frac{\Sigma\left(x-\bar{x}\right)^2}{n-1}}$

x	$\bar{x}$	$x - \bar{x}$	$\left(x - \bar{x}\right)^2$	$\sum\left(x - \bar{x}\right)^2$	$s = \sqrt{\frac{\Sigma\left(x-\bar{x}\right)^2}{n-1}}$
0.083 0.087 0.080	0.0833	- 0.0003 0.0037 - 0.0033	0.00000009 0.00001369 0.00001369	0.00002747	$\sqrt{\frac{0.00002747}{5-1}}$ = 0.**00262**
0.185 0.182 0.186	0.1843	0.0007 - 0.0023 0.0017	0.00000049 0.00000529 0.00000289	0.00000867	$\sqrt{\frac{0.00000867}{5-1}}$ = **0.00147**
0.380 0.382 0.382	0.3813	- 0.0013 - 0.0007 - 0.0007	0.00000169 0.00000049 0.00000049	0.00000267	$\sqrt{\frac{0.00000267}{5-1}}$ = **0.00082**
0.575 0.580 0.580	0.5783	- 0.0033 0.0017 0.0017	0.0000109 0.00000289 0.00000289	0.0000167	$\sqrt{\frac{0.0000167}{5-1}}$ = **0.00204**
0.800 0.795 0.800	0.7983	0.0017 - 0.0033 0.0017	0.00000289 0.00001089 0.00000289	0.00001667	$\sqrt{\frac{0.00001667}{5-1}}$ = **0.00204**

Plotting of graph using mean values

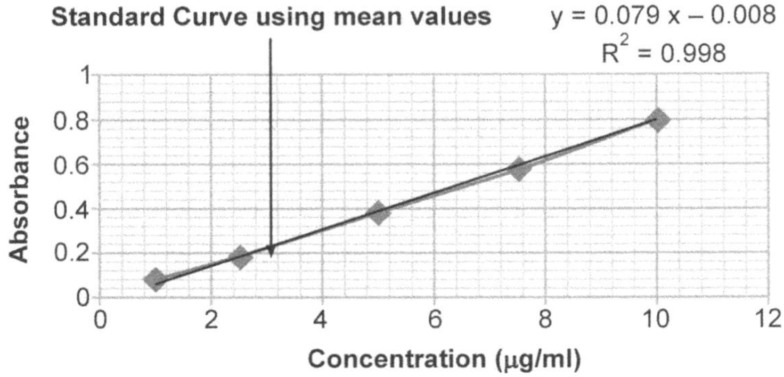

Dissolution rate

Various medium normally used to carry out the test are – 0.1N Hydrochloric acid, Phosphate buffer of pH 5.8, 7.2, etc., simulated gastric/intestinal fluid. Specific apparatus, called Dissolution test apparatus, is used to perform the test. The specifications for this apparatus and general method of test are mentioned in the Pharmacopoeias.

At different time intervals aliquot samples are drawn from the basket and the absorbance is measured to calculate the amount of drug present in the solution (amount released).

Example

In a dissolution test study on metronidazole tablet 100mg at pH 7.4 (PBS) the time schedule for withdrawals of sample and absorbance measured are given below. 1ml of sample was drawn from the basket (900ml), diluted to 10ml and measured the absorbance. Calculate cumulative amount released at different time interval and draw a graph to show the release pattern. Use the standard calibration curve shown in Example 6.

Sl. No	Time (min)	Abs. (y)
1	5	0.038
2	10	0.048
3	15	0.082
4	20	0.142

Contd...

Sl. No	Time (min)	Abs. (y)
5	25	0.171
6	30	0.237
7	35	0.243
8	40	0.285
9	45	0.301
10	50	0.405
11	55	0.465
12	60	0.590

Solution

Dilution of sample solution

Volume of diluted solution 10ml ≈ 1ml of sample drawn from 900ml.

Dilution factor = 10 × 900 = 9000

Concentration equivalent to absorbance was calculated from the standard calibration curve shown in Example 5;

The equation of the standard calibration curve is $y = 0.079x - 0.008$

(Where, y is absorbance and x is concentration, μg/ml)

or, $$x = \frac{y + 0.008}{0.079}$$

Amount of drug released from the tablet, a (μg) = Conc. (x) × Dilution factor (D.F.)

or, $$a\text{ (mg)} = \frac{\text{Conc.}(x)\times\text{Dilution factor (D.F.)}}{1000}$$

Here, the tablet strength is 100mg;

Hence, $\%\text{ release of drug} = \dfrac{\text{Amount of drug released} \times 100}{100}$

Sl. No	Time	Abs. (y)	Conc. ($x=\frac{y+0.008}{0.079}$)	Dilution factor	Amount of drug ($a=\frac{x\times DF}{1000}$)mg	% Cumulative Drug Release ($d=\frac{a\times 100}{\text{tablet strength}}$)
1	5 min	0.038	0.582μg/ml	9000	5.238mg	5.238
2	10 min	0.048	0.7088	9000	6.379	6.379
3	15 min	0.082	1.139	9000	10.25	10.25
4	20 min	0.142	1.898	9000	17.08	17.08
5	25 min	0.250	3.265	9000	29.38	29.38
6	30min	0.351	4.545	9000	40.91	40.91

Table contd...

Sl. No	Time	Abs. (y)	Conc. ($x=\frac{y+0.008}{0.079}$)	Dilution factor	Amount of drug ($a=\frac{x \times DF}{1000}$)mg	% Cumulative Drug Release ($d=\frac{a \times 100}{\text{tablet strength}}$)
7	35min	0.418	5.398	9000	48.59	48.59
8	40min	0.469	6.041	9000	54.37	54.37
9	45 min	0.520	6.687	9000	60.19	60.19
10	50min	0.563	7.226	9000	65.04	65.04
11	55min	0.605	7.764	9000	69.88	69.88
12	60 min	0.607	7.791	9000	70.12	70.12

Example

In a dissolution test on metronidazole tablet 200mg at pH 7.4 (PBS) the time schedule for withdrawals of sample and absorbance measured are given below. 1ml of sample was withdrawn from the basket (900ml), diluted to 10ml and measured the absorbance. Calculate the time taken for 60% and 90% release of the drug from the graph. Also show the pattern of drug release at different time intervals. Use the standard calibration curve shown in Example 6.

Sl. No	Time (min)	Abs. (y)
1	5	0.135
2	10	0.471
3	15	0.714
4	20	1.009
5	25	1.155
6	30	1.270
7	35	1.387
8	40	1.489
9	45	1.595
10	50	1.676
11	55	1.743
12	60	1.762

Solution

Dilution of sample solution

Volume of diluted solution 10ml $\approx$ 1ml of sample drawn from 900ml.

Dilution factor = $10 \times 900 = 9000$

Concentration equivalent to absorbance was calculated from the standard calibration curve shown in Example 6;

The equation of the standard calibration curve is; $y = 0.079x - 0.008$ (Where, y is absorbance and x is concentration, µg/ml) or, $$x = \frac{y + 0.008}{0.079}$$

Amount of drug released from the tablet, a (μg) = Conc. (x)×Dilution factor (D.F.)

or, $$a\ (\text{mg}) = \frac{\text{Conc.}(x)\times\text{Dilution factor (D.F.)}}{1000}$$

Here, the tablet strength is 200mg;

Hence, % release of drug = $\frac{\text{Amount of drug released} \times 100}{200}$

Sl. No	Time	Abs. (y)	Conc. ($x=\frac{y+0.008}{0.079}$)	Dilution factor	Amount of drug ($a=\frac{x\times DF}{1000}$)mg	% Cumulative Drug Release (d= $\frac{a\times 100}{\text{tablet strength}}$)
1	5 min	0.135	1.61μg/ml	9000	14.47mg	7.24
2	10 min	0.471	5.86	9000	52.78	26.39
3	15 min	0.714	8.94	9000	80.5	40.25
4	20 min	1.009	12.68	9000	114.16	57.08
5	25 min	1.155	14.53	9000	130.76	65.38
6	30min	1.270	15.98	9000	143.82	71.91
7	35min	1.387	17.46	9000	157.18	78.59
8	40min	1.489	18.75	9000	168.74	84.37
9	45 min	1.595	20.09	9000	180.38	90.19
10	50min	1.676	21.12	9000	190.08	95.04
11	55min	1.743	21.97	9000	197.76	98.88
12	60 min	1.762	22.20	9000	199.84	99.92

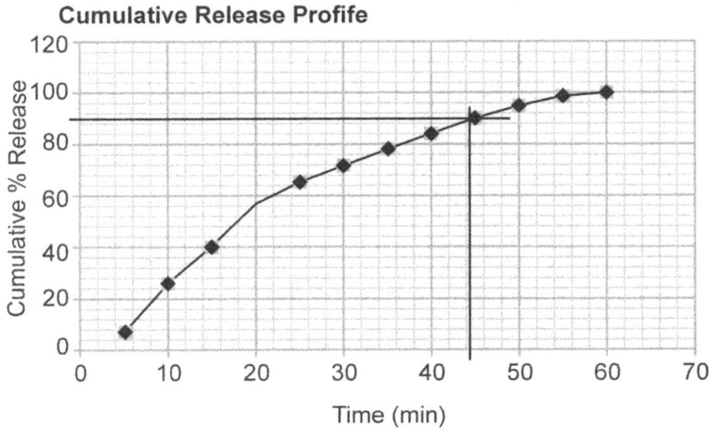

Time taken for release of 60% of the drug from the tablet, t_{60} is **21.8 min** and time taken for release of 90% of the drug from the tablet, t_{90} is **44.3 min** approximately.

Kinetics of Drug Release

Noyes-Whitney Rule

The rate of dissolution dM/dt is the amount dissolved per unit area per unit time, it can be expressed as;

$$dM/dt = KS\ (Cs - Ct)$$

Where K is a constant, M is the amount (mass) transferred with respect to time, t through dissolution, S is the solid (particle or tablet) surface area; Ct is the concentration at time, t and Cs is the equilibrium solubility of the solute at the experimental temperature. for most solids the rate of dissolution (dM/dt) can be expressed in units of $g/cm^2/sec$.

When Ct is less than 15% of the saturated solubility Cs, Ct has negligible influence on the dissolution rate. The dissolution of solid under such circumstance is said to occur under 'sink' condition. Usually the surface area, S is not constant except when (1) quantity of material present is more than the saturation solubility, (2) small amount of drug has dissolved (at initial stage of dissolution).

Nernst & Brunner Film Theory

Here the Fick's law of diffusion is used correlate the diffusion coefficient of the solute with the constant, K of the above Noyes-Whitney equation.

$$K = \frac{DS}{h\gamma}$$

Where D is the diffusion coefficient, S is the area of dissolving surface of the solid or area of the diffusion layer, γ is the volume of solution, and h is the thickness of the diffusion layer.

Assumption of Nernst & Brunner is that (1) the diffusion process at the surface is much faster than the transport process, and (2) a linear concentration gradient works at the layer of solution adhering to the solid surface.

As per Noyes-Whitney equation the *dissolution process follows first order reaction*.

Modeling of Release Kinetic

The release kinetics can be expressed in terms of three models;

- Statistical methods; e.g., exploratory data analysis method, repeated measures design, multivariate approach (MANOVA - multivariate analysis of variance)
- Model dependent method; e.g., zero order, first order, Higuchi, Korsmeyer-Peppas model, Hixson-Crowell, Baker-Lonsdale model, Weibull model, etc.
- Model independent methods; e.g., difference factor (f_1), similarity factor (f_2).

Zero-order model

Without disaggregation and slow release of drug from a dosage form is represented as;

$$Q_0 - Q_t = K_0t \quad \text{or, } Q_t = Q_0 + K_0t$$

Where Q_t is the amount of drug dissolved in time, t; Q_0 is the initial amount of drug in the solution (generally, $Q_0 = 0$) and K_0 is the zero order release constant (units of concentration/time).

In-vitro release kinetics can be determined by plotting the cumulative amount of drug released against time.

The dissolution of drug from various types of modified release dosage forms including some TDDS and matrix tablets containing drug with less solubility, osmotic systems.

Example

The results of dissolution test of a formulation are given below. Plot the graph and state at which order the drug is released.

Time(hr)	Cumulative drug release
0	0
0.5	17.567
1	23.224
2	32.226
3	43.922
4	51.558
5	66.545
6	73.556

Time(hr)	Cumulative drug release
7	82.667
8	86.607
9	90.184
10	96.511

Solution

The data given are plotted and the graph obtained is shown below,

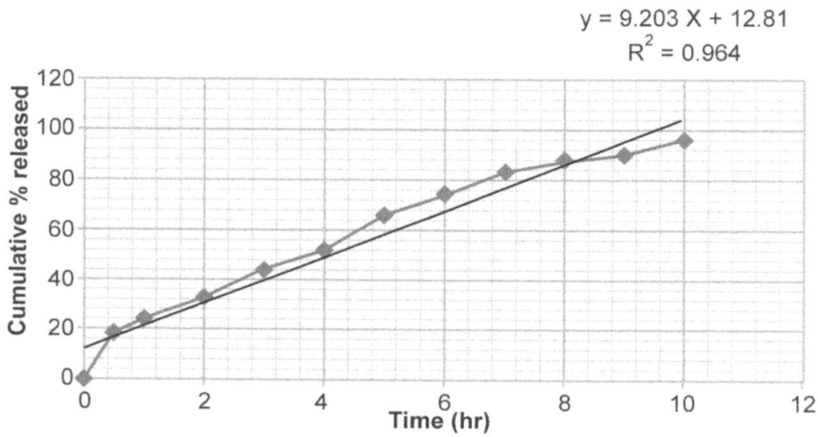

First Order Model

The release of the drug which followed first order kinetics can be expressed by the equation;

Or, $$\frac{dC}{dt} = -K \times c$$

log $$C = \log C_0 - Kt / 2.303$$

Where K is the first order rate constant, C_0 is the initial concentration of the drug, and t is the time.

The plot of log cumulative percent of drug remaining against time would be a straight line with a slope of – K/2.303.

Dosage forms containing water-soluble drugs in porous matrices would be suitable for this study.

Example

The results of dissolution test of a formulation are given below. Plot log cumulative percent of drug remaining against time and show whether the release follows first order.

Time(hr)	Cumulative drug release
0	0
0.5	17.567
1	23.224
2	32.226
3	43.922
4	51.558
5	66.545
6	73.556
7	82.667
8	86.607
9	90.184
10	96.511

Solution

According to first order release kinetics a plot of log cumulative percent of drug remaining against time is constructed. The cumulative amount remaining is calculated and shown in the table below.

Time(hr)	Cumulative % drug release	Cumulative %drug remaining	Log cum.% drug remaining
0	0	100	2
0.5	17.567	82.433	1.916101
1	23.224	76.776	1.885225
2	32.226	67.774	1.831063
3	43.922	56.078	1.748793
4	51.558	48.442	1.685222
5	66.545	33.455	1.524461
6	73.556	26.444	1.422327
7	82.667	17.333	1.238874
8	86.607	13.393	1.126878
9	90.184	9.816	0.991935
10	96.511	3.489	0.542701

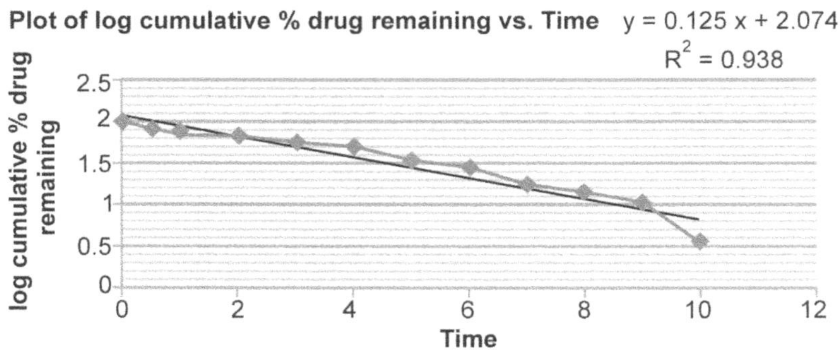

The R^2 value being 0.938, far away from 1.0 the release does not satisfactorily follow the first order kinetics.

Higuchi Model

Drug release from a matrix system can be expressed by Higuchi model. It is based on the following hypotheses;

- Initial drug concentration in the matrix is much higher than drug solubility;
- Drug diffusion takes place only in one dimension (edge effect must be negligible);
- Drug particles are much smaller than system thickness;
- Matrix swelling and dissolution are negligible;
- Drug diffusivity is constant; and
- Perfect sink conditions are always attained in the release environment.

The model equation given below is valid during all the time, except when there is total depletion of drug from the dosage form takes place.

$$f_t = Q = A\sqrt{D(2C - C_s)C_s t}$$

Where Q = the amount of drug released in time t per unit area A,

C = the drug initial concentration,

Cs = the drug solubility in the matrix media and D is the diffusivity of the drug molecules (diffusion coefficient) in the matrix substance.

When the dissolution takes place from a planar heterogeneous matrix system, where the drug concentration in the matrix is lower than its solubility and the release occurs through pores in the matrix, the equation used is;

$$f_t = Q = \sqrt{\frac{D\delta}{\tau}(2C - \delta C_s)C_s t}$$

Where D is the diffusion coefficient of the drug molecule in the solvent, δ is the porosity of the matrix, τ is the tortuisity (the dimensions of radius and branching of the pores and canals in the matrix) of the matrix and Q, A, Cs and t have the meaning explained earlier.

However, the Higuchi model can be simplified as;

$$f_t = Q = K_H\sqrt{t} = K_H \times t^{1/2}$$

Where, K_H is the Higuchi dissolution constant. *The dissolution rate is examined by plotting the cumulative percent drug release vs. square root of time.*

To describe the drug dissolution from several types of modified release pharmaceutical dosage forms including some transdermal systems and matrix tablets with water soluble drugs, this relationship can be used.

Example

The results of dissolution test of a formulation are given below. Plot the graph and state at which order the drug is released.

Time(hr)	Cumulative drug release
0	0
0.5	19.5
1	29.4
2	39.6
3	49.9
4	54.8
5	66.5
6	73.5
7	82.6
8	89.7
9	94.8
10	98.5

Solution

To examine whether the release kinetics fit Higuchi model or not, a plot of cumulative percent drug release vs. square root of time is to be drawn. If the R^2 value of the graph is nearest to 1.0, the release may be considered to fit Higuchi model.

Time(hr)	Square root of time	Cumulative % drug release
0	0	0
0.5	0.707107	19.5
1	1	29.4
2	1.414214	39.6
3	1.732051	49.9
4	2	54.8
5	2.236068	66.5
6	2.44949	73.5
7	2.645751	82.6
8	2.828427	89.7
9	3	94.8
10	3.162278	98.5

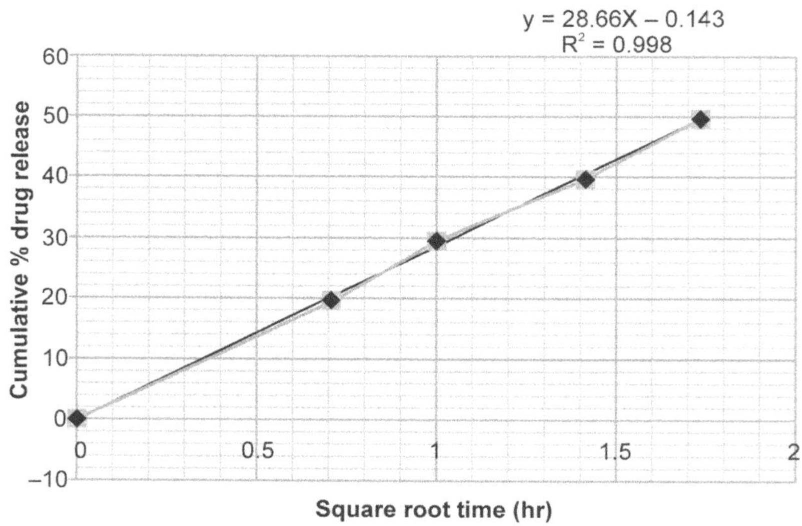

Since the value of R^2 is 0.998, nearest to 1.0, the release of drug follows Higuchi model.

Hixson-Crowell Model

Hixson and Crowell observed that the regular area of particles is proportional to the cube root of its volume. They derived an equation:

$$\kappa.t = \sqrt[3]{W_0} - \sqrt[3]{W_t} = W_0^{1/3} - W_t^{1/3}$$

Where W_0 is the initial amount of drug in the pharmaceutical dosage form, Wt is the amount of drug remaining in the pharmaceutical dosage form at time t and κ (kappa) is a constant incorporating the surface-volume relation. The equation describes the release from systems where there is a change in surface area and diameter of particles or tablets.

To determine the release kinetics, cube root of drug % remaining in matrix is to be plotted against time. This model is applicable to the dosage form such as tablets, where the dissolution occurs in planes parallel to the drug surface; if the tablet dimensions diminish proportionally, in such a manner that the initial geometrical form keeps constant all the time.

Example

The results of dissolution test of a formulation are given below. Plot the graph and state at which order the drug is released.

Time(hr)	Cumulative % drug release	Time(hr)	Cumulative % drug release
0	0	5	66.5
0.5	19.5	6	73.5
1	29.4	7	82.6
2	39.6	8	89.7
3	49.9	9	94.8
4	54.8	10	98.5

Solution

According to this model the release kinetics is to be evaluated by plotting cube root of cumulative % drug remaining against time. Hence, the required data is calculated and tabulated below for plotting the graph. If the R^2 value is 1 or approaching 1, the release kinetics would fit the Hixson and Crowell model.

Time (hr)	Cumulative % drug release	Cube root of Cumulative % drug remaining	Time (hr)	Cumulative % drug release	Cube root of Cumulative % drug remaining
0	0	4.641589	5	66.545	3.222209
0.5	17.567	4.352115	6	73.556	2.979264
1	23.224	4.250191	7	82.667	2.587962
2	32.226	4.077128	8	86.607	2.374794
3	43.922	3.827638	9	90.184	2.141139
4	51.558	3.645362	10	96.511	1.516702

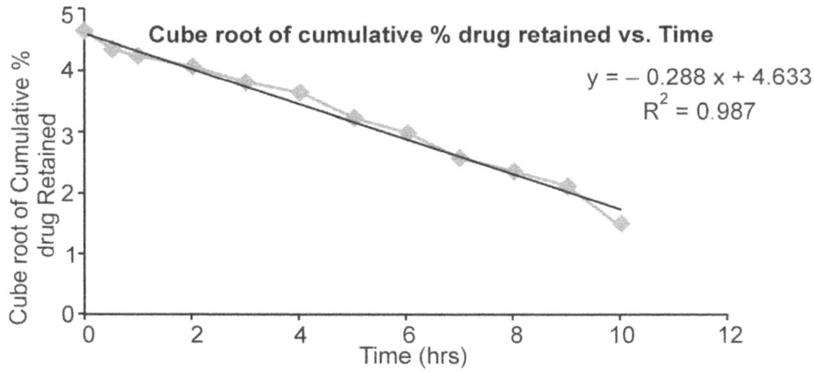

Since the R^2 value is 0.987, nearer to 1.0 the data fit the Hixson and Crowell model.

Korsmeyer-Peppas Model

This model is useful to describe drug release from a polymeric system equation. To find out the mechanism of drug release, first 60% drug release data were fitted in Korsmeyer-Peppas model.

$$\frac{M_t}{M_\infty} = kt^n$$

Where $\frac{M_t}{M_\infty}$ is the fraction of drug released at time t, k is the release rate constant and n is the release exponent. The n value characterizes different releases for cylindrical shaped matrices. In this model, the release mechanism of drug from polymeric film can be characterized by the value of n. For example,

- When the value of n = 0.5 and the rate of release is a function of time, $1/\sqrt{t}$ the release mechanism is the Fickian diffusion.

- When the value of n is within 0.45 to 0.89 (0.45 < n < 0.89), and the rate of release is a function of time, t^{n-1} it represents to a non-Fickian diffusion mechanism.
- When the value of n = 0.89, it shows Case II (relaxational) transport and the release follows zero-order kinetics.
- When the value of n is more than 0.89 and the rate of release is a function of time, t^{n-1} it indicates super case II transport.

The portion of the release curve, where Mt / M∞ < 0.6, is used to find out the exponent of n. *To determine the release kinetics, data obtained from in vitro drug release studies are to be plotted as log cumulative % drug release versus log time.*

Example

The results of dissolution test of a formulation are given below. Plot the graph and state at which order the drug is released.

Time(hr)	Cumulative % drug release	Time(hr)	Cumulative % drug release
0	0	5	66.545
0.5	17.567	6	73.556
1	23.224	7	82.667
2	32.226	8	86.607
3	43.922	9	90.184
4	51.558	10	96.511

Solution

According to this model the release kinetics is to be evaluated by plotting log of cumulative % drug release against log time. Hence, the required data is calculated and tabulated below for plotting the graph. If the R^2 value is 1 or approaching 1, the release kinetics would fit the Korsmeyer-Peppas model.

Time (hr)	log time	Cumulative % drug release	log of cumulative % drug release	Time (hr)	log time	Cumulative% drug release	log of Cumulative % drug release
0	0	∞	0	5	0.6989	73.5	1.823115
0.5	-0.3010	1.244698	1.4683	6	0.7781	82.6	1.866618
1	0	1.365937	1.5977	7	0.8451	89.7	1.917332
2	0.3010	1.508206	1.6981	8	0.9031	94.8	1.937553
3	0.4771	1.642682	1.7388	9	0.9542	98.5	1.955129
4	0.6020	1.712296	1.8228	10	1	99.7	1.984577

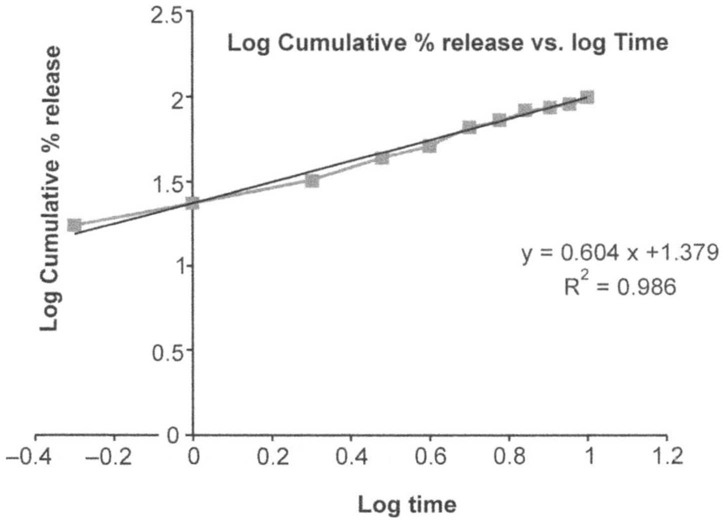

Since the R^2 value is 0.986, nearer to 1.0, it is expected to fit the Korsmeyer-Peppas model. The value of n being 0.604, (more than 0.45 but less than 0.89) the release of drug follows non-Fickian process.

Baker-Lonsdale Model

This model is derived from the Higuchi model and it describes the drug release from spherical matrices. The equation used is:

$$f_1 = \frac{3}{2}\left[1 - \left(1 - \frac{M_t}{M_\infty}\right)^{2/3}\right]\frac{M_t}{M_\infty} = k_t$$

Where k is the release rate constant and is the slope of the curve. *The in-vitro drug release kinetics can be determined by plotting* $d\left(\frac{M_t}{M_\infty}\right)/dt$ *against* $1/\sqrt{x}$. This equation is applicable for study of release kinetics from microcapsules and microspheres.

Weibull Model

This model is used to describe different dissolution processes with the help of the following equation:

$$M = M_0\left[1 - e^{-k(t-T)}\right]$$

Where M = the amount of drug dissolved as a function of time t,

M_0 = the total amount of drug released,

T = the lag time measured as a result of the dissolution process,

a is a scale parameter describing time dependence,

b = 1, and

k = $1/a$

The shape of the curve and value of b are closely related. When $b > 1$, curve is sigmoidal with a turning point; when $b = 1$, the curve is steeper; when $b < 1$, the curve is more steep than the previous case. The time required for dissolution of 50% and 90% of the drug from the formulation can be calculated by using the following equation;

$$t_{(50\% \text{ or } 90\% \text{ dissolved})} = \left(-a \times \ln \frac{M_0 - M}{M_0}\right)^{1/b} + T$$

This model is used to examine the release profile of matrix type of drug delivery systems.

Hopfenberg Model

This mathematical model is used to correlate the drug release through surface erosion till the surface area remains constant and to identify the mechanism of release from the optimized oily spheres using data derived from the composite profile, which essentially displayed site-specific biphasic release kinetics. The cumulative fraction of drug released from the polymer at time t can be described as:

$$\frac{M_t}{M_\infty} = 1 - \left(1 - \frac{k_0 t}{C_L a}\right)^n$$

Where, k_0 is the zero order rate constant (surface erosion process). C_L is the initial drug loaded throughout the system, a is the system's half thickness (i.e. the radius for a sphere or cylinder), and n is an exponent that varies with geometry n = 1, 2 and 3 for slab (flat), cylindrical and spherical geometry, respectively.

$$Y = \beta_0 + \beta_1 X_1 + \beta_2 X_2 + \ldots\ldots\ldots\ldots + \beta_n X_n$$

Gompertz Model

The *in-vitro* dissolution profile is usually expressed by a simple exponential model known as

Gompertz model:

$$X_{(t)} = X_{max} \exp [-\alpha e^{\beta \log t}]$$

Where $X_{(t)}$ = percent dissolved at time t divided by 100; X_{max} = maximum amount dissolved; α denotes the amount remains undissolved at time t = 1 and is considered as location or scale parameter; β = dissolution rate per unit of time and considered as shape parameter. This model has a steep increase in the beginning and then slowly covers to the asymptotic maximal dissolution. The model is useful for comparing the release profiles of drugs having good solubility and intermediate release rate.

Linear or First Order Regression Model

For determining the parameters of a linear system linear regression method is used. The empirical model that correlates the response variable to the independent variables is expressed by the following equation:

$$Y = \beta_0 + \beta_1 X_1 + \beta_2 X_2$$

Where Y is the response, X_1 and X_2 are the two independent variables. The parameter β_0 indicates the intercept of the plane. β_1 and β_2 are called partial regression coefficients; β_1 indicates the expected change in Y per unit change in X_1 when X_2 is kept constant; similarly β_2 indicates the expected change in Y per unit change in X_2 when X_1 is kept constant. The above equation can be rewritten as:

$$Y = \beta_0 + \beta_1 X_1 + \beta_2 X_2 + \ldots\ldots\ldots\ldots + \beta_n X_n$$

This is a multiple linear regression model with k regression variables.

APPENDIX 1: ATOMIC WEIGHT OF ELEMENTS

No.	Name of element	Symbol	Atomic No.	Atomic weight	Electronic configuration
1	Hydrogen	H	1	1.0079	$1s^1$
2	Helium	He	2	4.0026	$1s^2$
3	Lithium	Li	3	6.941	[He] $2s^1$
4	Beryllium	Be	4	9.0122	[He] $2s^2$
5	Boron	B	5	10.811	[He] $2s^2 2p^1$
6	Carbon	C	6	12.0107	[He] $2s^2 2p^2$
7	Nitrogen	N	7	14.0067	[He] $2s^2 2p^3$
8	Oxygen	O	8	15.9994	[He] $2s^2 2p^4$
9	Fluorine	F	9	18.9984	[He] $2s^2 2p^5$
10	Neon	Ne	10	20.1797	[He] $2s^2 2p^6$
11	Sodium	Na	11	22.9897	[Ne] $3s^1$
12	Magnesium	Mg	12	24.305	[Ne] $3s^2$
13	Aluminium	Al	13	26.9815	[Ne] $3s^2 3p^1$
14	Silicon	Si	14	28.0855	[Ne] $3s^2 3p^2$
15	Phosphorus	P	15	30.9738	[Ne] $3s^2 3p^3$
16	Sulphur	S	16	32.065	[Ne] $3s^2 3p^4$
17	Chlorine	Cl	17	35.453	[Ne] $3s^2 3p^5$
18	Argon	Ar	18	39.948	[Ne] $3s^2 3p^6$
19	Potassium	K	19	39.083	[Ar] $4s^1$
20	Calcium	Ca	20	40.078	[Ar] $4s^2$
21	Scandium	Sc	21	44.9559	[Ar] $3d^1 4s^2$
22	Titanium	Ti	22	47.867	[Ar] $3d^2 4s^2$
23	Vanadium	V	23	50.9415	[Ar] $3d^3 4s^2$
24	Chromium	Cr	24	51.9961	[Ar] $3d^5 4s^1$
25	Manganese	Mn	25	54.938	[Ar] $3d^5 4s^2$
26	Iron	Fe	26	55.845	[Ar] $3d^6 4s^2$

Table *Contd...*

No.	Name of element	Symbol	Atomic No.	Atomic weight	Electronic configuration
27	Cobalt	Co	27	58.9332	[Ar] $3d^7 4s^2$
28	Nickel	Ni	28	58.6934	[Ar] $3d^8 4s^2$
29	Copper	Cu	29	63.546	[Ar] $3d^{10} 4s^1$
30	Zinc	Zn	30	65.39	[Ar] $3d^{10} 4s^2$
31	Gallium	Ga	31	69.723	[Ar] $3d^{10} 4s^2 4p^1$
32	Germanium	Ge	32	72.64	[Ar] $3d^{10} 4s^2 4p^2$
33	Arsenic	As	33	74.9216	[Ar] $3d^{10} 4s^2 4p^3$
34	Selenium	Se	34	78.96	[Ar] $3d^{10} 4s^2 4p^4$
35	Bromine	Br	35	79.904	[Ar] $3d^{10} 4s^2 4p^5$
36	Krypton	Kr	36	83.8	[Ar] $3d^{10} 4s^2 4p^6$
37	Rubidium	Rb	37	85.4678	[Kr] $5s^1$
38	Strontium	Sr	38	87.62	[Kr] $5s^2$
39	Yttrium	Y	39	88.9059	[Kr] $4d^1 5s^2$
40	Zirconium	Zr	40	91.224	[Kr] $4d^2 5s^2$
40	Niobium	Nb	41	92.9064	[Kr] $4d^4 5s^1$
42	Molybdenum	Mo	42	95.94	[Kr] $4d^5 5s^1$
43	Technetium	Tc	43	98	[Kr] $4d^5 5s^2$
44	Ruthenium	Ru	44	101.07	[Kr] $4d^7 5s^1$
45	Rhodium	Rh	45	102.9052	[Kr] $4d^8 5s^1$
46	Palladium	Pd	46	106.42	[Kr] $4d^{10}$
47	Silver	Ag	47	107.8682	[Kr] $4d^{10} 5s^1$
48	Cadmium	Cd	48	112.411	[Kr] $4d^{10} 5s^2$
49	Indium	In	49	114.818	[Kr] $4d^{10} 5s^2 5p^1$
50	Tin	Sn	50	118.71	[Kr] $4d^{10} 5s^2 5p^2$
51	Antimony	Sb	51	121.76	[Kr] $4d^{10} 5s^2 5p^3$
52	Tellurium	Te	52	127.6	[Kr] $4d^{10} 5s^2 5p^4$
53	Iodine	I	53	126.9045	[Kr] $4d^{10} 5s^2 5p^5$
54	Xenon	Xe	54	131.293	[Kr] $4d^{10} 5s^2 5p^6$
55	Cesium	Cs	55	132.9052	[Xe] $6s^1$
56	Barium	Ba	56	137.327	[Xe] $6s^2$
57	Lanthanum	La	57	138.9052	[Xe] $5d^1 6s^2$
58	Cerium	Ce	58	140.116	[Xe] $4f^1 5d^1 6s^2$
59	Praseodymium	Pr	59	140.9072	[Xe] $4f^3 6s^2$
60	Neodymium	Nd	60	144.24	[Xe] $4f^4 6s^2$
61	Promethium	Pm	61	145	[Xe] $4f^5 6s^2$
62	Samarium	Sm	62	150.36	[Xe] $4f^6 6s^2$
63	Europium	Eu	63	151.964	[Xe] $4f^7 6s^2$
64	Gadolinium	Gd	64	157.25	[Xe] $4f^7 5d^1 6s^2$
65	Terbium	Tb	65	158.925	[Xe] $4f^9 6s^2$
66	Dysprosium	Dy	66	162.5	[Xe] $4f^{10} 6s^2$

Table *Contd...*

No.	Name of element	Symbol	Atomic No.	Atomic weight	Electronic configuration
67	Holmium	Ho	67	164.9303	[Xe] $4f^{11}\ 6s^2$
68	Erbium	Er	68	167.259	[Xe] $4f^{12}\ 6s^2$
69	Thulium	Tm	69	168.9342	[Xe] $4f^{13}\ 6s^2$
70	Ytterbium	Yb	70	173.04	[Xe] $4f^{14}\ 6s^2$
71	Lutetium	Lu	71	174.967	[Xe] $4f^{14}\ 5d^1\ 6s^2$
72	Hafnium	Hf	72	178.49	[Xe] $4f^{14}\ 5d^2\ 6s^2$
73	Tantalum	Ta	73	180.9479	[Xe] $4f^{14}\ 5d^3\ 6s^2$
74	Tungsten	W	74	183.84	[Xe] $4f^{14}\ 5d^4\ 6s^2$
75	Rhenium	Re	75	186.207	[Xe] $4f^{14}\ 5d^5\ 6s^2$
76	Osmium	Os	76	190.23	[Xe] $4f^{14}\ 5d^6\ 6s^2$
77	Iridium	Ir	77	192.217	[Xe] $4f^{14}\ 5d^7\ 6s^2$
78	Platinum	Pt	78	195.078	[Xe] $4f^{14}\ 5d^9\ 6s^1$
79	Gold	Au	79	196.9665	[Xe] $4f^{14}\ 5d^{10}\ 6s^1$
80	Mercury	Hg	80	200.59	[Xe] $4f^{14}\ 5d^{10}\ 6s^2$
81	Thallium	Tl	81	204.3833	[Xe] $4f^{14}\ 5d^{10}\ 6s^2 6p^1$
82	Lead	Pb	82	207.2	[Xe] $4f^{14}\ 5d^{10}\ 6s^2 6p^2$
83	Bismuth	Bi	83	208.9804	[Xe] $4f^{14}\ 5d^{10}\ 6s^2 6p^3$
84	Polonium	Po	84	209	[Xe] $4f^{14}\ 5d^{10}\ 6s^2 6p^4$
85	Astatine	At	85	210	[Xe] $4f^{14}\ 5d^{10}\ 6s^2 6p^5$
86	Radon	Rn	86	222	[Xe] $4f^{14}\ 5d^{10}\ 6s^2 6p^6$
87	Francium	Fr	87	223	[Rn] $7s^1$
88	Radium	Ra	88	226	[Rn] $7s^2$
89	Actinium	Ac	89	227	[Rn] $6d^1\ 7s^2$
90	Thorium	Th	90	232.0381	[Rn] $6d^2\ 7s^2$
91	Protactinium	Pa	91	231.0351	[Rn] $5f^2\ 6d^1\ 7s^2$
92	Uranium	U	92	238.0289	[Rn] $5f^3\ 6d^1\ 7s^2$
93	Neptunium	Np	933	237	[Rn] $5f^4\ 6d^1\ 7s^2$
94	Plutonium	Pu	94	244	[Rn] $5f^6\ 7s^2$
95	Americium	Am	95	243	[Rn] $5f^7\ 7s^2$
96	Curium	Cm	96	247	[Rn] $5f^7 6d^1 7s^2$
97	Berkelium	Bk	97	247	[Rn] $5f^9 7s^2$
98	Californium	Cf	98	251	[Rn] $5f^{10} 7s^2$
99	Einsteinium	Es	99	252	[Rn] $5f^{11} 7s^2$
100	Fermium	Fm	100	257	[Rn] $5f^{12} 7s^2$

Table *Contd...*

No.	Name of element	Symbol	Atomic No.	Atomic weight	Electronic configuration
101	Mendelevium	Md	101	258	$[Rn]\ 5f^{13}7s^2$
102	Nobelium	No	102	259	$[Rn]\ 5f^{14}7s^2$
103	Lawrencium	Lr	103	262	$[Rn]\ 5f^{14}7s^27p^1$
104	Rutherfordium	Rf	104	261	$[Rn]5f^{14}6d^27s^2$
105	Dubnium	Db	105	262	$[Rn]5f^{14}6d^37s^2$
106	Seaborgium	Sg	106	266	$[Rn]5f^{14}6d^47s^2$
107	Bohrium	Bh	107	264	$[Rn]5f^{14}6d^57s^2$
108	Hassium	Hs	108	277	$[Rn]5f^{14}6d^67s^2$
109	Meitnerium	Mt	109	268	$[Rn]5f^{14}6d^77s^2$
110	Darmstadtium	Ds	110	281	$[Rn]5f^{14}6d^97s^1$
111	Roentgenium	Rg	111	272	$[Rn]5f^{14}6d^{10}7s^1$
112	Coprnicium	Cn	112	285	$[Rn]5f^{14}6d^{10}7s^2$
113	Ununtrium	Unt	113	284	$[Rn]5f^{14}6d^{10}7s^27p^1$
114	Ununquadium	Uuq	114	289	$[Rn]5f^{14}6d^{10}7s^27p^2$
115	Ununpentium	Uup	115	288	$[Rn]5f^{14}6d^{10}7s^27p^3$
116	Ununhexium	Uuh	116	292	$[Rn]5f^{14}6d^{10}7s^27p^4$
117	Ununseptium	Uus	117	NA	$[Rn]5f^{14}6d^{10}7s^27p^5$
118	Ununoctium	Uuo	118	294	$[Rn]5f^{14}6d^{10}7s^27p^6$

APPENDIX 2: DENSITY OF WATER AT VARIOUS TEMPERATURES

Temperature (°C)	Pressure (Pa)	Density (gm/cm^3)	Saturation Vapor pressure (Pa)	Dynamic Viscosity (kg/m.s)
0.00	101325	0.99982	611	0.001792
1.00	101325	0.99989	657	0.001731
2.00	101325	0.99994	705	0.001674
3.00	101325	0.99998	757	0.001620
4.00	101325	1.00000	813	0.001569
5.00	101325	1.00000	872	0.001520
6.00	101325	0.99999	935	0.001473
7.00	101325	0.99996	1001	0.001429
8.00	101325	0.99991	1072	0.001386
9.00	101325	0.99985	1147	0.001346
10.00	101325	0.99977	1227	0.001308
11.00	101325	0.99968	1312	0.001271
12.00	101325	0.99958	1402	0.001236
13.00	101325	0.99946	1497	0.001202
14.00	101325	0.99933	1597	0.001170
15.00	101325	0.99919	1704	0.001139
16.00	101325	0.99903	1817	0.001109
17.00	101325	0.99886	1936	0.001081
18.00	101325	0.99868	2063	0.001054
19.00	101325	0.99849	2196	0.001028
20.00	101325	0.99829	2337	0.001003
21.00	101325	0.99808	2486	0.000979
22.00	101325	0.99786	2642	0.000955
23.00	101325	0.99762	2808	0.000933
24.00	101325	0.99738	2982	0.000911
25.00	101325	0.99713	3166	0.000891
26.00	101325	0.99686	3360	0.000871
27.00	101325	0.99659	3564	0.000852

Table *Contd...*

Temperature (^oC)	Pressure (Pa)	Density (gm/cm^3)	Saturation Vapor pressure (Pa)	Dynamic Viscosity (kg/m.s)
28.00	101325	0.99631	3779	0.000833
29.00	101325	0.99602	4004	0.000815
30.00	101325	0.99571	4242	0.000798
31.00	101325	0.99541	4491	0.000781
32.00	101325	0.99509	4754	0.000765
33.00	101325	0.99476	5029	0.000749
34.00	101325	0.99443	5318	0.000734
35.00	101325	0.99408	5622	0.000720
36.00	101325	0.99373	5940	0.000705
37.00	101325	0.99337	6274	0.000692
38.00	101325	0.99300	6624	0.000678
39.00	101325	0.99263	6991	0.000666
40.00	101325	0.99225	7375	0.000653
41.00	101325	0.99186	7777	0.000641
42.00	101325	0.99146	8198	0.000629
43.00	101325	0.99105	8639	0.000618
44.00	101325	0.99064	9100	0.000607
45.00	101325	0.99022	9582	0.000596
46.00	101325	0.98980	10085	0.000586
47.00	101325	0.98936	10612	0.000576
48.00	101325	0.98892	11161	0.000566
49.00	101325	0.98847	11735	0.000556
50.00	101325	0.98802	12335	0.000547
51.00	101325	0.98756	12960	0.000538
52.00	101325	0.98709	13612	0.000529
53.00	101325	0.98662	14292	0.000521
54.00	101325	0.98614	15001	0.000512
55.00	101325	0.98565	15740	0.000504
56.00	101325	0.98516	16510	0.000496
57.00	101325	0.98466	17312	0.000489
58.00	101325	0.98416	18146	0.000481
59.00	101325	0.98364	19015	0.000474
60.00	101325	0.98313	19919	0.000467
61.00	101325	0.98260	20859	0.000460
62.00	101325	0.98207	21837	0.000453
63.00	101325	0.98154	22854	0.000447
64.00	101325	0.98100	23910	0.000440
65.00	101325	0.98045	25008	0.000434
66.00	101325	0.97990	26148	0.000428
67.00	101325	0.97934	27332	0.000422
68.00	101325	0.97878	28561	0.000416
69.00	101325	0.97821	29837	0.000410
70.00	101325	0.97763	31161	0.000404
71.00	101325	0.97705	32533	0.000399
72.00	101325	0.97647	33957	0.000394

Table *Contd...*

Temperature (°C)	Pressure (Pa)	Density (gm/cm³)	Saturation Vapor pressure (Pa)	Dynamic Viscosity (kg/m.s)
73.00	101325	0.97588	35433	0.000388
74.00	101325	0.97528	36963	0.000383
75.00	101325	0.97468	38548	0.000378
76.00	101325	0.97408	40190	0.000373
77.00	101325	0.97346	41890	0.000369
78.00	101325	0.97285	43650	0.000364
79.00	101325	0.97223	45473	0.000359
80.00	101325	0.97160	47359	0.000355
81.00	101325	0.97097	49310	0.000351
82.00	101325	0.97033	51328	0.000346
83.00	101325	0.96969	53415	0.000342
84.00	101325	0.96904	55572	0.000338
85.00	101325	0.96839	57803	0.000334
86.00	101325	0.96773	60107	0.000330
87.00	101325	0.96707	62488	0.000326
88.00	101325	0.96641	64947	0.000322
89.00	101325	0.96574	67486	0.000319
90.00	101325	0.96506	70108	0.000315
91.00	101325	0.96438	72814	0.000311
92.00	101325	0.96370	75607	0.000308
93.00	101325	0.96301	78488	0.000304
94.00	101325	0.96231	81460	0.000301
95.00	101325	0.96162	84525	0.000298
96.00	101325	0.96091	87685	0.000295
97.00	101325	0.96020	90943	0.000291
98.00	101325	0.95949	94301	0.000288
99.00	101325	0.95878	97760	0.000285
100.00	101325	0.95805	101325	0.000282

Pressure: Atmospheric pressure at 101325 bar, i.e. normal atmospheric pressure on the sea level at 0°C.

Density: Ratio of the mass of water (kg) occupied in a volume of 1 cubic m.

Dynamic viscosity: The viscosity of a fluid characterizes the resistance to the movement of the fluid.

APPENDIX 3: COMMON LOGARITHMS

Table 1

Log10	Four-Place Common Logarithm										Proportional Parts								
	0	1	2	3	4	5	6	7	8	9	1	2	3	4	5	6	7	8	9
10	0000	0043	0086	0128	0170	0212	0253	0294	0334	0374	4	8	12	17	21	25	29	33	37
11	0414	0453	0492	0531	0569	0607	0645	0682	0719	0755	4	8	11	15	19	23	26	30	34
12	0792	0828	0864	0899	0934	0969	1004	1038	1072	1106	3	7	10	14	17	21	24	28	31
13	1139	1173	1206	1239	1271	1303	1335	1367	1399	1430	3	6	10	13	16	19	23	26	29
14	1461	1492	1523	1553	1584	1614	1644	1673	1703	1732	3	6	9	12	15	18	21	24	27
15	1761	1790	1818	1847	1875	1903	1931	1959	1987	2014	3	6	8	11	14	17	20	22	25
16	2041	2068	2095	2122	2148	2175	2201	2227	2253	2279	3	5	8	11	13	16	18	21	24
17	2304	2330	2355	2380	2405	2430	2455	2480	2504	2529	2	5	7	10	12	15	17	20	22
18	2553	2577	2601	2625	2648	2672	2695	2718	2742	2765	2	5	7	9	12	14	16	19	21
19	2788	2810	2833	2856	2878	2900	2923	2945	2967	2989	2	4	7	9	11	13	16	18	20
20	3010	3032	3054	3075	3096	3118	3139	3160	3181	3201	2	4	6	8	11	13	15	17	19
21	3222	3243	3263	3284	3304	3324	3345	3365	3385	3404	2	4	6	8	10	12	14	16	18
22	3424	3444	3464	3483	3502	3522	3541	3560	3579	3598	2	4	6	8	10	12	14	15	17
23	3617	3636	3655	3674	3692	3711	3729	3747	3766	3784	2	4	6	7	9	11	13	15	17
24	3802	3820	3838	3856	3874	3892	3900	3927	3945	3962	2	4	5	7	9	11	12	14	16
25	3979	3997	4014	4031	4048	4065	4082	4099	4116	4133	2	3	5	7	9	10	12	14	15
26	4150	4166	4183	4200	4216	4232	4249	4265	4281	4298	2	3	5	7	8	10	11	13	15
27	4314	4330	4346	4362	4378	4393	4409	4425	4440	4456	2	3	5	6	8	9	11	13	14
28	4472	4487	4502	4518	4533	4548	4564	4579	4594	4609	2	3	5	6	8	9	11	12	14
29	4624	4639	4654	4669	4683	4698	4713	4728	4742	4757	1	3	4	6	7	9	10	12	13
30	4771	4786	4800	4814	4829	4843	4857	4871	4886	4900	1	3	4	6	7	9	10	11	13
31	4914	4928	4942	4955	4969	4983	4997	5011	5024	5038	1	3	4	6	7	8	10	11	12
32	5051	5065	5079	5092	5105	5119	5132	5145	5159	5172	1	3	4	5	7	8	9	11	12
33	5185	5198	5211	5224	5237	5250	5263	5276	5289	5302	1	3	4	5	6	8	9	10	12
34	5315	5328	5340	5353	5366	5378	5391	5403	5416	5428	1	3	4	5	6	8	9	10	11
35	5441	5453	5465	5478	5490	5502	5514	5527	5539	5551	1	2	4	5	6	7	9	10	11
36	5563	5575	5587	5599	5611	5623	5635	5647	5658	5670	1	2	4	5	6	7	8	10	11
37	5682	5694	5705	5717	5729	5740	5752	5763	5775	5786	1	2	3	5	6	7	8	9	10
38	5798	5809	5821	5832	5843	5855	5866	5877	5888	5899	1	2	3	5	6	7	8	9	10
39	5911	5922	5933	5944	5955	5966	5977	5988	5999	6010	1	2	3	4	5	7	8	9	10
40	6021	6031	6042	6053	6064	6075	6085	6096	6107	6117	1	2	3	4	5	6	8	9	10
41	6128	6138	6149	6160	6170	6180	6191	6201	6212	6222	1	2	3	4	5	6	7	8	9
42	6232	6243	6253	6263	6274	6284	6294	6304	6314	6325	1	2	3	4	5	6	7	8	9
43	6335	6345	6355	6365	6375	6385	6395	6405	6415	6425	1	2	3	4	5	6	7	8	9
44	6435	6444	6454	6464	6474	6484	6493	6503	6513	6522	1	2	3	4	5	6	7	8	9
45	6532	6542	6551	6561	6571	6580	6590	6599	6609	6618	1	2	3	4	5	6	7	8	9
46	6628	6637	6646	6656	6665	6675	6684	6693	6702	6712	1	2	3	4	5	6	7	7	8
47	6721	6730	6739	6749	6758	6767	6776	6785	6794	6803	1	2	3	4	5	5	6	7	8
48	6812	6857	6830	6839	6848	6857	6866	6875	6884	6893	1	2	3	4	4	5	6	7	8
49	6902	6911	6920	6928	6937	6946	6955	6964	6972	6981	1	2	3	4	4	5	6	7	8

Table 2

Log10	Four-Place Common Logarithm 0	1	2	3	4	5	6	7	8	9	Proportional Parts 1	2	3	4	5	6	7	8	9
50	6990	6998	7007	7016	7024	7033	7042	7050	7059	7067	1	2	3	3	4	5	6	7	8
51	7076	7084	7093	7101	7110	7118	7126	7135	7143	7152	1	2	3	3	4	5	6	7	8
52	7160	7168	7155	7185	7193	7202	7210	7218	7226	7235	1	2	2	3	4	5	6	7	7
53	7243	7251	7259	7267	7275	7284	7292	7300	7308	7316	1	2	2	3	4	5	6	6	7
54	7324	7332	7340	7348	7356	7364	7372	7380	7388	7396	1	2	2	3	4	5	6	6	7
55	7404	7412	7419	7427	7435	7443	7451	7459	7466	7474	1	2	2	3	4	5	5	6	7
56	7482	7490	7497	7505	7513	7520	7528	7536	7543	7551	1	2	2	3	4	5	5	6	7
57	7559	7566	7574	7582	7589	7597	7604	7612	7619	7627	1	2	2	3	4	5	5	6	7
58	7634	7642	7649	7657	7664	7672	7679	7686	7694	7701	1	1	2	3	4	4	5	6	7
59	7709	7716	7723	7731	7738	7745	7752	7760	7767	7774	1	1	2	3	4	4	5	6	7
60	7782	7789	7796	7803	7810	7818	7825	7832	7839	7846	1	1	2	3	4	4	5	6	6
61	7853	7860	7868	7875	7882	7889	7896	7903	7910	7917	1	1	2	3	4	4	5	6	6
62	7924	7931	7938	7945	7952	7959	7966	7973	7980	7987	1	1	2	3	3	4	5	6	6
63	7993	8000	8007	8014	8021	8028	8035	8041	8048	8055	1	1	2	3	3	4	5	5	6
64	8062	8069	8075	8082	8089	8096	8102	8109	8116	8122	1	1	2	3	3	4	5	5	6
65	8129	8136	8142	8149	8156	8162	8169	8176	8182	8189	1	1	2	3	3	4	5	5	6
66	8195	8202	8209	8215	8222	8228	8235	8241	8248	8254	1	1	2	3	3	4	5	5	6
67	8261	8267	8274	8280	8287	8293	8299	8306	8312	8319	1	1	2	3	3	4	5	5	6
68	8325	8331	8338	8344	8351	8357	8363	8370	8376	8382	1	1	2	3	3	4	4	5	6
69	8388	8395	8401	8407	8414	8420	8426	8432	8439	8445	1	1	2	2	3	4	4	5	6
70	8451	8457	8463	8470	8476	8482	8488	8494	8500	8506	1	1	2	2	3	4	4	5	6
71	8513	8519	8525	8531	8537	8543	8549	8555	8561	8567	1	1	2	2	3	4	4	5	5
72	8573	8579	8585	8591	8597	8603	8609	8615	8621	8627	1	1	2	2	3	4	4	5	5
73	8633	8639	8645	8651	8657	8663	8669	8675	8681	8686	1	1	2	2	3	4	4	5	5
74	8692	8698	8704	8710	8716	8722	8727	8733	8739	8745	1	1	2	2	3	4	4	5	5
75	8751	8756	8762	8768	8774	8779	8785	8791	8797	8802	1	1	2	2	3	3	4	5	5
76	8808	8814	8820	8825	8831	8837	8842	8848	8854	8859	1	1	2	2	3	3	4	5	5
77	8865	8871	8876	8882	8887	8893	8899	8904	8910	8915	1	1	2	2	3	3	4	4	5
78	8921	8927	8932	8938	8943	8949	8954	8960	8965	8971	1	1	2	2	3	3	4	4	5
79	8976	8982	8987	8993	8998	9004	9009	9015	9020	9025	1	1	2	2	3	3	4	4	5
80	9031	9036	9042	9047	9053	9058	9063	9069	9074	9079	1	1	2	2	3	3	4	4	5
81	9085	9090	9096	9101	9106	9112	9117	9122	9128	9133	1	1	2	2	3	3	4	4	5
82	9138	9143	9149	9154	9159	9165	9170	9175	9180	9186	1	1	2	2	3	3	4	4	5
83	9191	9196	9201	9206	9212	9217	9222	9227	9232	9238	1	1	2	2	3	3	4	4	5
84	9243	9248	9253	9258	9263	9269	9274	9279	9284	9289	1	1	2	2	3	3	4	4	5
85	9294	9299	9304	9309	9315	9320	9325	9330	9335	9340	1	1	2	2	3	3	4	4	5
86	9345	9350	9355	9360	9365	9370	9375	9380	9385	9390	1	1	2	2	3	3	4	4	5
87	9395	9400	9405	9410	9415	9420	9425	9430	9435	9440	0	1	1	2	2	3	3	4	4
88	9445	9450	9455	9460	9465	9469	9474	9479	9484	9489	0	1	1	2	2	3	3	4	4
89	9494	9499	9504	9509	9513	9518	9523	9528	9533	9538	0	1	1	2	2	3	3	4	4
90	9542	9547	9552	9557	9562	9566	9571	9576	9581	9586	0	1	1	2	2	3	3	4	4
91	9590	9595	9600	9605	9609	9614	9619	9624	9628	9633	0	1	1	2	2	3	3	4	4
92	9638	9643	9647	9652	9657	9661	9666	9671	9675	9680	0	1	1	2	2	3	3	4	4
93	9685	9789	9694	9699	9702	9708	9713	9717	9722	9727	0	1	1	2	2	3	3	4	4
94	9731	9736	9741	9745	9750	9754	9759	9763	9768	9773	0	1	1	2	2	3	3	4	4
95	9777	9782	9786	9791	9795	9800	9805	9809	9814	9818	0	1	1	2	2	3	3	4	4
96	9823	9827	9832	9836	9841	9845	9850	9854	9859	9863	0	1	1	2	2	3	3	4	4
97	9868	9872	9877	9881	9886	9890	9894	9899	9903	9908	0	1	1	2	2	3	3	4	4
98	9912	9917	9921	9926	9930	9934	9939	9943	9948	9952	0	1	1	2	2	3	3	4	4
99	9956	9961	9965	9969	9974	9978	9983	9987	9991	9996	0	1	1	2	2	3	3	3	4

Table 2 Contd….

No	Four-Place Antilogarithms										Proportional Parts								
	0	1	2	3	4	5	6	7	8	9	1	2	3	4	5	6	7	8	9
0.00	1000	1002	1005	1007	1009	1012	1014	1016	1019	1021	0	0	1	1	1	1	2	2	2
0.01	1023	1026	1028	1030	1033	1035	1038	1040	1042	1045	0	0	1	1	1	1	2	2	2
0.02	1047	1050	1052	1054	1057	1059	1062	1064	1067	1069	0	0	1	1	1	1	2	2	2
0.03	1072	1074	1076	1079	1081	1084	1086	1089	1091	1094	0	0	1	1	1	1	2	2	2
0.04	1096	1099	1102	1104	1107	1109	1112	1114	1117	1119	0	1	1	1	1	2	2	2	2
0.05	1122	1125	1127	1130	1132	1135	1138	1140	1143	1146	0	1	1	1	1	2	2	2	2
0.06	1148	1151	1153	1156	1159	1161	1164	1167	1169	1172	0	1	1	1	1	2	2	2	2
0.07	1175	1178	1180	1183	1186	1189	1191	1194	1197	1199	0	1	1	1	1	2	2	2	2
0.08	1202	1205	1208	1211	1213	1216	1219	1222	1225	1227	0	1	1	1	1	2	2	2	3
0.09	1230	1233	1236	1239	1242	1245	1247	1250	1253	1256	0	1	1	1	1	2	2	2	3
0.10	1259	1262	1265	1268	1271	1275	1276	1279	1282	1285	0	1	1	1	1	2	2	2	3
0.11	1288	1291	1294	1297	1300	1303	1306	1309	1312	1315	0	1	1	1	2	2	2	2	3
0.12	1318	1321	1324	1327	1330	1334	1337	1340	1343	1346	0	1	1	1	2	2	2	2	3
0.13	1349	1352	1355	1358	1361	1365	1368	1371	1374	1377	0	1	1	1	2	2	2	3	3
0.14	1380	1384	1387	1390	1393	1396	1400	1403	1406	1409	0	1	1	1	2	2	2	3	3
0.15	1413	1416	1419	1422	1426	1429	1432	1435	1439	1442	0	1	1	1	2	2	2	3	3
0.16	1445	1449	1452	1455	1459	1462	1466	1469	1472	1476	0	1	1	1	2	2	2	3	3
0.17	1479	1483	1486	1489	1493	1496	1500	1503	1507	1510	0	1	1	1	2	2	2	3	3
0.18	1514	1517	1521	1524	1528	1531	1535	1538	1542	1545	0	1	1	1	2	2	2	3	3
0.19	1549	1552	1556	1560	1563	1567	1570	1574	1578	1581	0	1	1	1	2	2	3	3	3
0.20	1585	1589	1592	1596	1600	1603	1607	1611	1614	1618	0	1	1	1	2	2	3	3	3
0.21	1622	1626	1629	1633	1637	1641	1644	1648	1652	1656	0	1	1	2	2	2	3	3	3
0.22	1660	1663	1667	1671	1675	1679	1683	1687	1690	1694	0	1	1	2	2	2	3	3	3
0.23	1698	1702	1706	1710	1714	1718	1722	1726	1730	1734	0	1	1	2	2	2	3	3	4
0.24	1738	1742	1746	1750	1754	1758	1762	1766	1770	1774	0	1	1	2	2	2	3	3	4
0.25	1778	1782	1786	1791	1795	1799	1803	1807	1811	1816	0	1	1	2	2	2	3	3	4
0.26	1820	1824	1828	1832	1837	1842	1845	1849	1854	1858	0	1	1	2	2	3	3	3	4
0.27	1862	1866	1871	1875	1879	1884	1888	1807	1807	1901	0	1	1	2	2	3	3	3	4
0.28	1905	1910	1914	1919	1923	1928	1932	1936	1941	1945	0	1	1	2	2	3	3	4	4
0.29	1950	1954	1059	1963	1968	1972	1977	1982	1986	1991	0	1	1	2	2	3	3	4	4
0.30	1995	2000	2004	2009	2014	2018	2023	2028	2032	2037	0	1	1	2	2	3	3	4	4
0.31	2042	2046	2051	2056	2061	2065	2070	2075	2080	2084	0	1	1	2	2	3	3	4	4
0.32	2089	2094	2099	2104	2109	2014	2018	2023	2028	2033	0	1	1	2	2	3	3	4	4
0.33	2138	2143	2148	2153	2158	2163	2168	2173	2178	2183	0	1	1	2	2	3	3	4	4
0.34	2188	2193	2198	2203	2208	2213	2218	2223	2228	2234	1	1	2	2	3	3	4	4	5
0.35	2239	2244	2249	2254	2259	2265	2270	2275	2280	2286	1	1	2	2	3	3	4	4	5
0.36	2291	2296	2301	2307	2312	2317	2323	2328	2333	2339	1	1	2	2	3	3	4	4	5
0.37	2344	2350	2355	2360	2366	2371	2377	2382	2388	2393	1	1	2	2	3	3	4	4	5
0.38	2399	2404	2410	2415	2421	2427	2432	2438	2443	2449	1	1	2	2	3	3	4	4	5
0.39	2455	2460	2466	2472	2477	2483	2489	2495	2500	2506	1	1	2	2	3	3	4	5	5
0.40	2512	2518	2523	2529	2535	2541	2547	2553	2559	2564	1	1	2	2	3	4	4	5	5
0.41	2570	2576	2582	2588	2594	2600	2606	2612	2618	2624	1	1	2	2	3	4	4	5	5
0.42	2630	2636	2642	2649	2655	2661	2667	2673	2679	2685	1	1	2	2	3	4	4	5	6
0.43	2692	2698	2704	2710	2716	2723	2729	2735	2742	2748	1	1	2	3	3	4	4	5	6
0.44	2754	2761	2767	2673	2780	2786	2793	2799	2803	2812	1	1	2	3	3	4	4	5	6
0.45	2818	2825	2831	2838	2844	2851	2858	2864	2871	2877	1	1	2	3	3	4	5	5	6
0.46	2884	2891	2897	2904	2911	2917	2924	2931	2938	2944	1	1	2	3	3	4	5	5	6
0.47	2951	2958	2965	2972	2979	2985	2992	2999	3006	3013	1	1	2	3	3	4	5	5	6
0.48	3020	3027	3034	3041	3048	3055	3062	3069	3076	3083	1	1	2	3	4	4	5	6	6
0.49	3090	3097	3105	3112	3119	3126	3133	3141	3148	3155	1	1	2	3	4	4	5	6	6

Table 2 Contd....

Four-Place Antilogarithms											Proportional Parts								
No	0	1	2	3	4	5	6	7	8	9	1	2	3	4	5	6	7	8	9
50	6990	6998	7007	7016	7024	7033	7042	7050	7059	7067	1	2	3	3	4	5	6	7	8
51	7076	7084	7093	7101	7110	7118	7126	7135	7143	7152	1	2	3	3	4	5	6	7	8
52	7160	7168	7155	7185	7193	7202	7210	7218	7226	7235	1	2	2	3	4	5	6	7	7
53	7243	7251	7259	7267	7275	7284	7292	7300	7308	7316	1	2	2	3	4	5	6	6	7
54	7324	7332	7340	7348	7356	7364	7372	7380	7388	7396	1	2	2	3	4	5	6	6	7
55	7404	7412	7419	7427	7435	7443	7451	7459	7466	7474	1	2	2	3	4	5	5	6	7
56	7482	7490	7497	7505	7513	7520	7528	7536	7543	7551	1	2	2	3	4	5	5	6	7
57	7559	7566	7574	7582	7589	7597	7604	7612	7619	7627	1	2	2	3	4	5	5	6	7
58	7634	7642	7649	7657	7664	7672	7679	7686	7694	7701	1	1	2	3	4	4	5	6	7
59	7709	7716	7723	7731	7738	7745	7752	7760	7767	7774	1	1	2	3	4	4	5	6	7
60	7782	7789	7796	7803	7810	7818	7825	7832	7839	7846	1	1	2	3	4	4	5	6	6
61	7853	7860	7868	7875	7882	7889	7896	7903	7910	7917	1	1	2	3	4	4	5	6	6
62	7924	7931	7938	7945	7952	7959	7966	7973	7980	7987	1	1	2	3	3	4	5	6	6
63	7993	8000	8007	8014	8021	8028	8035	8041	8048	8055	1	1	2	3	3	4	5	5	6
64	8062	8069	8075	8082	8089	8096	8102	8109	8116	8122	1	1	2	3	3	4	5	5	6
65	8129	8136	8142	8149	8156	8162	8169	8176	8182	8189	1	1	2	3	3	4	5	5	6
66	8195	8202	8209	8215	8222	8228	8235	8241	8248	8254	1	1	2	3	3	4	5	5	6
67	8261	8267	8274	8280	8287	8293	8299	8306	8312	8319	1	1	2	3	3	4	5	5	6
68	8325	8331	8338	8344	8351	8357	8363	8370	8376	8382	1	1	2	3	3	4	4	5	6
69	8388	8395	8401	8407	8414	8420	8426	8432	8439	8445	1	1	2	2	3	4	4	5	6
70	8451	8457	8463	8470	8476	8482	8488	8494	8500	8506	1	1	2	2	3	4	4	5	6
71	8513	8519	8525	8531	8537	8543	8549	8555	8561	8567	1	1	2	2	3	4	4	5	5
72	8573	8579	8585	8591	8597	8603	8609	8615	8621	8627	1	1	2	2	3	4	4	5	5
73	8633	8639	8645	8651	8657	8663	8669	8675	8681	8686	1	1	2	2	3	4	4	5	5
74	8692	8698	8704	8710	8716	8722	8727	8733	8739	8745	1	1	2	2	3	4	4	5	5
75	8751	8756	8762	8768	8774	8779	8785	8791	8797	8802	1	1	2	2	3	3	4	5	5
76	8808	8814	8820	8825	8831	8837	8842	8848	8854	8859	1	1	2	2	3	3	4	5	5
77	8865	8871	8876	8882	8887	8893	8899	8904	8910	8915	1	1	2	2	3	3	4	4	5
78	8921	8927	8932	8938	8943	8949	8954	8960	8965	8971	1	1	2	2	3	3	4	4	5
79	8976	8982	8987	8993	8998	9004	9009	9015	9020	9025	1	1	2	2	3	3	4	4	5
80	9031	9036	9042	9047	9053	9058	9063	9069	9074	9079	1	1	2	2	3	3	4	4	5
81	9085	9090	9096	9101	9106	9112	9117	9122	9128	9133	1	1	2	2	3	3	4	4	5
82	9138	9143	9149	9154	9159	9165	9170	9175	9180	9186	1	1	2	2	3	3	4	4	5
83	9191	9196	9201	9206	9212	9217	9222	9227	9232	9238	1	1	2	2	3	3	4	4	5
84	9243	9248	9253	9258	9263	9269	9274	9279	9284	9289	1	1	2	2	3	3	4	4	5
85	9294	9299	9304	9309	9315	9320	9325	9330	9335	9340	1	1	2	2	3	3	4	4	5
86	9345	9350	9355	9360	9365	9370	9375	9380	9385	9390	1	1	2	2	3	3	4	4	5
87	9395	9400	9405	9410	9415	9420	9425	9430	9435	9440	0	1	1	2	2	3	3	4	4
88	9445	9450	9455	9460	9465	9469	9474	9479	9484	9489	0	1	1	2	2	3	3	4	4
89	9494	9499	9504	9509	9513	9518	9523	9528	9533	9538	0	1	1	2	2	3	3	4	4
90	9542	9547	9552	9557	9562	9566	9571	9576	9581	9586	0	1	1	2	2	3	3	4	4
91	9590	9595	9600	9605	9609	9614	9619	9624	9628	9633	0	1	1	2	2	3	3	4	4
92	9638	9643	9647	9652	9657	9661	9666	9671	9675	9680	0	1	1	2	2	3	3	4	4
93	9685	9789	9694	9699	9702	9708	9713	9717	9722	9727	0	1	1	2	2	3	3	4	4
94	9731	9736	9741	9745	9750	9754	9759	9763	9768	9773	0	1	1	2	2	3	3	4	4
95	9777	9782	9786	9791	9795	9800	9805	9809	9814	9818	0	1	1	2	2	3	3	4	4
96	9823	9827	9832	9836	9841	9845	9850	9854	9859	9863	0	1	1	2	2	3	3	4	4
97	9868	9872	9877	9881	9886	9890	9894	9899	9903	9908	0	1	1	2	2	3	3	4	4
98	9912	9917	9921	9926	9930	9934	9939	9943	9948	9952	0	1	1	2	2	3	3	4	4
99	9956	9961	9965	9969	9974	9978	9983	9987	9991	9996	0	1	1	2	2	3	3	3	4

APPENDIX 4

Dissociation Constants of some acidic and basic substances of pharmaceutical use at t °C

Name	Mol. formula	Step	t°C	pKa		Step	t°C	pKa
Acetamide	C_2H_5NO		25	15.1				
Acetanilide	C_8H_9NO		25	0.5				
Acetazolamide	$C_4H_6N_4O_3S_2$			7.2				
Acetic acid	$C_2H_4O_2$		25	4.76				
Acetoacetic acid	$C_4H_6O_3$		25	3.6				
Acetohydroxamic acid	$C_2H_5NO_2$			8.70				
Acetaldehyde	C_2H_4O		25	13.57				
N-Acetylglycine	$C_4H_7NO_3$		25	3.67				
Aconitine	$C_{34}H_{47}NO_{11}$			5.88				
Acrylic acid	$C_3H_4O_2$		25	4.25				
Adenine	$C_5H_5N_5$	1		4.3		2		9.83
Adenosine	$C_{10}H_{13}N_5O_4$	1	25	3.6		2	25	12.4
Adipamic acid	$C_6H_{11}NO_3$		25	4.63				
Adipic acid	$C_6H_{10}O_4$	1	18	4.41		2	18	5.41
2-Aminoadipic acid	$C_6H_{11}NO_4$	1	25	2.14		3	25	9.77
		2	25	4.21				
D-Adrenaline	$C_9H_{13}NO_3$	1	25	8.66		2	25	9.95
α-Alanine	$C_3H_7NO_2$	1	25	2.34		2	25	9.87
Aniline	C_6H_7N		25	4.87				
2-Fluoroaniline	C_6H_6FN		25	3.20				
3-Fluoroaniline	C_6H_6FN		25	3.59				
4-Fluoroaniline	C_6H_6FN		25	4.65				
2-Chloroaniline	C_6H_6ClN		25	2.66				
3-Chloroaniline	C_6H_6ClN		25	3.52				
4-Chloroaniline	C_6H_6ClN		25	3.98				
2-Bromoaniline	C_6H_6BrN		25	2.53				

Name	Mol. formula	Step	t°C	pKa		Step	t°C	pKa
3-Bromoaniline	C_6H_6BrN		25	3.53				
4-Bromoaniline	C_6H_6BrN		25	3.89				
2-Iodoaniline	C_6H_6IN		25	2.54				
3-Iodoaniline	C_6H_6IN		25	3.58				
4-Iodoaniline	C_6H_6IN		25	3.81				
2-Nitroaniline	$C_6H_6N_2O_2$		25	-0.25				
3-Nitroaniline	$C_6H_6N_2O_2$		25	2.46				
4-Nitroaniline	$C_6H_6N_2O_2$		25	1.02				
β-Alanine	$C_3H_7NO_2$	1	25	3.55		2	25	10.24
Allantoin	$C_4H_6N_4O_3$		25	8.96				
Allopurinol	$C_5H_4N_4O$			10.2				
Allyl alcohol	C_3H_6O		25	15.5				
Alloxanic acid	$C_4H_4N_2O_5$		25	6.64				
Allylamine	C_3H_7N		25	9.49				
3,5-Dibromo aniline	$C_6H_5Br_2N$		25	2.34				
2,4-Dichloroaniline	$C_6H_5Cl_2N$		22	2.05				
Aminoacetonitrile	$C_2H_4N_2$		25	5.34				
DL-2-Amino butanoic acid	$C_4H_9NO_2$	1	25	2.29		2	25	9.83
4-Aminobutanoic acid	C_4H_9NO2	1	25	4.03		2	25	10.55
3-Aminopropanenitrile	$C_3H_6N_2$		20	7.80				
2-Aminoethanesulfonic acid	$C_2H_8NO_3S$	1	25	1.5		2	25	9.06
Arginine	$C_6H_{14}N_4O_2$	1 2	25 25	1.82 8.99		3	25	12.48
L-Ascorbic acid	$C_6H_8O_6$	1	25	4.04		2	16	11.4
L-Asparagine	$C_4H_8N_2O_3$	1	20	2.1		2	20	8.80
Aspergillic acid	$C_{12}H_{20}N_2O_2$			5.5				
Glycylasparagine	$C_6H_{11}N_3O_4$	1	25	2.94		2	18	8.44
L-Aspartic acid	$C_4H_7NO_4$	1 2	25 25	1.99 3.90		3	25	9.90
Atenolol	$C_{14}H_{22}N_2O_3$			9.6				
Azaserine	$C_5H_7N_3O_4$			8.55				
Azetidine	C_3H_7N		25	11.29				
Barbital	$C_8H_{12}N_2O_3$		25	7.43				
Barbituric acid	$C_4H_4N_2O_3$		25	4.01				
Benzamide	C_7H_7NO		25	13				
Benzenethiol	C_6H_6S		25	6.62				
Benzoic acid	$C_7H_6O_2$		25	4.19				
1*H*-Benzotriazole	$C_6H_5N_3$		20	1.6				
Benzeneboronic acid	$C_6H_7BO_2$			8.83				

Name	Mol. formula	Step	t°C	pKa		Step	t°C	pKa
Benzylamine	C_7H_9N		25	9.34				
Betaine	$C_5H_{11}NO_2$		0	1.83				
Biguanide	$C_2H_7N_5$	1		11.52		2		2.93
Bromoacetic acid	$C_2H_3BrO_2$		25	2.90				
Bromocresol Green	$C_{21}H_{14}Br_4O_5S$			4.7				
Bromocresol Purple	$C_{21}H_{16}Br_2O_5S$			6.3				
3-Bromopropanoic acid	$C_3H_5BrO_2$		25	4.00				
3-Bromopyridine	C_5H_4BrN		25	2.84				
Bromothymol Blue	$C_{27}H_{28}Br_2O_5S$			7.0				
Brucine	$C_{23}H_{26}N_2O_4$	1		6.04		2		11.04
4-Cyanobutanoic acid	$C_4H_7NO_2$		25	2.42				
3-Methyl-1-butanamine	$C_5H_{13}N$		25	10.60				
2-Methyl-2-butanamine	$C_5H_{13}N$		19	10.85				
1,4-Butanediamine	$C_4H_{12}N_2$	1	25	10.80		2	25	9.63
1,2,3,4-Butanetetrol	$C_4H_{10}O_4$			13.9				
Butanoic acid	$C_4H_8O_2$		25	4.83				
2,4-Diaminobutanoic acid	$C_4H_{10}N_2O_2$	1 2	25 25	1.85 8.24		3	25	10.44
3-Hydroxybutanoic acid,(±)	$C_4H_8O_3$		25	4.70				
4-Hydroxybutanoic acid	$C_4H_8O_3$		25	4.72				
2-Methylbutanoic acid	$C_5H_{10}O_2$		25	4.80				
3-Methylbutanoic acid	$C_5H_{10}O_2$		25	4.77				
3-Butenoic acid	$C_4H_6O_2$		25	4.34				
Butylamine	$C_4H_{11}N$		25	10.6				
sec-Butylamine	$C_4H_{11}N$		25	10.56				
tert-Butylamine	$C_4H_{11}N$		25	10.68				
Dibutylamine	$C_8H_{19}N$		21	11.25				
2-Butynoic acid	$C_4H_4O_2$		25	2.62				
Carbamodithioic acid	CH_3NS_2		25	2.95				
Captopril	$C_9H_{15}NO_3S$	1		3.7		2		9.8
2-Thiophenecarboxylic acid	$C_5H_4O_2S$		25	3.49				
3-Thiophenecarboxylic acid	$C_5H_4O_2S$		25	4.1				
2-Furancarboxylic acid	$C_5H_4O_3$		25	3.16				
3-Furancarboxylic acid	$C_5H_4O_3$		25	3.9				

Name	Mol. formula	Step	t°C	pKa		Step	t°C	pKa
Carnosine	$C_9H_{14}N_4O_3$	1	20	2.73		2 3	20 20	6.87 9.73
Pyrocatechol	$C_6H_6O_2$	1	25	9.34		2	25	12.6
Cephalexin	$C_{16}H_{17}N_3O_4S$	1		5.2		2		7.3
Cephaloridine	$C_{19}H_{17}N_3O_4S_2$			3.2				
Citric acid	$C_6H_8O_7$	1 2	25 25	3.13 4.76		3	25	6.40
Isocitric acid	$C_6H_8O_7$	1 2	25 25	3.29 4.71		3	25	6.40
Clindamycin	$C_{18}H_{33}ClN_2O_5S$			7.6				
Codeine	$C_{18}H_{21}NO_3$		25	8.21				
Colchicine	$C_{22}H_{25}NO_6$		20	12.36				
Choline	$C_5H_{14}NO$		25	13.9				
Chloroacetic acid	C_2H_3ClO2		25	2.87				
2-Chlorobutanoic acid	$C_4H_7ClO_2$			2.86				
3-Chlorobutanoic acid	$C_4H_7ClO_2$			4.05				
4-Chlorobutanoic acid	$C_4H_7ClO_2$			4.52				
2-Chloropropanoic acid	$C_3H_5ClO_2$		25	2.83				
3-Chloropropanoic acid	$C_3H_5ClO_2$		25	3.98				
cis-Cinnamic acid	$C_9H_8O_2$		25	3.89				
trans-Cinnamic acid	$C_9H_8O_2$		25	4.44				
Cinnoline	$C_8H_6N_2$		20	2.37				
Creatine	$C_4H_9N_3O_2$	1	25	2.63		2	25	14.3
Creatinine	$C_4H_7N_3O$	1		44.8		2		9.2
o-Cresol	C_7H_8O		25	10.29				
m-Cresol	C_7H_8O		25	10.09				
p-Cresol	C_7H_8O		25	10.26				
trans-Crotonic acid	$C_4H_6O_2$		25	4.69				
Cyanic acid	CHNO		25	3.7				
Cyanamide	CH_2N_2		29	1.1				
Cyanoacetic acid	$C_3H_3NO_2$		25	2.47				
Cyanuric acid	$C_3H_3N_3O_3$	1 2		6.88 11.40		3		13.5
1,3-Cyclohexanedione	$C_6H_8O_2$		25	5.26				
Cyclohexylamine	$C_6H_{13}N$		25	10.64				
Cyclopropanecarboxylic acid	$C_4H_6O_2$		25	4.83				

Name	Mol. formula	Step	t°C	pKa		Step	t°C	pKa
1,1-Cyclopropanedicarboxylic acid	$C_5H_6O_4$	1	25	1.82		2	25	7.43
1-Propene-2,3-dicarboxylic acid	$C_5H_6O_4$	1	25	3.85		2	25	5.45
L-Cysteine	$C_3H_7NO_2S$	1	25	1.5		2 3	25 25	8.7 10.2
Cysteamine	C_2H_7NS	1	25	8.27		2	25	10.53
DL-Cysteic acid	$C_3H_7NO_5S$	1 2	25 25	1.3 1.9		3	25	8.70
Cytidine	$C_9H_{13}N_3O_5$	1		4.22		2		12.5
Cytosine	$C_4H_5N_3O$	1		4.60		2		12.16
1,3-Diamino-2-propanol	$C_3H_{10}N_2O$	1	20	9.69		2	20	7.93
1,5-Pentanediamine	$C_5H_{14}N_2$	1	25	10.05		2	25	10.93
Dichloroacetic acid	$C_2H_2Cl_2O2$		25	1.35				
2,4-Hexadienoic acid	$C_6H_8O_2$		25	4.76				
Diethylamine	$C_4H_{11}N$		25	10.84				
Dimethylamine	C_2H_7N		25	10.73				
Dimethylarsinic acid	$C_2H_7AsO_2$	1	25	1.57		2	25	6.27
N,N-Dimethylglycine	$C_4H_9NO_2$		25	9.89				
2,2-Dimethyl-1,3-dioxane-4,6-dione	$C_6H_8O_4$			5.1				
Diphenylamine	$C_{12}H_{11}N$		25	0.79				
Dopamine	$C_8H_{11}NO_2$	1	25	8.9		2	25	10.6
Emetine	$C_{29}H_{40}N_2O_4$	1		5.77		2		6.64
Epinephrine	$C_9H_{13}NO_3$	1	25	8.66		2	25	9.95
Norepinephrine	$C_8H_{11}NO_3$	1	25	8.64		2	25	9.70
d-Ephedrine	$C_{10}H_{15}NO$		10	10.14				
l-Ephedrine	$C_{10}H_{15}NO$		10	9.96				
Ergometrinine	$C_{19}H_{23}N_3O_{2s}$			7.3				
Erythromycin	$C_{37}H_{67}NO_{13}$			8.8				
1,2-Ethanediamine	$C_2H_8N_2$	1	25	9.92		2	25	6.86
Ethanimidamide	$C_2H_6N_2$		25	12.1				
Ethanolamine	C_2H_7NO		25	9.50				
Ethanol	C_2H_6O		25	15.5				
Ethoxyacetic acid	$C_4H_8O_3$		18	3.65				
Ethyl acetoacetate	$C_6H_{10}O_3$		25	10.68				
Ethylamine	C_2H_7N		25	10.65				
Ethylene glycolmonomethyl ether	$C_3H_8O_2$		25	14.8				

Name	Mol. formula	Step	t°C	pKa		Step	t°C	pKa
Ethyleneglycol	$C_2H_6O_2$		25	15.1				
Ethyleneimine	C_2H_5N		25	8.04				
Formaldehyde	CH_2O		25	13.27				
Formic acid	CH_2O_2		25	3.75				
Flucytosine	$C_4H_4FN_3O$			3.26				
Hydroflumethiazide	$C_8H_8F_3N_3O_4S_2$			8.90				
Fluoroacetic acid	$C_2H_3FO_2$		25	2.59				
β-*D*-Fructose	$C_6H_{12}O_6$		25	12.27				
Fumaric acid	$C_4H_4O_4$	1	25	3.02		2	25	4.38
Gallic acid	$C_7H_6O_5$		25	4.41				
α-*D*-Glucose	$C_6H_{12}O_6$		25	12.46				
L-Glutamic acid	$C_5H_9NO_4$	1 2	25 25	2.13 4.31		3		9.67
L-Glutamine	$C_5H_{10}N_2O_3$	1	25	2.17		2	25	9.13
L-γ-Carboxyglutamic acid	$C_6H_9NO_6$	1 2	25 25	1.7 3.2		3 4	25 25	4.75 9.9
Glutaric acid	$C_5H_8O_4$	1	18	4.32		2	25	5.42
3-Methylglutaric acid	$C_6H_{10}O_4$		25	4.24				
l-Glutathione	$C_{10}H_{17}N_3O_6S$	1 2	25 25	2.12 3.59		3 4	25 25	8.75 9.65
Glycine	$C_2H_5NO_2$	1	25	2.35		2	25	9.78
N-Propylglycine	$C_5H_{11}NO_2$	1	25	2.35		2	25	10.19
Glyceric acid	$C_3H_6O_4$		25	3.52				
Glycerol	$C_3H_8O_3$		25	14.15				
Glycocholic acid	$C_{26}H_{43}NO_6$			4.4				
Guanidine	CH_5N_3		25	13.6				
Glycocyamine	$C_3H_7N_3O_2$		25	2.82				
Glycolic acid	$C_2H_4O_3$		25	3.83				
Glycylalanine	$C_5H_{10}N_2O_3$		25	3.15				
N-Glycylglycine	$C_4H_8N_2O_3$	1	25	3.14		2		8.17
Glycylserine	$C_5H_{10}N_2O_4$	1	25	2.98		2	25	8.38
Glyoxylic acid	$C_2H_2O_3$		25	3.18				
Guanine	$C_5H_5N_5O$		40	9.92				
Haloperidol	$C_{21}H_{23}ClFNO_2$			8.3				
Hexanoic acid	$C_6H_{12}O_2$		25	4.85				
L-Histidine	$C_6H_9N_3O_2$	1 2	25 25	1.80 6.04		3	25	9.33
Histamine	$C_5H_9N_3$	1	25	6.04		2	25	9.75

Name	Mol. formula	Step	t°C	pKa		Step	t°C	pKa
Hippuric acid	$C_9H_9NO_3$		25	3.62				
DL-Homocysteine	$C_4H_9NO_2S$	1 2	25 25	2.22 8.87		3	25	10.86
L-Homoserine	$C_4H_9NO_3$	1	25	2.71		2	25	9.62
1-Hydroxy-1,1-diphosphonoethane	$C_2H_8O_7P_2$	1 2		1.35 2.87		3 4		7.03 11.3
Tris(hydroxymethyl)methy lamine	$C_4H_{11}NO_3$		20	8.3				
Hydroxypropanedioic acid	$C_3H_4O_5$	1		2.42		2		4.54
3-Hydroxypropanoic acid	$C_3H_6O_3$		25	4.51				
Hyoscyamine	$C_{17}H_{23}NO_3$		21	9.7				
Hypoxanthine	$C_5H_4N_4O$		25	8.7				
Imidazole	$C_3H_4N_2$		25	6.99				
2,4-Dimethylimidazole	$C_5H_8N_2$		25	8.36				
Iminodiacetic acid	$C_4H_7NO_4$	1		2.98		2		9.89
Indomethacin	$C_{19}H_{16}ClNO_4$			4.5				
Isopropylamine	C_3H_9N		25	10.63				
Iodoacetic acid	$C_2H_3IO_2$		25	3.18				
Isoxazole	C_3H_3NO		25	-2.0				
Lactic acid	$C_3H_6O_3$		25	3.86				
L-Leucine	$C_6H_{13}NO_2$	1	25	2.33		2	25	9.74
Isoleucine	$C_6H_{13}NO_2$	1	25	2.32		2	25	9.76
Norleucine	$C_6H_{13}NO_2$	1	25	2.33		2	25	9.8
Levodopa	$C_9H_{11}NO_4$	1 2	25 25	2.32 8.72		3 4	25 25	9.96 11.79
Linoleic acid	$C_{18}H_{32}O_2$		25	4.77				
Lysine	$C_6H_{14}N_2O_2$	1 2	25 25	2.16 9.06		3	25	10.54
Maleic acid	$C_4H_4O_4$	1	25	1.92		2	25	6.23
Malonic acid	$C_3H_4O_4$	1	25	2.85		2	25	5.70
Dimethylmalonic acid	$C_5H_8O_4$		25	3.15				
Malic acid	$C_4H_6O_5$	1	25	3.40		2	25	5.11
α-Maltose	$C_{12}H_{22}O_{11}$		21	12.05				
D-Mannose	$C_6H_{12}O_6$		25	12.08				
2-Mercaptoethanol	C_2H_6OS		25	9.72				
Methanol	CH_4O		25	15.5				
Methazolamide	$C_5H_8N_4O_3S_2$			7.30				
(Methylthio)acetic acid	$C_3H_6O_2S$		25	3.66				
Methanethiol	CH_4S		25	10.33				
L-Methionine	$C_5H_{11}NO_2$	1	25	2.13		2	25	9.27

Name	Mol. formula	Step	t°C	pKa		Step	t°C	pKa
2-Methylalanine	$C_4H_9NO_2$	1	25	2.36		2	25	10.21
Methylamine	CH_5N		25	10.66				
1-Methylimidazol	$C_4H_6N_2$		25	6.95				
Diethylmethylamine	$C_5H_{13}N$		25	10.35				
Methylmalonic acid	$C_4H_6O_4$	1	25	3.07		2	25	5.76
2-Methoxyethylamine	C_3H_9NO		25	9.40				
O-Methylhydroxyl amine	CH_5NO			12.5				
2-Methylpropanoic acid	$C_4H_8O_2$		20	4.84				
Morphine	$C_{17}H_{19}NO_3$	1	25	8.21		2	20	9.85
Apomorphine	$C_{17}H_{17}NO_2$	1		7.0		2		8.92
Morpholine	C_4H_9NO		25	8.50				
4-Methylmorpholine	$C_5H_{11}NO$		25	7.38				
Minoxidil	$C_9H_{15}N_5O$			4.61				
N-Ethylmorpholine	$C_6H_{13}NO$		25	7.67				
1-Naphthol	$C_{10}H_8O$		25	9.39				
2-Naphthol	$C_{10}H_8O$		25	9.63				
1-Naphthylamine	$C_{10}H_9N$		25	3.92				
2-Naphthylamine	$C_{10}H_9N$		25	4.16				
Nicotine	$C_{10}H_{14}N_2$	1	25	8.02		2	25	3.12
Nitromethane	CH_3NO_2		25	10.21				
Nitroacetic acid	$C_2H_3NO_4$		24	1.48				
Nitrobenzene	$C_6H_5NO_2$		0	3.98				
Nitroethane	$C_2H_5NO_2$		25	8.46				
Nitrofurantoin	$C_8H_6N_4O_5$			7.2				
Noradrenaline	$C_8H_{11}NO_3$	1	25	8.64		2	25	9.70
L-Norvaline	$C_5H_{11}NO_2$	1	25	2.32		2	25	9.81
DL-Norvaline	$C_5H_{11}NO_2$	1		2.36		2		9.72
Noscapine	$C_{22}H_{23}NO_7$			7.8				
L-Ornithine	$C_5H_{12}N_2O_2$	1 2	25 25	1.71 8.69		3	25	10.76
Oxalic acid	$C_2H_2O_4$	1	25	1.25		2	25	3.81
Oxaloacetic acid	$C_4H_4O_5$	1 2	25 25	2.55 4.37		3	25	13.03
Oxazole	C_3H_3NO		33	0.8				
5,5-Dimethyl-2,4-oxazolidinedione	$C_5H_7NO_3$		37	6.13				
2-Oxobutanoic acid	$C_4H_6O_3$		25	2.50				
2-Oxoglutaric acid	$C_5H_6O_5$	1	25	2.47		2	25	4.68
Papaverine	$C_{20}H_{21}NO_4$		2	6.4				
3-Pentanamine	$C_5H_{13}N$		17	10.59				

Name	Mol. formula	Step	t°C	pKa		Step	t°C	pKa
Pentanoic acid	$C_5H_{10}O_2$		20	4.83				
4-Methylpentanoic acid	$C_6H_{12}O_2$		18	4.84				
trans-3-Pentenoic acid	$C_5H_8O_2$		25	4.51				
5-Aminopentanoic acid	$C_5H_{11}NO_2$	1	25	4.27		2	25	10.77
5-Amino-4-oxopentanoic acid	$C_5H_9NO_3$	1	25	4.05		2	25	8.90
Pentylamine	$C_5H_{13}N$		25	10.63				
Phenylhydrazine	$C_6H_8N_2$		15	8.79				
Piperidine	$C_5H_{11}N$		25	11.12				
Piperazine	$C_4H_{10}N_2$	1	25	9.73		2	25	5.33
Phenol	C_6H_6O		25	9.99				
Phenol Red	$C_{19}H_{14}O_5S$			7.9				
2-Bromophenol	C_6H_5BrO		25	8.45				
3-Bromophenol	C_6H_5BrO		25	9.03				
4-Bromophenol	C_6H_5BrO		25	9.37				
2-Chlorophenol	C_6H_5ClO		25	8.56				
3-Chlorophenol	C_6H_5ClO		25	9.12				
4-Chlorophenol	C_6H_5ClO		25	9.41				
2-Fluorophenol	C_6H_5FO		25	8.73				
3-Fluorophenol	C_6H_5FO		25	9.29				
4-Fluorophenol	C_6H_5FO		25	9.89				
2-Nitrophenol	C_6H5NO_3		25	7.23				
3-Nitrophenol	$C_6H_5NO_3$		25	8.36				
4-Nitrophenol	$C_6H_5NO_3$		25	7.15				
o-Phenylenediamine	$C_6H_8N_2$	1	20	4.57				
m-Phenylenediamine	$C_6H_8N_2$	1	20	5.22		2	20	2.50
p-Phenylenediamine	$C_6H_8N_2$	1	20	6.31		2	20	2.97
2,3-Dichlorophenol	$C_6H_4Cl_2O$		25	7.44				
2,4,6-Trinitrophenol	$C_6H_3N_3O_7$		24	0.42				
2,5-Dinitrophenol	$C_6H_4N_2O_5$		15	5.15				
2,4-Dinitrophenol	$C_6H_4N_2O_5$		25	4.07		2	25	6.9
5-Nitropyrimidinamine	$C_4H_4N_4O_2$		20	0.35				
Phenobarbital	$C_{12}H_{12}N_2O_3$	1		7.3		2		11.8
Phenylbutazone	$C_{19}H_{20}N_2O_2$			4.5				
L-Proline	$C_5H_9NO_2$	1	25	1.95		2	25	10.64
2-Iodophenol	C_6H_5IO		25	8.51				
3-Iodophenol	C_6H_5IO		25	9.03				
4-Iodophenol	C_6H_5IO		25	9.33				
2-Aminophenol	C_6H_7NO	1	20	4.78		2	20	9.97
3-Aminophenol	C_6H_7NO	1	20	4.37		2	20	9.82

Name	Mol. formula	Step	t°C	pKa		Step	t°C	pKa
4-Aminophenol	C_6H_7NO	1	20	5.48		2	20	10.30
2-Methoxyphenol	C_7H_8OS		25	9.53				
3-Methoxyphenol	C_7H_8OS		25	9.98				
4-Methoxyphenol	C_7H_8OS		25	9.65				
Phthalic acid	$C_8H_6O_4$	1	25	2.94		2	25	5.43
Isophthalic acid	$C_8H_6O_4$	1	25	3.70		2	25	4.60
Physostigmine	$C_{15}H_{21}N_3O_2$	1		6.12		2		12.24
Terephthalic acid	$C_8H_6O_4$	1	25	3.54		2	25	4.34
Phthalazine	$C_8H_6N_2$		20	3.47				
Phenazine	$C_{12}H_8N_2$		20	1.20				
Phenolphthalein	$C_{20}H_{14}O_4$		25	9.7				
Piperine	$C_{17}H_{19}NO_3$		18	12.22				
trans-4-Hydroxyproline	$C_5H_9NO_3$	1	25	1.82		2	25	9.66
1,3-Propanediamine	$C_3H_{10}N_2$	1	25	10.55		2	25	8.88
1,2-Propanediamine (±)	$C_3H_{10}N_2$	1	25	9.82		2	25	6.61
Propanoic acid	$C_3H_6O_2$		25	4.87				
2,2-Dimethylpropanoic acid	$C_5H_{10}O_2$		20	5.03				
2-Propanone oxime	C_3H_7NO		25	12.42				
Propargyl alcohol	C_3H_4O		25	13.6				
1-Methylpiperidine	$C_6H_{13}N$		25	10.38				
Propylamine	C_3H_9N		25	10.54				
2,2-Dimethylpropylamine	$C_5H_{13}N$		25	10.15				
2-Propynoic acid	$C_3H_2O_2$		25	1.84				
Protriptyline	$C_{19}H_{21}N$			8.2				
1*H*-Purine	$C_5H_4N_4$	1	20	2.30		2	20	8.96
1,7-Dihydro-6Hpurine-6-thione	$C_5H_4N_4S$	1		7.77		2		11.17
Pyrazine	$C4H_4N_2$		20	0.65				
Pyrazinecarboxamide	$C_5H_5N_3O$			0.5				
2-Methylpyrazine	$C_5H_6N_2$		27	1.45				
Pyrazinecarboxamide	$C_5H_5N_3O$			0.5				
Methylaminopyrazine	$C_5H_7N_3$		25	3.39				
1H-Pyrazole	$C_3H_4N_2$		25	2.49				
Pyridazine	$C_4H_4N_2$		20	2.24				
2,5-Pyridinediamine	$C_5H_7N_3$		20	6.48				
2-Pyridinamine	$C_5H_6N_2$		20	6.82				
3-Pyridinamine	$C_5H_6N_2$		25	6.04				
4-Pyridinamine	$C_5H_6N_2$		25	9.11				
Pyridine	C_5H_5N		25	5.23				

Name	Mol. formula	Step	t°C	pKa		Step	t°C	pKa
2-Methylpyridine	C_6H_7N		25	6.00				
3-Methylpyridine	C_6H_7N		25	5.70				
4-Methylpyridine	C_6H_7N		25	5.99				
2-Pyridinecarboxaldehyde	C_6H_5NO		25	12.68				
4-Pyridinecarboxaldehyde	C_6H_5NO		30	12.05				
Pyridine-1-oxide	C_5H_5NO		24	0.79				
2-Chloropyridine	C_5H_4ClN		25	0.49				
3-Chloropyridine	C_5H_4ClN		25	2.81				
4-Chloropyridine	C_5H_4ClN		25	3.83				
2-Fluoropyridine	C_5H_4FN		25	-0.44				
4-Nitropyridine	$C_5H_4N_2O_2$		25	1.61				
2-Methoxypyridine	C_6H_7NO		20	3.28				
3-Methoxypyridine	C_6H_7NO		25	4.78				
4-Methoxypyridine	C_6H_7NO		25	6.58				
Xanthopterin	$C_6H_5N_5O_2$		20	6.59				
Pteridine	$C_6H_4N_4$		20	4.05				
2-Amino-4-hydroxypteridine	$C_6H_5N_5O$	1	20	2.27		2	20	7.96
2-Pyridinol	C_5H_5NO	1	20	0.75		2	20	11.65
3-Pyridinol	C_5H_5NO	1	20	4.79		2	20	8.75
4-Pyridinol	C_5H_5NO	1	20	3.20		2	20	11.12
2(1H)-Pyridinone	C_5H_5NO	1	20	0.75		2	20	11.65
Pyrimidine	$C_4H_4N_2$		20	1.23				
2,4,6-Pyrimidinetriamine	$C_4H_7N_5$		20	6.84				
2-Pyrimidinamine	$C_4H_5N_3$		20	3.45				
4-Pyrimidinamine	$C_4H_5N_3$		20	5.71				
N-Methylpyridinamine	$C_6H_8N_2$		20	9.65				
Pyrocatechol	$C_6H_6O_2$	11	25	9.34		2	25	12.6
L-Pyroglutamic acid	$C_5H_7NO_3$		25	3.32				
1*H*-Pyrrole-3-carboxylic acid	$C_5H_5NO_2$		20	5.00				
Pyrrolidine	C_4H_9N		25	11.31				
N-Methylpyrrolidine	$C_5H_{11}N$		25	10.46				
1,2-Dimethylpyrrolidine	$C_6H_{13}N$		26	10.20				
Pyrrole	C_4H_5N		25	-3.8				
1*H*-Pyrrole-2-carboxylic acid	$C_5H_5NO_2$		20	4.45				
1*H*-Pyrrole-3-carboxylic acid	$C_5H_5NO_2$		20	5.00				
Pyruvic acid	$C_3H_4O_3$		25	2.39				

Name	Mol. formula	Step	t°C	pKa		Step	t°C	pKa
Quinazoline	$C_8H_6N_2$		29	3.43				
Quinine	$C_{20}H_{24}N_2O_2$	1	25	8.52		2	25	4.13
Hydroquinine	$C_{20}H_{26}N_2O_2$			5.33				
Quinidine	$C_{20}H_{24}N_2O_2$	1	20	5.4		2	20	1
Quinoline	C_9H_7N		20	4.90				
Isoquinoline	C_9H_7N		20	5.40				
2-Quinolinol	C_9H_7NO		20	-0.31		2	20	11.76
3-Quinolinol	C_9H_7NO		20	4.28		2	20	8.08
4-Quinolinol	C_9H_7NO		20	2.23		2	20	11.28
6-Quinolinol	C_9H_7NO	1	20	55.15		2	20	8.90
8-Quinolinol	C_9H_7NO	1	25	4.91		2	25	9.81
7-Isoquinolinol	C_9H_7NO	1	20	5.68		2	20	8.90
Quinoxaline	$C_8H_6N_2$		20	0.56				
p-Hydroquinone	$C_6H_6O_2$	1	25	9.85		2	25	11.4
Resorcinol	$C_6H_6O_2$	1	25	9.32		2	25	11.1
L-Ribose	$C_5H_{10}O_5$		25	12.22				
D-2-Deoxyribose	$C_5H_{10}O_4$		25	12.61				
Reserpine	$C_{33}H_{40}N_2O_9$			6.6				
Riboflavin	$C_{17}H_{20}N_4O_6$			1.7				
Rifampin	$C_{43}H_{58}N_4O_{12}$	1		1.7		2		7.9
Saccharin	$C_7H_5NO_3S$		18	11.68				
Sarcosine	$C_3H_7NO_2$	1	25	2.21		2	25	10.1
Sebacic acid	$C_{10}H_{18}O_4$	1		4.59		2		5.59
L-Serine	$C_3H_7NO_3$	1	25	2.19		2	25	9.21
Solanine	$C_{45}H_{73}NO_{15}$		15	6.66				
Strychnine	$C_{21}H_{22}N_2O_2$		25	8.26				
Succinic acid	$C_4H_6O_4$	1	25	4.21		2	25	5.64
Methylsuccinic acid	$C_5H_8O_4$	1	25	4.13		2	25	5.64
Succinimide	$C_4H_5NO_2$		25	9.62				
Sucrose	$C_{12}H_{22}O_{11}$		25	12.7				
Sulfathiazole	$C_9H_9N_3O_2S_2$			7.2				
Sulfamethazine	$C_{12}H_{14}N_4O_2S$	1		7.4		2		2.65
Sulfisoxazole	$C_{11}H_{13}N_3O_3S$			5				
Benzenesulfinic acid	$C_6H_6O_2S$		20	1.3				
Benzenesulfonic acid	$C_6H_6O_3S$		25	0.70				
2-Aminobenzenesulfonic acid	$C_6H_7NO_3S$		25	2.46				
3-Aminobenzenesulfonic acid	$C_6H_7NO_3S$		25	3.74				

Name	Mol. formula	Step	t°C	pKa		Step	t°C	pKa
4-Aminobenzenesulfonic acid	$C_6H_7NO_3S$		25	3.23				
Dihydroxytartaric acid	$C_4H_6O_8$		25	1.92				
DL-Tartaric acid	$C_4H_6O_6$	1	25	3.03		2	25	4.37
meso-Tartaric acid	$C_4H_6O_6$	1	25	3.17		2	25	4.91
L-Tartaric acid	$C_4H_6O_6$	1	25	2.98		2	25	4.34
Taurocholic acid	$C_{26}H_{45}NO_7S$			1.4				
Hydrochlorothiazide	$C_7H_8ClN_3O_4S_2$	1		7.9		2		9.2
Thebaine	$C_{19}H_{21}NO_3$		15	6.05				
Theophylline	$C_7H_8N_4O_2$		25	8.77				
Thiazole	C_3H_3NS		25	2.52				
2-Thiazolamine	$C_3H_4N_2S$		20	5.36				
Thioacetic acid	C_2H_4OS		25	3.33				
Theobromine	$C_7H_8N_4O_2$		18	7.89				
Thioglycolic acid	$C_2H_4O_2S$		25	3.68				
Thiourea	CH_4N_2S		25	- 1				
L-Thyroxin	$C_{15}H_{11}I_4NO_4$	1 2	25 25	2.2 6.45		3	25	10.1
L-Threonine	$C_4H_9NO_3$	1	25	2.09		2	25	9.10
Thymine	$C_5H_6N_2O_2$		25	9.94				
Nitrilotriacetic acid	$C_6H_9NO_6$	1 1	20 20	3.03 3.07		3	20	10.70
1,2,3-Triaminopropane	$C_3H_{11}N_3$	1	20	9.59		2	20	7.95
1,3,5-Triazine-2,4,6-triamine	$C_3H_6N_6$		25	5.00				
1H-1,2,3-Triazole	$C_2H_3N_3$		20	1.17				
1H-1,2,4-Triazole	$C_2H_3N_3$		20	2.27				
Trichloroacetaldehyde	C_2HCl_3O		25	10.04				
2,2,2-Trichloroethanol	$C_2H_3Cl_3O$		25	12.24				
Trichloroacetic acid	$C_2HCl_3O_2$		20	0.66				
Triethylenediamine	$C_6H_{12}N_2$	1		3.0		2		8.7
Trifluoroacetic acid	$C_2HF_3O_2$		25	0.52				
2,2,2-Trifluoroethanol	$C_2H_3F_3O$		25	12.37				
Trimethoprim	$C_{14}H_{18}N_4O_3$			6.6				
Trimethylamine	C_3H_9N		25	9.80				
Trimethylamine oxide	C_3H_9NO		20	4.65				
Tryptamine	$C_{10}H_{12}N_2$		25	10.2				
Tryptophan	$C_{11}H_{12}N_2O_2$	1	25	2.46		2	25	9.41
5-Hydroxytryptamine	$C_{10}H_{12}N_2O$	1	25	9.8		2	25	11.1

Name	Mol. formula	Step	t°C	pKa		Step	t°C	pKa
Tyramine	$C_8H_{11}NO$	1	25	9.74		2	25	10.52
Tyrosine	$C_9H_{11}NO_3$	1 2	25 25	2.20 9.21		3	25	10.46
Uracil	$C_4H_4N_2O_2$		25	9.45				
Urea	CH_4N_2O		25	0.10				
Tetramethylurea	$C_5H_{12}N_2O$			2				
Uric acid	$C_5H_4N_4O_3$		12	3.89				
L-Valine	$C_5H_{11}NO_2$	1	25	2.29		2	25	9.74
Verapamil	$C_{27}H_{38}N_2O_4$			8.6				
Veratridine	$C_{36}H_{51}NO_{11}$			9.54				
Xanthopterin	$C_6H_5N_5O_2$		20	6.59				
D-Xylose	$C_5H_{10}O_5$		18	12.14				

Example: If pKa of acetic acid is 4.75, find out the value of Ka.

$$pKa = -\log Ka$$
$$= -\log 4.75$$
$$= 1.76 \times 10^{-4}$$

www.ingramcontent.com/pod-product-compliance
Ingram Content Group UK Ltd.
Pitfield, Milton Keynes, MK11 3LW, UK
UKHW061536190726
13845UKWH00006B/129

9 789386 819918